Radiology Education

Rethy K. Chhem · Kathryn M. Hibbert
Teresa Van Deven (Eds.)

Radiology Education

The Scholarship of Teaching and Learning

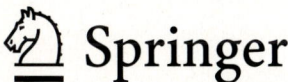

Rethy K. Chhem
Professor & Chair
Department of Medical Imaging
Schulich School of Medicine and Dentistry
University of Western Ontario
London,ON
Canada N6A 5C1

Teresa Van Deven
Curriculum and Pedagogy Support
Centre for Education in Medical Imaging
Schulich School of Medicine and Dentistry
University of Western Ontario
London, ON
Canada N6A 5C1

Kathryn M. Hibbert
Director
Centre for Education in Medical Imaging
Assistant Professor
Department of Medical Imaging
Schulich School of Medicine and Dentistry
University of Western Ontario
London, ON
Canada N6A 5C1

ISBN: 978-3-540-68987-4   e-ISBN: 978-3-540-68989-8

DOI: 10.1007/978-3-540-68989-8

Library of Congress Control Number: 2008928775

Cover design: Frido Steinen-Broo, e-Studio Calamar, Spain

Printed on acid-free paper

9 8 7 6 5 4 3 2 1

springer.com

Foreword

This is a book about scholarship in the broadest sense. The writing of this book has shown how through scholarship we can bring together academics, practitioners, scientists, radiologists, and administrators from around the world to begin the kinds of conversations that promise to move us to a new way of thinking about and enacting radiology education.

Over the past century, we have witnessed tremendous change in biomedical science and the scope of this change has demanded new approaches to medical education. The most significant of the changes in medical education has been a fundamental paradigm shift from a *teacher-centered approach* to a *student-centered approach*. This shift, combined with the explosion of knowledge, has pressed medical schools to undertake major curricular and institutional reform. At the same time, progress in medical education research methods has led to innovative approaches to support the improvement of learning methods and evaluation.

Over the past several years there has also been a shift toward thinking about and planning for medical education beyond the undergraduate level to include postgraduate and continuing medical education, but also to consider learning within the professional environment and the development of professional continuous education. Viewing medical education as a continuum that spans from the first year of medical school until retirement introduces new ways to conceptualize the teaching and learning needs that address lifelong learning demands that extend over 30 or 40 years.

To add complexity to the demands, we have to consider the changing role and function of radiology in the twenty-first century. Given the historic advancement of knowledge, coupled with technological development, radiology as a specialty has progressively reached a tremendous scope during its golden age. These advancements have called for a redefinition of the boundaries of this specialty. As a consequence, medical imaging has positioned itself as an important component at the core of any medical curriculum. It has also become a very popular specialty among medical students and consequently has led to innovative residency training and research program initiatives. These initiatives often serve as models for general medical education curriculum design and implementation. There is no question

that current medical students, residents, colleagues, and patients have benefited much
more from this revised curriculum than the curriculum I experienced during my own training
a couple of decades ago.

Although I am reassured by the quality of the current radiology education content,
I remain worried and uncomfortable about some of the other professional competencies.
For example, what is the best way to teach residents how to obtain informed consent
from a patient before undertaking a complex interventional procedure? How can we help
our medical students to develop the processes of self-assessment, communication, and
collaboration with other health professionals even within our own radiology department?
When I observe a general lack of respect for colleagues or a radiologist who takes refuge
in the comfort of his/her subspecialty (thereby not offering general radiology
services), I wonder, *Have I failed in my role as a teacher? Have I not been a good
role model?* Clearly, accumulating radiological content knowledge and skills as a superb
medical expert is not sufficient. To be accountable to our patients, and to society generally, requires more than diagnostic and therapeutic skills. Patients today are often much
more sophisticated and informed about their own illness and expect to communicate as
partners in their health care team. Patients want quick access to medical imaging facilities despite scarce health care resources. As taxpayers, they exercise their right to make
demands on universities and teaching hospitals to meet their needs. Schools of medicine
and continuous medical education providers should adopt mechanisms to accurately assess
the characteristics and needs of the populations they serve. Economic, social, and demo-
graphic parameters should all be taken into consideration by medical curriculum designers
in order to meet societal needs. These parameters include aging process, chronic disease,
poverty, vulnerable population, multicultural society, system of beliefs, globalization and
ecohealth system, scarce resources, and interprofessional collaboration.

Finally, zero tolerance for nonethical and irresponsible behavior should be assumed as
the core value of medical education. Advances in technology and changing societal needs
have meant that radiology has ceased to be a pure "contemplative" activity, and instead the
radiologist's role has evolved into that of an attending physician with full responsibility
for the entire spectrum of patient management. Beyond the clinical role then, radiologists
should be engaged in debate on the key issues that affect society. Increasingly, there is an
expectation that a physician should embrace the role of community leader. The skills
necessary to take up that role must be integrated as fundamental learning outcomes during
the design of curriculum, at all levels of medical education.

This book calls upon radiologists to expand their role beyond limited understandings
of themselves as simply a clinical service provider and to engage in dialogue, scholarship,
and educational activities rooted in professional responsibility and accountability toward
the community. Rethy Chhem, the senior editor of this collection, has demonstrated such
a commitment to societal needs throughout his entire career. It is not surprising to see
that he has taken up the challenge of producing a book that expands the understanding of
the scholarship of teaching and learning in medicine, with a special focus on radiology
education. The chapters included in this book highlight a path that has been taken by a
few pioneers in radiology education, and also offer innovative ideas that may help medical educators in their commitment to train and educate radiologists equipped as "medical
experts" with full social responsibility. Rethy Chhem and his coeditors Kathy Hibbert and

Teresa Van Deven are to be congratulated for having gathered leaders and experts in radiology education across the globe to come together to share their expertise in this exciting and promising field. This book promised to fill a void, as there is currently no book available that addresses radiology education from a scholarship of teaching and learning perspective. Let the dialogue begin!

Montreal, PQ, Canada   **Louise M. Samson**
April 2008

Acknowledgements

We wish to thank the radiology faculty and residents of the Department of Medical Imaging, Schulich School of Medicine and Dentistry University of Western Ontario for welcoming us into their departments and for their valuable input along the way. We thank our Deans for their enthusiastic support; we thank, Dr. Carol Herbert, Dean of the Schulich School of Medicine & Dentistry, University of Western Ontario and Dr. Julia O'Sullivan, Dean of the Faculty of Education, University of Western Ontario. We also wish to thank the following Research Assistants for their contributions to this work: Sarah Flynn, Hongfang Yu, Senlin Yang, Lucy Karanja, Jennifer Neil and Holly Ellinor. We would like to acknowledge the support of a Faculty Support for Research in Education grant from the Schulich School of Medicine & Dentistry, University of Western Ontario.

Rethy Chhem

I would like to thank Dr. Louise Samson, President of the Royal College of Physicians and Surgeons for both her support of this project and for graciously writing the Forward to our book. As always, I thank my family for their encouragement and continual support: my wife, Yanny, my daughters, Sirika and Kanika and my son, Siriwat.

Kathy Hibbert

I read a quote once that seems appropriate to include here: "Don't ask yourself what the world needs. Ask yourself what makes you feel like you have come alive. And then go and do that. Because what the world needs is people who have come alive." Thank you to my colleagues Rethy Chhem, Teresa Van Deven, Sharon Rich, Roz Stooke and Rachel Heydon, and to my family, Bill, Darren and Ali for their friendship and support—all things that make me feel like I have come alive. Thanks too, to all of the wonderful physicians and residents that we have worked with to complete this book.

Teresa Van Deven

First and foremost I thank the radiology physicians and residents from the three hospital sites in London, Ontario, for taking the steps towards these dialogues around scholarship. These dialogues have truly constituted the beginnings of this book. I thank my colleagues and mentors who have helped to cultivate not only my own sense of scholarship but also the passion to pursue this work: Dr. Kathy Hibbert, Dr. Rethy Chhem, Dr. Suzanne Majh-anovich, Dr. Allan Pitman, Dr. Geoffrey Milburn and Father Francisco de las Heras . I thank and cherish those in my life who have so enthusiastically encouraged my new jour-ney into medical education: Kate Danielle, Joan, Louis, Kimberly, Richard James, and Brooklyne.

Contents

Introduction
Transforming Radiology Education Through Scholarship...................................... 1
C.P. Herbert, J. O'Sullivan

Part I   Education for Non-Educators

1   The Genesis and Application of Radiology Education:
Mind the Gap.. 5
T. Van Deven, K. Hibbert, R.K. Chhem

    1.1   Introduction.. 6
    1.2   Border Crossings.. 6
    1.3   Communities of Professional Practice 7
    1.4   Building a New Home but Living the Same Old Life
            Within It 8
    1.5   Cultivating Scholarship 9
            References.. 11

2   Scholarship in Radiology Education.. 13
R.K. Chhem

    2.1   What is Scholarship in Radiology Education?..................... 14
    2.2   Why Expand Scholarship in Medical Imaging? 18
    2.3   How to Expand Scholarship in Medical Imaging Education?............ 19
    2.3.1   Academic Leadership 19
    2.3.2   Faculty Members.. 20
    2.3.3   Specific Educational Structures 21
    2.4   Conclusion 22
            References.. 23

**3   Today's Radiology Student: What Every Radiology
     Training Program Director Needs to Know** 25
     J. Amann, S. Kribs, K. Hibbert, M. Landis

     3.1   Imagine 25
     3.2   The Context 26
     3.3   Today's Radiology Student 27
     3.4   The Role of Radiologists as Teachers 29
     3.5   Leadership and the RTPD 30
     3.5.1   What Is the Profile of a RTPD? 30
     3.5.2   Responsibilities of the RTPD 31
     3.5.2.1 Overall Program: Setting the Stage 31
     3.5.2.2 Building a Culture To Support Resident Education 31
     3.5.2.3 Meeting Accreditation Requirements 32
     3.5.2.4 Faculty Development 32
     3.5.2.5 Resident Advocacy 32
     3.6   The Role of Radiology Educators 33
     3.7   The Role of the RTC 33
     3.8   Radiology Training and the Trainee: A Case for Level-Specific
              Curricula from a Resident's Perspective 33
     3.9   The Ideal Academic Environment for Postgraduate
              Radiology Residents 35
              References 38

4   Teaching and Learning: Defining the Scholarship of Teaching 39
     T. Van Deven, K. Hibbert, H.C. Ellinor

     4.1   Narrative 39
     4.2   Introduction: What do We Mean by "Scholarship of Teaching?" 40
     4.3   Creating the Conditions to Foster "Scholarship in Teaching" 41
     4.3.1   The "Series" 42
     4.3.1.1 "Anatomy of the Curriculum" 42
     4.3.1.2 Theories of Teaching and Learning 43
     4.3.1.3 Assessment and Evaluation 44
     4.3.1.4 Creating a Culture that Supports Mentorship 46
     4.4   The Centre for Education in Medical Imaging:
              A Collaborative Effort 47
              References 48

5   Interdisciplinary Learning: A Stimulant for Reflective Practice 51
     S.J. Rich

     5.1   Interdisciplinary Learning: A Century of Growth 52
     5.2   The Context Today 53
     5.3   Interdisciplinary Learning and Learner Engagement 54
     5.4   Interdisciplinary Learning: It Is and It Is Not 55

5.5   Interdisciplinary Teaching and Learning as Meaning Making
        and an Entrée to Reflective Practice   57
5.6   Interdisciplinary Learning and Reflective Practice   58
5.7   Interprofessional Education and Interdisciplinarity   60
        References...   61

6   Feedback in Radiologic Education..   63
       R.B. Gunderman, K.B. Williamson

6.1   Lack of Feedback   64
6.2   Disparagement versus Feedback..   65
6.3   The Never-Satisfied Educator..   66
6.4   Teachable Moments   67
6.5   The Spirit of Inquiry...   68
6.6   Conclusion   69
        References...   69

7   The Role of Mentoring in Professional Education...   71
       R. Garvey

7.1   Introduction: A Glimpse into the UK Health Service Story.............   71
7.2   What Is Mentoring?   74
7.3   Descriptions of Mentoring Through History......................................   74
7.4   Why Is Mentoring Powerful?...   77
7.5   CPD and Mentoring...   77
7.6   Connections with Practice..   79
7.7   Making the Transition..   80
7.7.1   Defining the Purpose and Scope   80
7.7.2   Diagnosis..   80
7.7.3   Implementation..   81
7.8   Expanded Understanding of the Mentoring Role   83
7.8.1   Conditions for Success in Mentoring..   83
7.9   Conclusions   84
        References...   84

8   Radiological and Biomedical Knowledge Integration:
       The Ontological Way   87
       R. Arp, C. Romagnoli, R.K. Chhem, J.A. Overton

8.1   Introduction...   87
8.2   Domain Ontology..   89
8.3   Formal Ontology   94
8.4   Constructing a Radiology Ontology...   96
8.4.1   Steps in Constructing a RadO...   96
8.4.1.1   Step 1: Determine the Purpose of the RadO   96
8.4.1.2   Step 2: Provide an Explicit Statement of the Intended
          Subject Matter of the RadO   97

8.4.1.3   Step 3: Determine the Most Basic Universal Terms
          and Relations Dealt with in the RadO.. 97
8.4.1.4   Step 4: Construct a List of Terms for the RadO,
          Starting with the Most Basic Terms 98
8.4.1.5   Step 5: Put the Terms in a Taxonomic Hierarchy Complete
          with Appropriate Relationships 99
8.4.1.6   Step 6: Regiment the Information in Order
          To Ensure Logical and Scientific Coherence 99
8.4.1.7   Step 7: Regiment the Information To Ensure Compatibility
          with Other Relevant Ontologies... 100
8.4.1.8   Step 8: Concretize This Information in a Computer-Tractable
          Format, Such As Protégé 101
8.4.1.9   Step 9: Implement the RadO in Some Specific
          Computing Context.. 101
8.4.2   Basic Formal Ontology... 101
          References.. 103

Part II   Educational Insights From Practitioners

9   Educational Insights About Professional Ethics in Radiology.................... 107
     L. Brazeau-Lamontagne

     9.1   Introduction 107
     9.2   Radiologists Are Physicians... 108
     9.3   What Is Included in Radiology Ethics? 110
     9.4   Learning Professional Ethics in Radiology......................... 112
     9.4.1   Learning Professional Ethics... 112
     9.4.2   Ethics in Daily Radiology Practice 113
     9.5   Consent in Radiology 114
     9.6   Professional Confidentiality 115
     9.7   The End-of-Life Issues.. 116
     9.8   Personal Convictions 117
     9.9   Resource Allocation... 118
     9.10   Collegiality 119
     9.11   Conclusions 121
               References 121

**10   Learning in Practice: New Approaches to Professional
      Development for Radiologists**.. 123
      I.J. Parboosingh, B.P. Wood, L.M. Samson, C.M. Campbell

      10.1   A Department of Radiology Narrative 123
      10.2   Learning Habits Emphasized During Residency................ 124
      10.3   Programs Supporting Professional Development
                and Practice Enhancement: A Historical Perspective........ 124
      10.4   Practice Models the Lifelong-Learning Curriculum.......... 125
      10.5   Reflective Practice Drives the Learning Processes 126

10.5.1	Knowing-in-Action	126
10.5.2	Reflection-in-Action	126
10.5.3	Reflection-on-Action	127
10.5.4	Research Supports Reflection in Practice	127
10.6	Embedding Learning in a Practice Environment	127
10.6.1	Communities of Practice	127
10.6.2	Interprofessional Collaborative Learning	128
10.7	Working Towards a Culture of Learning	129
10.8	Practice Assessment and Performance Enhancement	130
10.9	Management of Learning in Practice	131
10.9.1	Information Sources	131
10.9.2	Learning Plans and Projects	132
10.9.3	Networks	132
10.9.4	Recognition of Expertise	132
10.10	Conclusions	132
	References	133

11 Acquiring Competencies in Radiology: The CanMEDS Model 135

R.K. Chhem, L.M. Samson, J.R. Frank, J. Dubois

11.1	Introduction and History of CanMEDS	135
11.2	What Is Educational Competency?	136
11.3	What Is Outcome-Based Education?	137
11.4	What is CanMEDS?	138
11.5	CanMEDS and Radiology Competencies	138
11.5.1	Medical Expert	139
11.5.2	Communicator Role	139
11.5.3	Collaborator Role	140
11.5.4	Manager Role	140
11.5.5	Health Advocate Role	141
11.5.6	Scholar Role	141
11.5.7	Professional Role	142
11.6	Evaluation	142
11.7	Challenges for Implementation of the Competency Framework of CanMEDS	142
	References	144

12 Technologies for Teaching: Exploring the Use of PACS, Databases, and Teaching Files 145

R.N. Rankin

12.1	Introduction	145
12.2	Information Availability and Its Currency	147
12.3	Information Use to Suit the Learning Opportunity	148
12.4	Feedback for Students and Teachers	148
12.5	The Record of Expertise	149
12.6	Summary	150
	References	150

**13 Portable Imaging Systems for Interactive Teaching of Radiography,
      Computed Tomography and Ultrasound Imaging Principles**...................... 151
J.J. Battista, T.L. Poepping

13.1   Introduction 151
13.2   Small-Scale Imaging Systems 153
13.2.1   Optical CT Imaging System 153
13.2.2   Ultrasound Imaging System 155
13.3   Educational Sessions 156
13.3.1   CT Imaging Experiments 156
13.3.1.1   Image Reconstruction.. 156
13.3.1.2   Spatial Resolution... 158
13.3.1.3   Contrast Resolution 160
13.3.2   Ultrasound Imaging Experiments 160
13.3.2.1   Acoustic Velocity (Speed of Sound)... 161
13.3.2.2   Reverberations.. 162
13.3.2.3   Attenuation 163
13.3.2.4   Acoustic Impedance, Reflection and Scatter 164
13.3.2.5   In Vitro and In Vivo Imaging.. 165
13.4   Summary and Conclusion... 165
13.5   Conflict of Interest Statement.. 167
            Acknowledgements... 167
            References 168

**14 Medical Education Research: Challenges and Opportunities
      in the Scholarship of Discovery**.. 169
J. Collins

14.1   Introduction 171
14.2   Challenges in Medical Education Research................................... 172
14.3   Funding of Medical Education Research 173
14.4   Characteristics of Successful Medical Education
            Research Centers.. 176
14.5   Trends in Medical Education Research 177
14.6   Opportunities in Medical Education Research 179
14.7   The Future of Radiology Education Research.............................. 180
14.8   Summary... 182
            References 183

**15 Developing a Radiology Curriculum for a New Medical
      School in Singapore** 187
Kiang-Hiong Tay, Robert Kamei, Bien-Soo Tan

15.1   Preamble 187
15.2   Background for Setting Up a New Medical School........................ 188
15.3   Duke-NUS Graduate Medical School Curriculum......................... 188
15.4   Radiology in Duke-NUS Graduate Medical School:
            Getting Started 190

15.5	Defining the Role of Radiology in the Graduate Medical School Curriculum	191
15.5.1	Using Radiology to Teach	191
15.5.2	Teaching of Radiology	191
15.6	Developing the Radiology Program for Duke-NUS	192
15.7	TeamGMS and Self-Directed Learning	193
15.8	Radiology and the Research Year	194
15.9	Graduate Medical School Radiology Faculty	194
15.10	Moving Forward	195
	References	195

16 Leadership in Radiology Education   197
R.B. Gunderman

16.1	Level One: Failures in What We Do	198
16.2	Level Two: Failures in Who We Are	198
16.3	Level Three: Failures of Who We Want To Be	199
	References	200

17 The Business of Radiology Education Scholarship   201
L.A. Matheson

17.1	Introduction	201
17.2	A Review of the Literature	202
17.3	Establishing the Right Team	203
17.4	Infrastructure and Support Considerations	204
17.4.1	Space	204
17.4.2	Information Technology	205
17.4.3	Human Resources	206
17.4.4	Overview of Business-Planning Considerations	207
17.5	Funding and Budgeting	208
17.6	What has been Learned	208
17.7	The Vision for the Future	209
	References	209

Part III Radiology Education Global Outreach

**18 Radiology Education in Southeast Asia:
Current Status and Pedagogical Challenges**   213
Shih-chang Wang

18.1	Introduction	213
18.2	Regional Overview	214
18.3	Socioeconomic and Political Factors	217
18.4	Regional Pedagogical Approaches	218
18.5	National Radiology Education Programmes	221
18.5.1	Singapore	221
18.5.2	Malaysia	225

18.5.3   Indonesia.. 226
18.5.4   Thailand 227
18.5.6   Myanmar... 228
18.5.7   Other Countries... 229
18.6   Pedagogical Challenges in Radiology Education 230
             Acknowledgements... 232
             References 232

**19   Training of Ultrasound Doctors and Educational Reform
         in West China Hospital of Sichuan University, China** 233
         L. Yan

19.1   Introduction 233
19.2   Chinese Medical Education 236
19.3   Reforming Chinese Medical Education 238
19.3.1   Degree Programs.. 239
19.3.2   Continuing Medical Education.. 239
19.4   Training Program for Ultrasound Residents
             in West China Hospital, Chengdu, China.................................... 239
19.4.1   General Information 239
19.4.2   Current Training Plan 240
19.4.3   Challenges 240
19.5   Medical Imaging Technician Education and Training Program
             at Sichuan University Affiliated with West China Hospital 240
19.5.1   Background 240
19.5.2   Present Status 241
19.6   Conclusions 241
             Acknowledgments 241
             References 242

**20   Teaching Radiology at the Angkor Hospital for Children
         in Siem Reap, Cambodia** 243
         M. Fortier

20.1   The Community 243
20.2   Health and Imaging Needs of the Community 244
20.3   Implementation-Transition 244
20.4   Providing Opportunities To Make the Transition 246
             References 247

21   Teaching Radiology in Latin America: Images from Peru 249
         R. DelCarpio-O'Donovan

21.1   Narrative 249
21.2   Language as a Cornerstone of Cultural Teaching
             and Learning... 250
21.3   Technology: The Necessity for Adaptability................................ 250

	21.4	Considering Your Audience	251
	21.4.1	Medical Students..	251
	21.4.2	Radiology Residents..	253
	21.4.3	Nonradiologists (Other Physicians)	254
	21.5	Topics and Border Crossing...	254
	21.5.1	The Power of Humor	255
	21.5.2	Reciprocal Learning	255
	21.6	Recommendations..	255
	21.7	Summary..	256
		Acknowledgments	257
		References	257

22   Using the World Wide Web to Develop Competencies
Around the Globe **259**
C. Daniels

	22.1	Introduction	259
	22.2	Effectiveness of Digital Radiology Learning Resources................	260
	22.3	The Educational Framework..	260
	22.4	Practical Measures...	261
	22.5	Implications for the Facilitator of Distributive Learning................	268
	22.6	The Role of the Sponsoring Organization..	268
	22.7	Conclusion..	269
		References	270

23   The Role of a Learned Society in the Promotion
and Dissemination of Knowledge.. **273**
P.A. Peetrons

	23.1	Introduction	273
	23.2	Musculoskeletal Ultrasound Society	274
	23.3	Groupement des Echographistes	
		de L'Appareile Locomoteur	278
	23.4	Role of the Learned Societies...	279
		References	280

24   Radiology Education in the Faculty of Medicine at Cairo University
(Kasr Al-Ainy Hospital)... **283**
S.N. Saleem, Y.Y. Sabri, A.S. Saeed

	24.1	Introduction and Historic Background...	283
	24.2	Modern Kasr Al-Ainy Hospital Facilities...	284
	24.3	Radiology Department of Kasr Al-Ainy Hospital:	
		Personnel, Equipment, and Clinical Services	285
	24.4	Radiology Department's Teaching Duties	285
	24.4.1	Radiology Education for Undergraduates...	286
	24.4.2	Radiology Education for Postgraduate Studies	286

24.4.2.1   Residency...   286
24.4.2.2   MSc in Radiology (Part I): 6 Months   287
24.4.2.3   MSc in Radiology (Part II): 18 Months.............................   289
24.4.2.4   MD in Radiology   290
24.4.2.5   Postgraduate Examinations (MSc Part II and MD).........   291
24.4.3   Continuing Medical Education...   291
24.4.4   Education Resources in the Radiology Department.........   292
24.5   Radiology Department of Kasr Al-Ainy Hospital
            and the World   293
24.6   Radiology Department of Kasr Al-Ainy Hospital:
            Stated Mission...   293
24.7   Looking to the Future...   294
24.8   Summary...   294
            References   294

Index   295

List of Contributors

Justin Amann
Department of Medical Imaging
University of Western Ontario
London, ON
Canada

Robert Arp
National Center for Biomedical Ontology
University at Buffalo
New York
USA

JerryJ. Battista
Professor, Department of Medical
Biophysics
The University of Western Ontario,
London, ON
Canada

Lucie Brazeau-Lamontagne
Department of Radiology
Centre Hospitalier Universitaire
de Sherbrooke
Sherbrooke, QC
Canada

Craig M. Campbell
Director, Office of Professional Affairs
Royal College of Physicians and Surgeons
of Canada
Ottawa, ON
Canada

Rethy K. Chhem
Department of Medical Imaging
Schulich School of Medicine and Dentistry
University of Western Ontario
London, ON
Canada

Jannette Collins
Department of Radiology
University of Wisconsin School of Medicine
and Public Health
Madison, WI
USA

Cupido Daniels
Diagnostic Medical Physics Division
Department of Radiology
Dalhousie University
Halifax, Nova Scotia
Canada

Raquel DelCarpio
Department of Neurology and Neurosurgery
McGill University Health Centre
Montreal, QC
Canada
and
Interim Radiologist-in-Chief
Montreal General Hospital
McGill University Health Centre
Montreal, QC
Canada

Josée Dubois
Faculté de medicine
Radiologie, oncologie et médecine
nucléaire
Centre de Recherche du CHU
Sainte-Justine
Montreal, QC
Canada

Holly C. Ellinor
Administrative Assistant
Centre for Education in Medical Imaging
Schulich School of Medicine
and Dentistry
University of Western Ontario
London, ON
Canada

Marielle Fortier
Department of Medical Imaging
Schulich School of Medicine
and Dentistry
University of Western Ontario
London, ON
Canada

Jason R Frank
Office of Education – CanMEDS
Royal College of Physicians and Surgeons
of Canada
Ottawa, ON
Canada

Bob Garvey
The Coaching and Mentoring
Research Unit
Sheffield Hallam University
Howard Street
Sheffield
UK

Richard B. Gunderman
Education Division
Department of Radiology
Indiana University School of Medicine
Indianapolis
USA

Carol P. Herbert
Schulich School of Medicine
and Dentistry
University of Western Ontario
London, ON
Canada

Kathy Hibbert
Centre for Education in
Medical Imaging
Department of Medical Imaging
Schulich School of Medicine
and Dentistry
University of Western Ontario
London, ON
Canada

Kiang Hiong Tay
Education Faculty
Duke-National University of Singapore
Graduate Medical School
Jalan Bukit Merah
Singapore

Robert Kamei
Duke-National University of Singapore
Graduate Medical School
Jalan Bukit Merah
Singapore

Stewart Kribs
Department of Medical Imaging
University of Western Ontario
London, ON
Canada

Mark Landis
Department of Medical Imaging
University of Western Ontario
London, ON
Canada

Lori A. Matheson
Department of Medical Imaging
University of Western Ontario,
London, ON
Canada

Julia O'Sullivan
Faculty of Education
University of Western Ontario
London, ON
Canada

James A Overton
Department of Philosophy
University of Western Ontario
London, ON
Canada

I. John Parboosingh
Obstetrics & Gynecology, and Medical
Education
University of Calgary
Calgary, AB
Canada

Philippe A. Peetrons
Department of Radiology
Centre Hospitalier Molière Longchamp
Brussels
Belgium

Tammie L. Poepping
Department of Physics & Astronomy
The University of Western Ontario
London, ON
Canada

Richard N. Rankin
Department of Medical Imaging
Schulich School of Medicine
and Dentistry
University of Western Ontario
London, ON
Canada

Sharon J. Rich
Faculty of Education
University of New Brunswick
Fredericton and Saint John, NB
Canada

Cesare Romagnoli
Department of Medical Imaging
University of Western Ontario

London, ON
Canada

Youssriah Y. Sabri
Diagnostic Radiology
Kasr Al Ainy Hospital
Cairo University
Egypt

Ahmed Sami Saeed
Diagnostic and Interventional
Radiology
Kasr Al Ainy Hospital
Cairo University
Egypt

Sahar N. Saleem
Department of Diagnostic Radiology
Kasr Al-Ainy Hospital
Cairo University
Egypt
and
University of Western Ontario
(Education in Radiology and MRI)
London, ON
Canada

Louise M. Samson
President, Royal College of Physicians
& Surgeons of Canada
Ottawa, ON
Canada

Wang Shih-chang
Parker-Hughes Chair of Diagnostic
Radiology
Discipline of Imaging
University of Sydney
Department of Radiology
Westmead Hospital, Westmead NSW 2145
Australia

Bien-Soo Tan
Department of Diagnostic Radiology
Singapore General Hospital
Outram Road
Singapore 169608
Singapore

Teresa Van Deven
Centre for Education in Medical Imaging
Schulich School of Medicine and Dentistry
University of Western Ontario
London, ON
Canada

Kenneth B. Williamson
Education Division
Department of Radiology
Indiana University School of Medicine
Indianapolis, IN
USA

Beverly P. Wood
Radiology, Pediatrics and
Medical Education
Keck School of Medicine
University of Southern California
Los Angeles, CA
USA

Luo Yan
Ultrasonic Diagnosis Department
West China Hospital
Sichuan University
China

Introduction

Transforming Radiology Education Through Scholarship

C.P. Herbert, J. O'Sullivan

Clinical education for health professionals is an interesting division of adult education, undergoing both evolution and revolution, as it develops from traditional experiential and opinion-based approaches to encompass more evidence-informed educational practices. While traditional approaches to preceptor-based education remain dominant, there is increasing interest in engaging in the type of scholarly work necessary for establishing an evidence base to drive better educational practices. The ultimate goal is to ensure that health professionals are not only well trained but are also well prepared for lifelong learning, respectful and appreciative of colleagues from other health professions, knowledgeable about new technology, including simulation and Web-based learning opportunities, and broadly educated to enable participation in their community and leadership in health care. This book places radiology education squarely on the theory-driven, evidence-informed end of the continuum.

We understand the need for interdisciplinary approaches to address complex questions. We have fostered the development of the Centre for Scholarship in Radiology Education across our two faculties of medicine and dentistry and education, because of our commitment to ensuring that the expertise in education can inform health professional education, and in turn that the practical realities and needs of clinical learners can inform research in education and contribute to the advancement of knowledge in both fields. We are proud that the Centre is spearheading the discussion across disciplinary and geographical boundaries to create an overview of scholarship in radiology education with practical elements included to guide those who develop curriculum.

The first section of this book is a primer of educational theory and principles, emphasizing the essential need for scholarship in radiology education that will provide the evidence base necessary to inform effective practice. Convincing argument is made that leads the clinical educator-reader to the conclusion that today's radiology students are adult learners, who should be provided with learning opportunities that engage them fully in considering

C.P. Herbert (✉)
Schulich School of Medicine and Dentistry, University of Western Ontario,
London, ON, Canada N6A 5C1

Radiology Education. R.K. Chhem et al. (Eds.)
DOI: 10.1007/978-3-540-68989-8, © Springer-Verlag Berlin Heidelberg 2009

what should be learned, developing their individual learning objectives and goals, planning and monitoring their learning experiences, and demonstrating competency at appropriate intervals throughout their practice lifetime.

Interdisciplinary learning and mentoring are described from a historical perspective that emphasizes the context and relevance of both approaches. Mentoring is presented as complementary to formal educational content and described in practical terms, including, for example, the characteristics of successful mentors. Similarly, interdisciplinary learning is identified as a "rich" and active learning process that stimulates learners to reflect on or think about their practice, identify inconsistencies in their own knowledge base and between their and other learners' knowledge, challenge their prior beliefs and assumptions, seek solutions, and reconstruct their knowledge.

In Part 2 the perspectives of radiology practitioners on professional development, ethics, evidence-based decision-making, and the application of technology to learning in practice are presented. In the chapters on radiology education and scholarship, the theoretical underpinnings are outlined along with a business perspective: "how to do it". Similarly, the chapter on research in medical education reviews challenges and trends in clinical education scholarship generally, as well as detailing the characteristics of some successful educational research centres. The chapter on a radiology curriculum for a new medical school in Singapore brings theory to life, with description of how to educate radiologists but also, importantly, how imaging is an indispensable tool for teaching medicine.

In the "new" radiology, digital imaging is shown to transform clinical data into databases for research and teaching. Learners can use tabletop imaging instruments to learn medical physics, and to become familiar with radiography, computed tomography, and ultrasound images, free of the pressure of the clinical setting.

In Part 3 global approaches to radiology education are considered, with examples from Southeast Asia, China, French-speaking countries, Cambodia, Latin America, and Egypt. Included here are specific examples of tools for successful curriculum delivery to medical students, residents, radiologists, and other physicians. An interesting discussion of the use of the World Wide Web in distributive learning moves the discourse from the narrow perspective of individual curricula to the possibility of worldwide shared curriculum approaches. Similarly, we become aware of the role of professional organizations in leading change, by promoting and disseminating general competencies such as the CanMEDS roles as well as direct teaching of new techniques, with the example of ultrasound workshops.

Overall, this book achieves its goal of bridging theory and practice, by presenting theoretically driven practical approaches to educational scholarship and education in radiology. Importantly it offers encouragement, lessons learned, and evidence-informed advice to help others establish and sustain a culture of scholarship within their own particular domain.

The Genesis and Application of Radiology Education: Mind the Gap

1

T. Van Deven, K. Hibbert, R.K. Chhem

> *I'd rather stand on the edge of a cliff,*
> *And hang my toes over a bit,*
> *And then jump when they dared me even if it scares me to death.*
> *I'd rather build my wings on the way down,*
> *Do my best not to fall to the ground.*
> *And then laugh at my mistakes because they are only lessons I've learned.*
> *Paul Brandt, Risk, 2007.*

Fittingly perhaps, this book emerged from a conversation among a network of scholars in diagnostic radiology and nuclear medicine who shared a deep passion and respect for the power that a "scholarship of teaching and learning" dialogue offered to this neglected field. The First Annual International Conference on Scholarship in Radiology Education, London, Ontario, Canada, proved to be an excellent forum to extend the conversation and invite voices from interested scholars around the world. As we shared our work, it became immediately clear that we were struggling with common issues and constraints. Residents and radiologists alike commented that the conference served to publicly "name" their challenges, and they were buoyed by the ideas generated in the ensuing dialogue around building capacity for change. Over the next several months, as we worked with radiologists in our own department and elsewhere, we realized that in our approach toward optimizing the role and function of education in the radiology department, we were both embodying and enacting the scholarship we were promoting with our colleagues.

A unique feature of this book is that we invited our authors to begin with a "narrative" as "both a mode of thought and an expression of a culture's world view" (Bruner 1996, xiv). Since we were an eclectic group of scholars interested in overlapping themes, we believed that the concept of narrative would help the reader situate each chapter in an appropriate context to encourage meaning making. Not all authors responded with a narrative. For many, the notion of writing in narrative form was significantly outside the mode of written

T. Van Deven (✉)
Centre for Education in Medical Imaging, Schulich School
of Medicine and Dentistry, University of Western Ontario, London, ON, Canada N6A 5C1
E-mail: tvandev@uwo.ca

Radiology Education. R.K. Chhem et al. (Eds.)
DOI: 10.1007/978-3-540-68989-8, © Springer-Verlag Berlin Heidelberg 2009

1

expression in which they were either trained or comfortable. That is alright. Education, as Bruner reminds us, "is a complex pursuit of fitting a culture to the needs of its members and of fitting its members and their ways of knowing to the needs of the culture."

We have experienced this dance before. We fondly recall setting up a room in preparation for a talk we had been invited to give. We had organized the room so that all of the chairs were positioned in small groups so that our participants could have an opportunity to engage in small-group dialogues and activities. While we were occupied with the technology, the attendees filed into the room, and literally "took" their seats, placing them squarely back into rows. This is but one example that clearly demonstrates that many of us have been conditioned to be "received knowers," passively sitting and receiving information, preferably in the form of recipes for success. This book is not a "cookbook." You will not find simple recipes here that can be dropped into a department and served. Rather, we hope that the stories you find within these pages will stimulate an appetite for working with colleagues in your respective departments to integrate scholarship into your routine "diet" of activity in a way that holds great promise to improve the overall academic health of the department, the employees, and most importantly improved outcomes for patient care. We begin by sharing our story.

1.1
Introduction

In *Educating Medical Teachers*, Miller (1980) considers what would happen if "professionals in education and educators in medicine joined forces". In 2006, such a union occurred between radiologists in the Department of Medical Imaging at the Schulich School of Medicine and Dentistry, and educators in the Faculty of Education, The University of Western Ontario, Canada. Like many institutions in search of academic renewal, we drew upon Boyer's (1990) framework for scholarship in order to begin conversations about giving scholarship a more "efficacious meaning" (Glassick 2000). Boyer has suggested that the process of engaging with scholars beyond the traditional disciplinary boundaries may stimulate discussions that reveal insights not previously seen through our traditional disciplinary lens. In this chapter, we examine some of what we have learned along the way.

1.2
Border Crossings

Crossing academic borders, we discovered, is a little bit like walking across a suspension bridge: tentative and shaky at times, thrilling at others. As teachers, we understood that we brought with us a specific educational discourse that may not be familiar to our medical colleagues. Likewise, we understood that the language used in medicine is something we are learning to acquire over time. In this book we are bringing the language of radiologists and the language of educators together through a scholarly endeavor, and as we do this, we cannot help but both shape and be shaped by the other.

When we began this work, the beauty and potential of this mutual reciprocity was not immediately evident. Some of our colleagues in the education faculty asked when we were going to get a "real job." Similarly, some of our medical colleagues did not seem to understand what we might "teach" without the content knowledge of radiology. Initially, therefore, some interpreted our role as being aligned with others in the hospital setting who were deemed "Education Coordinators," but who functioned in a clerical role; for example, one radiologist suggested that we could convert his teaching files from analogue to digital. As we delved further into the medical education literature, we were both comforted and amused by stories from those who have gone before us. Educational pioneer Charles W. Dohner described his path-finding phase into the new field of medical education as akin to being "viewed by some as a second-class citizen" (Irby and Wilkerson 2003). He remarks that he "came in scared … [as if] walking unarmed into a den of lions" (Irby and Wilkerson 2003). In time, he discovered ways in which he could function within the medical culture and in doing so he began to see himself in a new way:

> [I am]…an ambassador from another land, not a second class citizen, and I bring some theories about teaching and learning, and some teaching methodologies to share. If we can develop a collaborative relationship, we can work together to improve medical education (Irby and Wilkerson 2003).

Another medical educator, Hilliard Jason, suggests that PhD educators considering a career in medical education must see themselves as anthropologists and take the time to explore the culture of medicine. He argues that they must be adaptable and able to translate educational discourse into the discourse, climate, and characteristics of the medical setting, and perhaps most importantly "the PhD educator needs to understand the strengths and risks of passion" (Wilkerson and Anderson 2004). Hilliard contends that when he began his career in medical education, he could "not have imagined that there would be careers in medical education, let alone somebody wanting to pay attention to those of us who were nutty enough to make careers of that activity" (Wilkerson and Anderson 2004). Mindful of the experiences of those who have gone before us, and situated at an institution actively encouraging interdisciplinary collaboration, we forged ahead.

1.3
Communities of Professional Practice

Communities of practice are "groups of people who share a concern or a passion for something they do and learn how to do it better as they interact regularly" (Wenger, http://www.ewenger.com/theory/index.htm). "Meaning" in this setting is generated through the negotiation of two main components, *participation* and *reification*. Communities of professional practice are keys to the organization's competence and to the evolution of professional competence. In our context, we had the enthusiastic support from both the Dean of Education and the Dean of the Schulich School of Medicine and Dentistry. Historically, faculties of education have been criticized for their sense of isolation from other disciplines; in 1957, Lyman wrote: "One of the greatest and one of the most unavoidable single mistakes that have been made in education is [its] isolation.... It seems as if each level delights in its isolation, for it does all it can to strengthen and maintain its apartness" (Lyman 1957). Supportive leadership is critical and can have profound implications for the ways in which members engage in their professional practice. Engaging in interdisciplinary scholarly dialogue between radiologists and educators fosters a shift in both identity (seeing themselves as scholars) and behavior (acting in ways that the institution recognizes as scholarly).

1.4
Building a New Home but Living the Same Old Life Within It

Building a "community of professional practice" is one key to realizing a shift in both identity and action. To ignore the community and the professional culture, implementing new curriculum changes would be akin to Miller's example of building a new home:

> ...while the architecture may be different and even admirable, it means nothing if the people within are living the "same old life....

> If [any] aspect of education is to be altered then the actors, not merely the stage setting probably need attention as well (Miller 1980).

We understood this well. We knew that as educators it would be inappropriate for us to conduct a "needs assessment" and then offer a "fix" based on a view from the outside-in. We recognized that there was an enormous gap between the training and subsequent expectations between educators and radiologists and that our work would need to begin addressing that gap in ways that might serve to narrow the chasm (see Table 1.1). Despite requests for a "workshop" that could simply give radiologists the teaching tools that they needed in an hour, we insisted on crafting an educational series in which we attempted to integrate radiology examples from their practice to stimulate dialogue and demonstrate "theory in action" (Schon). We understood that real change must occur from the ground up and that our role was to "foster doubt, to facilitate discovery, and to nourish change" (Miller 1980).

"Ground-up" initiatives must be supported by strong leadership and vision to be successful. In our "needs assessment" we found pockets of innovative and successful scholarship but also noted that with conflicting and sometimes competing agendas scholarship was not sufficiently supported or shared in any meaningful way. For faculty and residents to engage in scholarship broadly, institutions must be willing to value and reward all forms of scholarship equally: teaching, research, integration, and application. The literature is replete with calls for scholarship to be recognized in the broadest sense and rewarded accordingly, but despite these calls "discovery" continues to occupy its privileged position

Table 1.1 The chasm between training and subsequent expectations

	Educators	Radiologists
Educated and trained	– To teach, to develop lessons and curriculum	– To practice medicine, radiology
	– To assess and evaluate	
Expected	– To teach, to develop lessons and curriculum	– To teach, to develop lessons and curriculum
	– To assess and evaluate	– To assess and evaluate

in academia, leaving attention to the other areas woefully neglected. This book includes contributions from authors who work broadly across all levels of scholarship. Bringing their contributions together is another way in which we aim to stimulate dialogue.

1.5
Cultivating Scholarship

As early as 1876, German surgeon Theodor Billroth voiced his concerns about medical pedagogy noting that the "importance of form and method must not be underestimated. On the contrary, we must acknowledge their great pedagogical significance, and therefore spare no effort to perfect them" (Billroth 1924). He contends that scholars are the foundation on which learning, structures, and greatness rest and that this can only be accomplished "if the soil from which they have grown has been properly cultivated" (Billroth 1924). Cultivating scholarship within medical education has been a mission undertaken by many. In 1901, the President of the Association of American Medical Colleges argued that we "must introduce better methods of teaching; we must study medical pedagogy" (Sanazaro 1964). Fifty years later, the same sentiments can be heard:

> While the medical sciences have been rich inviting fields for experimentation and research, medical education is still virgin terrain waiting for equally meticulous inquiry into the art of effective teaching and its materials (Klapper 1950).

Reportedly, a 1955 experiment at the University of Buffalo was the first to hire professional educators in a medical school. Since then, "virtually every medical school and specialty in medicine now employs professional educators to assist with curriculum revision, train faculty to teach, conduct standardized patient programs, or assist with evaluating students and educational programs" (Hitchcock 2002).

When we began this partnership, we were necessarily concerned for radiologists because of the significant "gap" illustrated in Table 1.1. Our participation in the partnership has illustrated an additional gap however. The presence of educators within faculties of medicine is clearly not a new initiative and yet, in many departments, its effects are not translating into practice. As we engage with our medical colleagues it sometimes feels like we are attempting a new way of dancing together; while we have not met with overt resistance, the power of the old dance steps are so familiar and comfortable we had to practice our routine several times before we caught some members "humming our tune" and dancing the new dance. Our "dance card" is not full yet, but we have received increasing numbers of invitations to tango.

In this book, we aim to build community by including diverse voices of scholars, philosophers, academics, scientists, radiologists, residents, educationalists, and administrators working with radiology or in related and complementary disciplines. In this first section, we address "education for noneducators." In Chap. 2, Rethy Chhem brings a unique perspective as one who holds both medical and educational expertise to offer an overview of what scholarship in radiology education entails, and how we might find ways to expand scholarship in medical imaging. In Chap. 3, we bring together the perspectives of a novice radiology training program director (Justin Amann), an experienced radiology training program director (Stewart Kribs), an educationalist (Kathy Hibbert), and a resident (Mark Landis) to consider how we might strengthen the program for residents. In Chap. 4, Teresa Van Deven, Kathy Hibbert, and Holly Ellinor offer insight into the activities and insights gleaned as they formed a Centre for Education in Medical Imaging and began their interdisciplinary work. In Chap. 5, Sharon Rich picks up this thread, and provides an in-depth look at interdisciplinary learning and the power it promises in terms of learner engagement and reflective practice. We devoted Chap. 6 to the topic of feedback as a critical component of assessment and evaluation. In this chapter, Richard Gunderman and Kenneth Williamson outline some common practices and opportunities to provide meaningful feedback. In Chap. 7, Bob Garvey addresses the important role of mentoring in professional education, offering a historical overview and conditions for developing successful mentoring practices. Finally, in the last chapter of this section, Robert Arp, Cesare Ramagnoli, Rethy Chhem, and James Overton introduce a framework for constructing a radiology ontology.

In Part 2, which we have named "educational insights from practitioners," we invited contributions from those working in the field in order to stimulate dialogue around specific issues. Lucie Brazeau-Lamontagne opens this section with a discussion on what ought to be considered in professional ethics in radiology. Following that, John Parboosingh, Beverly Wood, Louise Samson, and Craig Campbell focus on learning in practice and the importance of interprofessional collaborative learning in the practice environment. We devote Chap. 11 to the Canadian CanMEDS framework, as has served as a model that has inspired application in the global context, and that is referred to frequently throughout the book. Rethy Chhem, Louise Samson, Jason Frank, and Josée Dubois review the model as a process for acquiring competencies in radiology. Given the dominant place that technology holds in the medical imaging sciences, in Chap. 12 Richard Rankin examines the use of picture archiving and communication systems, databases, and teaching files in radiological practice. This is followed by the description of an innovative project Jerry Battista and Tammie Poepping in Chap. 13, in which they outline their portable imaging systems and the potential for this innovation to improve interactive teaching.

In Chap. 14, Jannette Collins provides an in-depth review of medical education research generally, followed by a look at what the future may hold for radiology education research specifically. Her work presents useful information for those preparing to embark on research activities in the field. Kiang Hiong Tay, Bien Soo Tan, and Robert Kamei outline their experiences starting a graduate medical school in Singapore in Chap. 15. In particular, they focus on defining the role of radiology within the Graduate Medical School curricula. In Chap. 16, Richard Gunderman writes about leadership in radiology education and scholarship, demonstrating how learning from our failures can be the springboard for success. Finally, in Chap. 17, Lori Matheson outlines what is involved at the business end of scholarship, the need to build an effective team and consider infrastructure and support issues to develop a solid business plan to support desired scholarship activity.

Finally, in Part 3, we look to our colleagues around the world to learn about global outreach initiatives. Awareness and attention to what is happening in radiology education around the world informs and extends our understanding of radiology education scholarship, and invites discussion at a broader level. We begin this section with Chap. 18, in which Shih-chang Wang provides a detailed overview of radiology education programs in Southeast Asia, noting the pedagogical challenges and contrasts faced by our colleagues in that part of the world. Luo Yan adds to this picture in Chap. 19, presenting her experiences training ultrasound physicians in western China.

In Chaps. 20 and 21, Marielle Fortier and Raquel DelCarpio, respectively, discuss their experiences traveling from Canada to work, teach, and ultimately learn through outreach in Cambodia and Peru. In Chap. 22, Cupido Daniels writes about the role of the World Wide Web as a means and a mode of developing competencies through digital resources. In Chap. 23, Philippe Peetrons presents his experience participating in the formation of learned societies as a way to address a lack of training in musculoskeletal ultrasound in French-speaking countries, and discovers the societies to be an excellent venue for developing sophisticated pedagogical practices with participants. Finally, our book concludes with Chap. 24, in which Sahar Saleem, Youssriah Sabri, and Ahmed Sami Saeed review the radiology education program at the University of Cairo, a reminder to those of us who practice in the western world of the wisdom afforded by those with a significant history.

It has often been stated that radiologists have minimal patient contact. We agree with Fielding et al that it "may be time to change the emphasis from patient contact to patient impact. It is a rare patient who does not undergo an imaging examination for diagnosis" (Fielding 2007). Our partnership between the Faculty of Education and the Radiology Department has shown us the strength that can be found in a culture of reciprocity – by borrowing from both cultures, we believe we can enhance our own understanding, confidence and competence and therefore gain a degree of satisfaction from the recognition that we are preparing a new generation of health care professionals better able to meet the challenges of the profession.

References

Billroth T (1924) The medical sciences in the German universities. Macmillan, New York
Boyer EL (1990) Scholarship reconsidered: Priorities of the professoriate. The Carnegie Foundation for the Advancement of Teaching, New York
Bruner J (1996) The culture of education. Cambridge, Mass. Harvard University Press.

1

Fielding JR et al (2007) Choosing a specialty in medicine: Female medical students and radiology. Am J Radiol 188:897–900

Glassick CE (2000) Boyer's expanded definitions of scholarship, the standards of assessing scholarship, and the elusiveness of the scholarship of teaching. Acad Med 75:808

Hitchcock MA (2002) Introducing professional educators into academic medicine: Stories of exemplars. Adv Health Sci Educ 7:211–221

Irby DM, Wilkerson L (2003) Charles W. Dohner, PhD: An evaluator and mentor in medical education. Adv Health Sci Educ 8:63–73

Klapper P (1950) Medical education as education. J Assoc Am Med Coll 25:314

Lyman RA (1957) Disaster in pedagogy. N Eng J Med 257(11):504–507

Miller GE (1980) Educating medical teachers. Harvard University Press, Cambridge

Sanazaro P (1964) The renaissance of AAMC interest in medical education. Med Educ 39:229

Schon D (1983) The reflective practitioner: How professionals think in action. New York: Basic Books.

Wilkerson L, Anderson W (2004) Hilliard Jason, MD, EdD: A medical student turned educator. Adv Health Sci Educ 9:325–335

Scholarship in Radiology Education

R.K. Chhem

When one performs a Google search using the keywords "scholarship," "radiology," and "education" the results are quite surprising. For many people it appears, the term "scholarship" refers only to monetary support for the educational and training programs in radiology. For others, it refers to funding used to sponsor residents and fellows to attend professional conferences. When the same keywords were used for a PubMed search, 144 articles were identified. Most of the PubMed articles deal with residents and fellows training in radiology and its many subspecialties. This body of literature indicates the practice of educational scholarship within academic departments of radiology (i.e., the systematic documentation of teaching, learning, and assessment of learning outcomes). Only one article expresses the concept of scholarship in its full meaning within the community of academic radiologists. For the authors,

> …the contributions of educators to the viability and growth of the specialty require equal legitimacy to research in academic recognition. Development of educators and documentation of educational activities are key elements in achieving academic status for scholarly activity (Wood and May 2006).

From these cursory observations, it appears that there is a principal need to first define the term "scholarship" in the sense that we are using it in this book, where the goal is to promote and enhance the concept and formal implementation of scholarship in the teaching and learning of radiology within academic departments of radiology. Once the concept of educational scholarship is clearly defined, like-minded radiologists (who are already practicing teaching under this paradigm) may find opportunities to engage with the ideas and experiences of others through this endeavor.

R.K. Chhem
Department of Medical Imaging, Schulich School of Medicine
and Dentistry, University of Western Ontario, London, ON, Canada N6A 5C1
E-mail: rethy.chhem@lhsc.on.ca

Radiology Education. R.K. Chhem et al. (Eds.)
DOI: 10.1007/978-3-540-68989-8, © Springer-Verlag Berlin Heidelberg 2009

2.1
What is Scholarship in Radiology Education?

According to Merriam-Webster's online dictionary, the term "scholarship" is defined in the following order: (1) a grant-in-aid to a student (as by a college or foundation); (2) the character, qualities, activity, or attainments of a scholar; (3) a fund of knowledge and learning (drawing on the *scholarship* of the ancients). In this book scholarship would refer to either the second or the third meaning as given above. For a more comprehensive understanding of the application of the term "scholarship" as it applies to academia, we draw upon Ernest Boyer's work. Boyer popularized the concept of scholarship as it applied to academic activities in the American higher education system, which has increasingly permeated into many medical schools' academic paradigms (Boyer 1990). According to Boyer, the work of the professoriate can be divided into four overlapping functions, namely, the scholarship of discovery, integration, application, and teaching (Boyer 1990) (Table 2.1. Boyer's work stimulated a surge of interest and growth in the body of knowledge on scholarship, and in 1997, Glassick et al. (1997) followed it up with another notable work on the topic, *Scholarship Assessed*, which builds on Boyer's foundation.

Notably, in Boyer's conceptual framework of scholarship, the equitable inclusion of the four areas does not in any way minimize the importance of discovery.

According to Beattie (2000), the scholarship of discovery "should not be minimized as new models of scholarship are recognized, described, evaluated and rewarded" (p. 873). There is no argument that the scholarship of discovery must be sustained as the advancement of specialized knowledge is constantly required. Discovery of knowledge plays a vital role as the "process, the outcomes and especially the passion of discovery enhance

Table 2.1 Boyer's four areas of scholarship

Discovery	To discover is a key element in scholarship. For scholarship to be sustained, the advancement of specialized knowledge is required. Discovery contributes not only to knowledge but also to the intellectual climate of a college, university or department
Integration	To interpret, to draw together and to bring new insights to bear on original research
	Integration advocates a capacity to look for new relationships between the parts and the whole
Application	To ask questions: How can knowledge be applied? How can it serve the interests of the department, university, community, the world?
	Application addresses the issue of the interaction between theory and practice
Teaching	To move teaching beyond a routine function to be viewed as an endeavour that not only transmits knowledge but also transforms and extends it

From Boyer (1990)

the meaning of the effort of the institution itself" (see p. 9 in Glassick 1997). Integration becomes true scholarship when novel insights, both interpretative and interdisciplinary, are discovered. According to Glassick et al. (1997), the scholarship of integration makes connections between the disciplines by "altering the contexts in which people view knowledge and offsetting the inclination to split knowledge into ever more esoteric bits and pieces....The scholarship of integration seeks to interpret, draw together and bring new insights to bear on original research" (p. 9). Integration advocates a capacity to synthesize and to look for new relationships between the parts and the whole. Application looks at how knowledge can be applied and how can it serve the interests of the larger community. Scholarship of application has to "prove its worth not on its own terms, but by the service to the nation and the world" (Hanlin, in Derek Bok 1990, p. 103). The common aspect of scholarship of application is the dissemination of useful, testable, and reproducible information to others. In terms of clinical expertise, what constitutes the scholarship of application? This could apply to patient-oriented research such as clinical trials, drug or physical therapy, or case-controlling studies such as the relationship between smoking and lung cancer. Application looks at how intervention works when applied to humans.

According to Shapiro and Coleman (2000), in the case of clinicians who see many patients and become experts in clinical evaluation, their experiences constitute expertise but not necessarily scholarship. The authors add, however, that if clinicians "systematically assess the effectiveness of different techniques and communicate these findings in a way that allows others to benefit from that expertise" (p. 896) then that is scholarship. The dominant view of scholarship appears to place research and theory as hierarchically superior relative to practice; practice has been predominantly viewed as the passive recipient of knowledge. The scholarship of application dictates that theory and practice are complementary and mutually enriching. Teaching is often viewed as "a routine function, tacked on, something almost anyone can do" (see p. 23 in Boyer 1990). Boyer argues that teaching needs to be viewed as a dynamic endeavor that goes beyond the transmission of knowledge to transform and extend knowledge. Glassick et al. (1997) contend that scholarly teaching "initiates students into the best values of the academy, enabling them to comprehend better and participate more fully in the larger culture" (p. 9).

While there is a strong and well-established infrastructure to assess and reward the scholarship of discovery, there is an urgent need for mechanisms to review and advance the scholarship of teaching. There is a need to develop a strong infrastructure that can provide a systematic examination of the degree to which there is support and recognition for faculty as educators. Glassick proposes six standards for judging excellence of scholarship that include clear goals, adequate preparation, appropriate methods, significant results, effective presentation, and reflective critique (Glassick 2000) (Table 2.2).

For most faculty members, the scholarship of discovery is not only the most prestigious and "noble" function, but practically speaking it is the kind of scholarship that is rewarding during the promotion and tenure process. The scholarship of discovery is highly regarded because it "contributes to the intellectual climate of a college or university, not to mention its role in enhancing the track record of scholars, further increasing the likelihood that

2

Table 2.2 Glassick et al.'s six standards of assessment of scholarly work

Standard	Does the scholar
Clear goals	– State basic purpose of work? – Define objectives that are realistic? Achievable? – Identify the important questions in the field?
Adequate preparation	– Show an understanding of existing scholarship within the field? (ex: literature review) – Bring skills to the body of work? – Bring resources that allow the project to move forward?
Appropriate methods	– Utilize a methodology that is appropriate to goals? – Apply methods effectively? – Modify procedures in response to changing circumstances?
Significant results	– Achieve the goal? – Does the work add consequentially to the field? – Address areas for further exploration?
Effective presentation	– Utilize a suitable style and organization to present the work? – Utilize a suitable forum to communicate and share findings with an audience? – Present the findings with clarity and integrity?
Reflective critique	– Critically evaluate the work? – Bring appropriate breadth of evidence to the critique? – Use evaluation to improve quality of the work?

From Glassick et al. (1997)

they would secure a research grant. In medicine and radiology, scholarship of discovery activities includes an original research project, followed by publication in a high-impact peer-reviewed journal. An example of scholarship of integration is the use of specialized knowledge across the medical discipline with the goal of educating the nonspecialist. This includes the organization of imaging rounds for cancer specialists and the publication of a critical review of the indication of computed tomography angiography in cardiac diseases or a book chapter on musculoskeletal ultrasound in sports injuries. Scholarship of application consists in using knowledge for the benefit of individuals, institutions, and society. This includes the validation of a new 1 test in disease detection or the use of an image-guided interventional procedure to extract a ureteral stone. The last but not the least of these four types of scholarship is the scholarship of teaching, which is the focus of this book. It is important to emphasize that although we are focusing on teaching because it has been seriously neglected, it remains one component of the whole and we are promoting a program that synthesizes all four elements equally. Our efforts are directed at helping radiology departments understand the scholarship of teaching and learning as an integral part of the larger picture of academic scholarship.

The scholarship of teaching is curiously the least understood and practiced in academic radiology departments. It is worth remembering that the word doctor, as Gunderman et al. (2003) point out, comes from the Latin *doctoris*, which means "teacher." Indeed, we all teach radiology to medical students both informally and formally. We train and supervise residents in radiology and nuclear medicine, and fellows as well. Sometimes we participate in the assessment process during the examinations organized by the school of medicine or professional licensing bodies, submit multiple-choice questions to examination databases participating in objective structured clinical examination or objective structured practical examination, or rarely serve on curriculum committees. Exceptionally, a very few of us would publish a research paper on the process of teaching and learning itself. Finally, while we often consult PubMed to enlighten our daily radiology practice, few would consult a book on educational theories or strategies or learning objectives established by the curriculum office before lecturing an auditorium full of medical students. The difference between the very professional, scientifically rigorous way in which we embrace our clinical practice and the "amateurish" way we approach teaching is remarkable. An expanded body of medical imaging knowledge and medical sciences has led to a crowded curriculum for the 5-year residency that cannot be sustained without attention to the scholarship of teaching and learning.

This situation calls for a reassessment of the way we teach and learn radiology at the present time and in the future. We must reconsider the current approach to addressing the growing curriculum if we hope to keep the content and duration of radiology or nuclear medicine residency programs within a reasonable scope, breath, and time. Expanding the scholarship of medical imaging, which has traditionally predominantly recognized activities of discovery, integration, and application of knowledge, to include equal recognition of the scholarship of teaching is a pressing necessity if we hope to cope with the incoming tide of new knowledge and if radiology is to ride the crest of these inevitable changes.

The scholarship in outreach is the last but not the least important activity that measures the impact of scholarship on the community at local, regional, and global levels. Lerner et al. define "applied developmental science" as a scholarship that seeks to advance the integration of developmental research with actions – policies and programs – that promote positive development and/or enhance the life chances of vulnerable children and families (Lerner et al. 2000). Sandmann et al. recommend that scholars engage in community-based projects (defined as the scholarship of outreach), as an additional dimension within the many missions in academia. These authors suggest that community outreach provides an excellent opportunity to learn about the scholar's own work (Sandmann et al. 2000). These two separate projects share the same foundation, that is to foster the scholarship in outreach, and may become a model for sharing radiology teaching and learning experience with colleagues from developing countries such as China, Cambodia, or Peru as documented elsewhere in this book. In order to be accepted as a scholarly activity, outreach projects must be guided by a question that leads to knowledge discovery, integration, application, transmission, or preservation. Following on from Glassik's model, the scholarship of outreach must be guided by clear goals, appropriate methods, significant results, effective communication, and reflective critique (Sandmann et al. 2000). In fact the scholarship of outreach may become a "fifth dimension" of scholarly activities complementing the four others defined by Boyer.

2

2.2
Why Expand Scholarship in Medical Imaging?

The "ecosystem" of medical imaging is changing rapidly because of the acceleration of knowledge discovery in medical imaging in particular and in biomedical science in general. The new ecosystem of medical imaging includes, among others, the ability to map the human genome with its implications in life science and medical practices, the development of information technology (imaging informatics), and the availability of huge databases and powerful computers (computer grids, ultradense storage, and databases that integrate clinical, laboratory, and imaging data as well as DNA/protein sequences, advanced data mining, and pattern-discovery algorithms) (Thrall 2005; Branstetter 2007a, b; Garlatti and Sharples 1998). These medical and technological breakthroughs have already altered the pattern of medical practice. New medical imaging methods (molecular imaging, cell imaging, functional imaging, etc.) are now available, and most of them are already in operation in clinical practices. Progress in pharmacogenetics will soon lead to a new way of treating patients in the form of personalized medicine, not to mention the hope of an effective adult and embryonic stem-cell therapy for certain diseases. At the core of these tremendous changes stands medical imaging, which is becoming a sort of "medical GPS" that detects, targets, and destroys abnormal molecules or cells. To reach this goal, radiology educators may have to think about redesigning the medical imaging curriculum to equip future physicians and radiologists, and nuclear medicine physicians as well with a body of knowledge that meets the demands of medical practice in the postgenomic and digital eras (Thrall 2005).

Another technology that has revolutionized the way radiologists "read their films" is the widespread use of picture archiving and communication systems, which is addressed elsewhere in this book. The interpretation of a huge number of images, which can reach a few thousand in one computed tomography study, called also for a new way to interpret medical images. Computer-assisted diagnosis has already become operative in some advanced medical imaging centers. Equally important, there will be a major paradigm shift for radiologists who are used to the anatomical dimension of the human body to move towards a functioning interpretation of medical imaging. Finally, molecular imaging is looming on the horizon and may soon become available for some selected clinical situations. Again here radiologists have to move from organ to cells then to molecules (Hoffman and Gambhir 2007).

These medical and technological advances have already blurred the boundaries between "radiology" and nuclear medicine. Hybrid imaging, which is now already in operation, has actually "merged" the two specialties. This raises the question as to how to train physicians to become specialists who can operate in this new environment. Here again there is a need for innovation of the curriculum that needs to include new parameters imposed by the new medical imaging ecosystem (Hoffman and Gambhir 2007; Gunderman et al. 2002; Williamson et al. 2004).

Besides the issues related to curriculum content that would equip specialists to practice in this changing and expanding environment, the scholarship of teaching/learning must take into consideration the educational requirements of accreditation agencies such as the American Board of Radiology, the American Board of Nuclear Medicine, and the Royal College of Physicians and Surgeons of Canada, keeping in mind the specific requirements of, for example, the Canadian system of CanMEDS.

The issues mentioned above have addressed some of the complexities involved in the organization of teaching and learning in the context of a profession. In addition, curriculum planning must also take into consideration societal needs as the ultimate goal of any biomedical research in general and medical imaging in particular. Finally, the globalization of biomedical research and education with numerous transnational research and educational projects merits consideration in the planning and establishment of medical imaging residency programs.

A last word on the expanding role of medical imaging teaching is the humanitarian needs to address the teaching/learning of the medical imaging specialty in developing countries that have been taken up by outreach programs established by universities, learned professional societies, or governmental international organizations such as the International Atomic Energy Agency.

2.3
How to Expand Scholarship in Medical Imaging Education?

As in all endeavors, an innovative approach to teaching scholarship requires a combination of factors in order to be successful. At the top of the academic organization, there is a need for staunch support from the dean of the medical school, who will advocate and engage with peers, colleagues, administrators, and students as well as embarking on that journey. At the operational level, the academic chair of radiology needs to secure the support of members in the department. Not all members will be convinced at the early phase of the development of an auspicious environment for teaching scholarship to blossom. However, a few will respond enthusiastically and the majority will either follow or remain neutral with respect to the new initiative. The next crucial step is to recruit professional educationists willing to interact with radiologists; radiologists who bring a very different background in education and training to their commitment to teach their own specialty, despite the lack of a formal qualification in educational principles. Finally, the department chair must be able to secure the resources necessary to sustain a "business plan" to foster and practice the scholarship of teaching and learning.

2.3.1
Academic Leadership

In order to foster, to value, and to implement the scholarship of teaching unfailing support is required from the academic senior leadership team, including the provost, the dean of the medical school, and the radiology department chair. Leadership support must be translated into a business plan that includes sufficient resources, such as administrative, academic (educationists appointed within the clinical department and/or clinical radiologists with a formal qualification in education), equipment, space and supplies, and operational funding as well. In addition to senior leadership support, Fincher et al. suggest that clinicians and basic scientists must form coalitions with other educators to advocate changes needed to enhance teaching scholarship, through policy-setting committees (Fincher et al. 2000).

2.3.2
Faculty Members

Most academic departments of radiology invite faculty members to serve on educational committees (undergraduate and postgraduate) depending on their declared interest in and dedication to teaching. Although few have any formal training in education, their "passion for teaching" forms a necessary but insufficient requirement to do the work of developing and implementing a curriculum based on sound educational principles. As a result, programs tend to resemble an amalgam of presentations centered around the "medical expert" role, but devoid of any overarching vision or understanding of curriculum design, which includes, for example, plans for appropriate pedagogical strategies or meaningful assessment and evaluation. Educationalists are able to bring this knowledge and expertise to the department to work collaboratively on the macro issues that surround planning, and then on the micro issues that involve teaching.

It is important for educationalists to document all teaching and educational activities as a means of assessing and responding to the varying needs of the department, to build evidence to support scholarly activities, and as a way of generating exemplars to share across the department with committees experiencing similar challenges. The documentation also serves additional purposes. First, it allows each faculty member to build a teaching portfolio that reflects his/her own career development. Second, the collection of portfolios across the departmental faculty members can be assessed to reflect improved excellence in teaching within the department, a crucial tool for measurement of performance during the annual review. The development of a "scholarship-in-education" portfolio (Wood and May 2006) should include:

> Teaching and evaluation activities
> Educational program directorship
> Educational research (presentations, seminars, publications)
> Grants in education
> Educational awards
> Educational services (committees, councils, organizations, etc.)
> Advising, resident and graduate student supervision
> Curriculum development
> Outreach activities and
> Professional development

The "educational portfolio" model has been adopted as recognized criteria for promotion in many academic institutions (Hafler and Lovejoy 2000). For Simpson et al., "educational excellence requires documentation of the quantity and quality of education activities. Documenting a scholarly approach requires demonstrating evidence of drawing from and building on the work of others, and documenting scholarship requires contributing public display, peer review and dissemination; both involve engagement with the community of educators" (Simpson et al. 2007).

Beyond the establishment of faculty career development among physicians and basic scientists, it is crucial to include professional educationists within a clearly defined structure dedicated for the support of scholarly activities in radiology education. This is the fundamental point that needs to be emphasized within the endeavor. Physicians and basic scientists have been educated and trained to produce scholarly works in their respective clinical and scientific fields. Few of these faculty members have had any formal training in education such as curriculum design or development, philosophy and theories of education, cognitive psychology, measurements and assessment, etc. Hence, there is crucial need for the inclusion of professionals educationists within the radiology department. Ideally, in order to build a sustainable team, the educationalists would require a faculty appointment with a clear path for career development similar to those held by the clinicians and scientists in the field.

2.3.3
Specific Educational Structures

There are many types of structures within a medical school or a university that are dedicated to the development of teaching scholarship. An academy of/for medical educators is one example, with models from the University of California, San Francisco and from the UK (Bligh and Brice 2007; Cooke et al. 2007; Sandars and McAreavey 2007).

The overall aim [is] to develop and sustain medical education as an academic discipline. This is an important milestone in the journey of ensuring that medical education becomes a recognized professional discipline in the UK. Our experience suggests that few educators apply the same degree of scholarship to medical education as they do to their other professional discipline, such as being a physician or being a general medical practitioner. The potential of the new academy to improve the quality of medical education will be determined by its membership and their understanding of the nature of the scholarship of medical education (Sandars and McAreavey 2007).

These structures have been established to foster teaching scholarship in medical education in general. We have developed our own model, focusing exclusively on teaching/learning scholarship in radiology/nuclear medicine. For the first time in the history of the department, the Faculty of Education has entered into a partnership with the Department of Medical Imaging, Schulich School of Medicine and Dentistry, University of Western Ontario (http://www.edu.uwo.ca/cedrnm/). The purpose of the interdisciplinary collaboration is to support the vision of optimizing the role and function of education in radiology/nuclear medicine. This center has three main goals:

1. Strengthen curriculum design and implementation (including IT) in response to educational needs
2. Support and guide "the art of teaching" for faculty and residents at both practical and theoretical levels
3. Advance educational scholarship in medical imaging education through research

These three goals are the operational translation of the scholarship of teaching and learning as defined above. Within less than 2 years, the center was involved in several academic activities that included curriculum design and implementation as well as in supporting and guiding "the art of teaching" for faculty members and residents:

2

In practical terms, the educators from our center:

> Serve on the Department of Radiology's Resident Training Committee, both at undergraduate and et postgraduate levels
> Participate in Schulich's faculty and staff development courses in all applicable areas (for example, Web conferencing or CanMEDS roles)
> Attend the biannual department meeting of the Department of Medical Imaging
> Attend journal club meetings, citywide and grand rounds to gain understanding of the radiology/nuclear medicine resident's experience

In theoretical terms the educators:

> Met with various medical students showing an interest in radiology education to discuss the possibility of their involvement with the center's activities
> Met with the Associate Dean of Undergraduate Medical Education to gain understanding of the initial knowledge base of radiology residents
> Met with various members of the department on a one-on-one basis to discuss teaching methods and solutions and mentoring and to review their course materials
> Met with the chief residents from the areas of both radiology and nuclear medicine to discuss the role of the center and what can be offered to them specifically
> Met with members of the Schulich School of Medicine and Dentistry's Research Office to discuss funding possibilities and application

The center contributed to the advancement of scholarship in medical imaging education by:

> Establishing an educational series, developed and presented to residents, faculty, radiologists, and nuclear medicine scientists on the topics of anatomy of curriculum, teaching and learning theories, assessment and evaluation, and building a culture for mentorship
> Presenting the aforementioned educational series by invitation locally, nationally, and internationally (at the Duke-National University of Singapore Medical School)
> Applying for and receiving funding for radiology education research
> Establishing and organizing the First Annual Scholarship in Radiology Education conference, which was hosted jointly by the Schulich School of Medicine and Dentistry and the Faculty of Education, University of Western Ontario
> Launching the Society for Scholarship in Radiology Education

2.4
Conclusion

In this chapter we have defined what scholarship is in academic radiology, identified the categories, explored why and how we should expand scholarship in this clinical field, and stressed the importance of the scholarship of teaching in radiology departments. In order to achieve excellence in educational scholarship in radiology, there is a need to invest substantially in building intellectual capacity (educationists and radiologist-educators, resident-educators) and in developing adequate infrastructures. Exploring scholarship in radiology education is in its infancy and calls for a broader consultation and debate among educators and radiologists in order to expand the understanding of its concept and its implication in order to integrate its values into the training of radiologists to meet the accelerating changes of the practice of radiology.

References

Beattie DS (2000) Expanding the view of scholarship. Acad Med 75:871–876

Bligh J, Brice J (2007) The academy of medical educators: A professional home for medical educators in the UK. Med Educ 41:625–627

Bok DC (1990) Universities and the future of America. Duke University Press, Durham

Boyer EL (1990) Scholarship reconsidered: Priorities of the professoriate. Jossey-Bass, San Francisco

Branstetter BF IV (2007a) Basics of imaging informatics part 1. Radiology 243:656–667

Branstetter BF IV (2007b) Basics of imaging informatics part 2. Radiology 244:78–84

Cooke M, Irby DM, Debas HT (2007) The UCSF Academy of Medical Educators. Acad Med 78:666–672

Fincher RM, Simpson DE, Mennin SP, Rosenfeld GC, Rothman A, McGrew MC, Hansen PA, Mazmanian PE, Turnbull JM (2000) Scholarship in teaching: An imperative for the 21st century. Acad Med 75:887–894

Garlatti S, Sharples M (1998) The use of a computerized brain atlas to support knowledge-based training in radiology. Artif Intell Med 13:181–205

Glassick CE (2000) Reconsidering scholarship. J Public Health Manag Pract 6:4–9

Glassick CE, Huber MT, Maeroff G (1997) Scholarship assessed: Evaluation of the professoriate. Jossey-Bass, San Francisco

Gunderman RB, Kang YP, Fraley RE, Williamson KB (2002) Teaching the teachers. Radiology 222:599–603

Gunderman RB, Siddiqui AR, Heitkamp DE, Kipfer HD (2003) The vital role of radiology in the medical school curriculum. Am J Roentgenol 180:1239–1242

Hafler JP, Lovejoy FH Jr (2000) Scholarly activities recorded in the portfolios of teacher-clinician faculty. Acad Med 75:649–652

Hoffman JM, Gambhir SS (2007) Molecular imaging: The vision and opportunity for radiology in the future. Radiology 244:39–47

Lerner RM, Fisher CB, Weinberg RA (2000) Toward a science for and of the people: promoting civil society through the application of developmental science. Child Dev 71:11–20

Sandars J, McAreavey MJ (2007) Developing the scholarship of medical educators: a challenge in the present era of change. Postgrad Med J 83:561

Sandmann LR, Foster-Fishman PG, Lloyd J, Rauhe W, Rosaen C (2000) Managing critical tensions: How to strengthen the scholarship component of outreach. Change 32:45–52

Shapiro ED, Coleman DL (2000) The scholarship of application. Acad Med 75:895–898

Simpson D, Fincher RM, Hafler JP, Irby DM, Richards BF, Rosenfeld GC, Viggiano TR (2007) Advancing educators and education by defining the components and evidence associated with educational scholarship. Med Educ 41:1002–1009

2

Thrall JH (2005) Reinventing radiology in the digital age: part I. The all-digital department. Radiology 236:382–385

Williamson KB, Gunderman RB, Cohen MD, Frank MS (2004) Learning theory in radiology education. Radiology 233:15–18

Wood BP, May W (2006) Academic recognition of educational scholarship. Acad Radiol 13:254–257

Today's Radiology Student: What Every Radiology Training Program Director Needs to Know

3

J. Amann, S. Kribs, K. Hibbert, M. Landis

3.1
Imagine

Imagine that you have left a meeting with the Chair of the Radiology Department. Somehow you were persuaded to accept a new role as Director of Radiology Training. What exactly have you just agreed to? Feeling both apprehension and excitement, your mind begins to explore what you know and what you do not know about this role. You are certainly familiar with the position itself – after all, you are a radiologist, you have been a resident, and you have watched your colleague in another hospital serve in the role for the past 5 years. Now it is your turn. You make a mental note to visit the outgoing Director and find out what support and resources are in place that you need to become aware of in order to prepare for this new role. Since all programs have a residency, you consider that you will likely receive some direction from the Postgraduate Education (PGE) Office. Since all medical academic centers in Canada offering radiology programs are accredited by the same governing body (The Royal College of Physicians of Surgeons of Canada), you know that you will have provincial and national counterparts to call on for advice. You feel at once both overwhelmed and comforted by this thought and begin to wonder where you are going to find the time for all of this "networking" when you still have your own clinical work to do. You take a deep breath. You refocus on the various teaching hospitals within your own network, and you quickly recognize how important it will be to have a strong site director at each site that you can count on. In a very busy teaching hospital, you will need everyone to contribute to the academic mission through teaching rounds, reading cases, or offering weekly afternoon academic sessions. At the same time, you have to

J. Amann (✉)
Department of Medical Imaging,
University of Western Ontario, London, ON, Canada N6A 5C1
E-mail: jamann@uwo.ca

Radiology Education. R.K. Chhem et al. (Eds.)
DOI: 10.1007/978-3-540-68989-8, © Springer-Verlag Berlin Heidelberg 2009

3

provide leadership to radiology residents who come with knowledge, skills, and values that are somewhat different from those shared by their predecessors. What are these differences and how can you leverage them to result in positive learning experiences? What exactly have you just agreed to?

3.2
The Context

Understanding the context within which we practice can have profound implications for how we approach and design our responses to challenges. Acknowledging, for example, that the social environment or "informal" curriculum of a teaching hospital can profoundly influence its residents' values and professional identities may be the first step in understanding that teaching is part of every interaction that residents encounter in their residency. Recognizing this fact invokes an urgency to approach resident training in a way that engages all of the members of a radiology department. Even those who are not assigned to any formal "teaching" are inculcating the next generation of radiologists into a particular professional culture. What are they learning when we are not looking?

Similarly, residents bring a diverse body of knowledge, culture, and experience into the learning environment which necessarily influences and shapes that environment. The radiology pedagogue must consider his/her role in new ways. During the undergraduate medical education years, students typically develop fairly sophisticated skills as independent learners. Today's students are, for the most part, technologically savvy and capable of using the Internet and other digital databases to locate information quickly from a variety of sources. They also tend to be more global in their thinking and their experiences. Access to such a wealth of information brings both benefits and new challenges. In a teaching setting, it can foster a climate in which the primary source of information shifts. Rather than first attempting to seek information from textbooks or a more experienced mentor or colleague, residents can also locate information electronically. This shift creates a new set of needs (i.e., the ability to assess the relevance and credibility of the source of the information they are locating) and a new set of circumstances (i.e., reduced collaboration between residents and radiologists). Are preceptors and faculty aware of the sources of information that residents and clerks may be accessing? Does the availability of multiple sources of information lead to new opportunities for reciprocal learning between teacher and student?

The shift from undergraduate medical education to residency training is not a smooth one for many students. Some argue that "the transition from medical school to internship is a sudden confrontation with responsibilities for which students have only been partially trained" (Ten Cate et al. 2004). Consider, for example, the different skills involved for residents (accustomed to working on their own with radiologists in the department in small groups or individually) when they placed in situations where they must orally give evidence, describe a case, defend a differential diagnosis, or explain their reasoning. There is a notable difference between developing proficiency as passive receivers of knowledge and becoming active consumers and generators of knowledge.

The level of responsibility given to medical students is carefully monitored and controlled, as they do not have a license to practice. However, once a trainee transitions to an intern or resident, he/she earns the ability to practice medicine independently with graded responsibility. Interns and residents are now allowed to write orders and make medical decisions which will affect patient care. They must know their own limitations and seek help and guidance when appropriate. Trainees need direction, support, and encouragement from their program director to make this transition. Similarly, residents are confronted with a less-structured learning environment than they experienced in medical school. Most medical schools have a well-defined curriculum and students are examined to ensure they learn the material. In residency, learning is much less structured and there are greater clinical and nonclinical demands, including research, administrative duties, and family responsibilities. These other responsibilities compete for a resident's time to study and learn. While the interest to learn must come from within, the program director can help by providing a challenging, stimulating environment which encourages self-directed learning.

It is widely acknowledged that "the development of interpretive skills is universally emphasized in radiology residency programs" (Musick and Gunderman 2004). However, "a variety of non-interpretive skills are required for radiologists to function as well-rounded and competent physicians." In residency training, critical thinking, assessment, synthesis, evaluation, and application of understanding become paramount. In other words, by fostering an approach that views the resident not only as "trainee," but also as a "scholar," we better prepare our future radiologist with the requisite skills not only to perform the role but also to actively participate in the profession, in research, and in education to ensure a bright future for the profession.

All of these issues point to a requirement that the training of the radiology resident ought to be a shared responsibility. In the spirit of sharing responsibility, this chapter includes the voices of Justin Amann, the new Radiology Training Program Director, (RTPD) Stewart Kribs, the past RPTD, Kathy Hibbert, Director of the Centre for Education in Medical Imaging, and Mark Landis, a resident in our department. Each author brings a slightly different perspective to the conversation, but all are committed to creating a meaningful, pedagogically sound program. Writing this chapter together has provided a means to articulate and share our goals and responsibilities to help see that to fruition.

3.3
Today's Radiology Student

Who are today's radiology students? How is their training necessarily different now from what it was a decade ago or two decades ago? What are the implications of these differences for our teaching? "In reality, *all* learners come with varied backgrounds and clinical experiences, and they will approach the same patient and clinical problem with different cognitive needs, motives to learn, and learning skills and strategies, as well as variable needs for external guidance" (Ten Cate et al. 2004).

According to Musick and Gunderman (2004), "from the beginning of training, medical students and residents feel pressure to memorize as much information as possible … [believing that] the only way we can excel is to prove that we know more than others."

3

Similarly, medicine is a culture in which very high standards for excellence permeate every layer of the resident's experience. While this is a laudable goal, it can lead to unintended outcomes such as:

> Residents learn to seek only one "right" answer rather than searching for possibilities and recommendations.
> Residents may be less likely to raise questions or discuss interesting/difficult cases with their colleagues if a competitive environment exists.
> Residents may actively work to hide their errors rather than bring them out into the open to use them as opportunities for meaningful learning.
> Residents lose the opportunity to reinforce their learning through teaching their colleagues.

Teaching has always been a core component of radiology training. However, rapid advances in technology demand innovative responses. As we say goodbye to analog, we say goodbye to the consistent practice of simply writing notes on the film sleeve. Digital images require new learning that goes beyond approaching images to make differential diagnoses. Those activities are now compounded with decisions about how to compress the image, how to select and store it for an examination or teaching file, how to include it in an accessible database, how to import it to PowerPoint, and how to decide what information should be included and in what way?

According to Toms (2008), "the profile of radiology continues to rise as large sums of public money are being invested in a national implementation of picture archiving and communication systems (PACS) and [advanced imaging] services (CT, PET/CT, MR)" (p. 113). Ongoing advances in technology present both a blessing and a curse as radiologists are perpetually working to adapt to the changes, update their own knowledge and skills in response, and integrate the changes into their practice. Although technology has afforded radiologists the opportunity to increase the number of images it is possible to read any given day, the number of requests for readings has increased even faster. This creates a context in which requests for service completely overwhelm the radiologists available to provide them. In this scenario, it is not surprising to see a breakdown in the teacher–student relationship vis-à-vis the desired degree of teaching, supervision, or interaction.

According to Howell (2004),
…the practice of medicine is a 24h, 7-day commitment. The learning process for residents can be a grueling endeavor. However, the practice of medicine has historically been viewed as a sacred, social obligation, and professional honor, so that individuals in training willingly submitted to what may be described as a never ending learning obligation, in the process, providing physician services to those they tended.

The times have changed – for reasons that include social, political, cultural, and technological influences to name a few. Recent studies have suggested that excessive fatigue may contribute to a risk in patient care. Residents themselves have become more political by forming their own provincial bargaining collectives, which allows them a voice in decisions that concern their training. A high value is placed on making time for leisure and family activities. Remarkably, there are even Web sites (e.g., slacker stories; Anonymous 2008) devoted to residents counseling other residents on *how you can get away with more than you think* on rotation.

Similarly, the profession is changing. It is no longer sufficient to simply gain expertise in medical knowledge of areas such as anatomy, physiology, and pathology. Radiologists, like all medical professionals, must now demonstrate competencies in multiple areas that include, for example, skill in communication, collaboration, professionalism, advocacy, and scholarship. To ensure that these competencies are developed, students must be prepared for a learning environment that will privilege more than memorization. Expanding radiology education to address the scholarship of teaching and learning targets this goal. Similarly, looking for opportunities to integrate the competencies into the overall curriculum is precisely why the CanMEDS framework emerged, as is discussed further in Chap. 11.

3.4
The Role of Radiologists as Teachers

In an academic teaching hospital setting there is an expectation that everyone needs to participate in the academic mission of the department. If each radiologist gave a bit of time, it would not only be better for all of the residents, it would also reduce the stress created when a small number of individuals are trying to carry the workload on their own. This expectation and commitment is integral to offering a successful radiology training program.

There are many avenues to participate in teaching within a radiology department: teaching during radiology rotations, presenting didactic lectures, organizing conferences, offering rounds, serving as a role model or mentor, participating in Journal Club, and sharing self-directed learning materials. Indeed, Thind and Barter (2008) argue that "radiology departments, more than almost any other area of the hospital, rely on a degree of collaborative team working between individuals and professions for their effective performance." Even residents themselves ought to be included in the academic mission where appropriate. Including the residents in the educational mission can "improve resident teaching skills, teaching confidence, and knowledge acquisition" (Khasgiwala et al. 2007), but can also offer an opportunity to both experience and understand the academic side of the profession.

In order for such an inclusive model to be successful, "the teaching responsibilities of all departments must be officially recognized and funded in job planning" (see p. 116 in Dixon 2008). Similarly, teaching services that span a range from preclinical and clinical undergraduate to postgraduate teaching need to be shared and staffed with those appropriately prepared for what they are teaching.

Since teaching is not overtly financially supported nor visibly linked to patient care, not all radiologists commit time and effort to this area. It becomes important for each site team to come together and organize their time so that everyone is contributing in some way. For example, some staff radiologists may be able to model excellence in patient care, others may be able to model excellence in presenting cases, and someone else may offer exemplary report writing. What is important is that everyone is contributing.

One of the most effective components to consider when looking at program renewal is the mechanisms in place for clear communication and feedback. Feedback is a key component to monitor and evaluate students' learning. If it is not employed consistently or effectively, then residents miss out on one of the most meaningful learning experiences in their training. Training in communication and providing feedback should be an integral part of

3

the Department of Radiology's professional development plan. Indeed, it has been one of the early areas that our department's Centre for Education addressed in its first 2 years.

3.5
Leadership and the RTPD

3.5.1
What Is the Profile of a RTPD?

The RTPD is a faculty member who heads the Diagnostic Radiology Residency Program and chairs the Diagnostic Radiology Residency Program Committee. In Canada, radiology residency training is overseen by The Royal College of Physicians and Surgeons of Canada (http://rcpsc.medical.org). There are three individuals to whom the RTPD reports:

1. Dean, PGE Committee
   The Post-Graduate Dean oversees all of the residency programs at the university and ensures standards for training are met.
2. University Chair, Department of Radiology
   The Radiology Chair oversees the academic mission of the Department of Radiology. Diagnostic radiology residency training is one of several academic mandates of the department; others include undergraduate radiology education, fellowship training, and research.
3. Hospital Chief, Department of Radiology

The Hospital Chief (who may also be the University Chair) reports to the Medical Advisory Committee of the hospital. The Chief is responsible for the provision of clinical care, teaching, and research in the radiology department in the hospital.

Beyond this reporting structure, the RTPD interacts with many other individuals. These include the radiology residents, the radiology faculty, medical students, administrative personnel, radiology department staff, and individuals (residents, faculty, etc.) from other residency programs. The program also interacts with various organizations, including licensing bodies and professional associations.

The many responsibilities of the RTPD and the ongoing changes of the trainer/training requirements dictate that certain support systems be in place for that role. The increased demands on the role require strong leadership and support at the level of the College (information shared by radiology training directors across the country), the institution (PGE Office), the university department (Chair), each of the sites (strong chief at each site), and residents themselves (resident chiefs) in order to foster a team that can adequately address current challenges, as well as those that develop over time.

The RTPD is responsible for ensuring the educational needs of residents are met. There are various individuals and organizations who stipulate how this should be done. It is essential that RTPDs receive adequate support to carry out their roles. Delegation of responsibilities is essential. Administrative, teaching, and research responsibilities should be shared among many individuals, with the RTPD coordinating these efforts. A capable, efficient program assistant can manage the day-to-day running of a radiology residency program. The RTPD is dependent on support from the Chief, Chair, and Post-Graduate Dean to run the program, meet training standards, and adapt the program to changes in education or technology. The strength of a residency program represents the sum of the strengths of the individuals contributing to its educational goals.

The RTPD must be given time free from clinical duties to complete certain aspects of the job. There should be financial compensation for the role that allows his/her practice group to justify this time off. Ideally, funding would come from the university, or be spread out over all the practice groups involved in the training program. This would alleviate the burden on any one practice group.

3.5.2
Responsibilities of the RTPD

The responsibilities of a RTPD are many and varied, and can be categorized in ways that address the overall program, the culture of the department, accreditation requirements, faculty development, and his/her serving as an advocate for residents.

3.5.2.1
Overall Program: Setting the Stage

One of the primary responsibilities of a RTPD begins with recruitment of residents. This process begins at the undergraduate education level, by ensuring that medical students first become exposed to engaging teachers in radiology in a way that will pique interest in pursuing radiology as a specialty. Secondly, the RTPD will participate in the formalized programs for recruitment; in Canada, this is through the Canadian Resident Matching Service (CaRMs), the Ministry of Health (MOH) Re-entry Program, transfers, the International Medical Graduate (IMG) Program, and the Foreign Medical Graduate (FMG) Program. Once the "bodies" are secured, the RTPD liaises with the radiology practice groups at the various sites to ensure that rotation schedules are coordinated, and to optimize the use of local resources (both human and equipment) for maximal learning opportunities. Similarly, it is necessary to coordinate the teaching calendars at the various sites, and ensure that new modalities and applications of imaging are integrated into the curriculum. Important also is the implementation of a formal education system for residents in use of PACS teaching software workstations (postprocessing), and relevant Web sites (schedules, on-call reports).

3.5.2.2
Building a Culture To Support Resident Education

Organizing the functional components of a program is necessary but insufficient to ensure a successful educational experience for residents. As workload and knowledge demands increase, it is vital that the RTPD fosters a culture that encourages teamwork and healthy working relationships among residents and also between residents and staff or other clinical services.

3

3.5.2.3
Meeting Accreditation Requirements

One of the primary responsibilities of the role of the RTPD is to ensure that the program evolves in such a way that it continues to meet the specialty training requirements of the national education body (Royal College of Physicians and Surgeons in Canada). This means that the RTPD must review carefully recommendations made during past accreditation reviews, and develop a plan to address weaknesses. Addressing the weaknesses may require changes in the overall program, policies, curriculum, or process of monitoring progress. To achieve these objectives, the RTPD serves as Chair of the Resident Training Committee (RTC). Since the RTC includes representation from each of the various sites, the resident group, the Chair of the Department, and the Centre for Education in Radiology and Nuclear Medicine, an ongoing dialogue and sharing of information, new policies, curriculum development, and future planning can be communicated.

3.5.2.4
Faculty Development

The RTPD is in a unique position to review feedback from the accrediting body, alongside teaching and course reviews, in a context of ongoing dialogue with those the program is intended to serve: the residents. From this vantage point, the RTPD may identify faculty development needs that the program would benefit from. The RTPD must therefore become familiar with the faculty development programs offered through the institution, the department, and beyond that may offer faculty information and assistance to help guide them in both the art of teaching, and in strengthening their curriculum development. In addition, with advances in technology demanding continual adaptation and renewal, opportunities to upgrade technical skills may be required. The information must be made widely available to faculty so that they may attend where possible.

Part of the mandate of our department's Centre for Education is to guide faculty in the "art" of teaching. It is important then for the RTPD to work closely with the educationalists to assess the needs of the department in an ongoing way, and respond to those needs in fluid and flexible ways. The faculty support that we have developed together to date is described in more detail in Chap. 4.

3.5.2.5
Resident Advocacy

One of the key responsibilities of the RTPD is that of resident advocacy. Primarily, the RTPD is concerned that each resident satisfies the goals and objectives of training. This starts with the RTPD acting as a mentor/role model or directing residents to appropriate individuals who may serve in that capacity. Since one of the goals of the program is to encourage each resident to realize his/her potential, the RTPD also assists residents with career planning that may include arranging for fellowships or future positions.

It is likely that the RTPD will be involved in negotiating conflicts between residents, staff, and clinical services. To some extent, potential conflict can be alleviated by ensuring a system in which clear expectations, ongoing communication, and timely feedback and evaluation are provided to residents and staff. In addition, consistent application of policies and procedures can minimize conflict. The RTPD must therefore demonstrate exceptional listening skills, judicious decision-making abilities, and leadership qualities.

Finally, the RTPD must attend to the pyschosocial aspects of training, and include opportunities for residents to come together as a cohort through social events such as a resident barbeque, ski day, or golf afternoon.

3.6
The Role of Radiology Educators

The role of radiologists serving as "radiology educators" is multilayered, helping the resident to learn by:

- Daily development of medical expert skills
- Mentoring as a scholar, patient advocate, communicator, collaborator, professional, and manager
- Leading regular teaching rounds
- Serving as a mentor, supervisor, or colleague
- Giving formal academic half-day teaching sessions using a variety of formats, (e.g., didactic, quizzes, games, challenges)
- Stimulating interest and participation in scholarly pursuits (e.g., research, teaching).

3.7
The Role of the RTC

The role of the RTC is to:

- Guide ongoing assessment and change in the program
- Ensure the learning needs of the residents are met
- Ensure the requirements of training are met
- Provide a forum for residents, clinical departments, researchers, and the university to ensure that the academic mission is being achieved

3.8
Radiology Training and the Trainee: A Case for Level-Specific Curricula from a Resident's Perspective

As already mentioned, radiology training programs are based on frameworks organized by a collective agreement set out between national governing bodies, e.g., the Royal College of

Physicians and Surgeons in Canada and the American Board of Radiology in the USA, and the university-affiliated departments of radiology. Their mandates are shared in that the overarching goal is to develop rather undifferentiated medical graduates into expert consultants in all areas of medical imaging. Benchmarks and quality are assessed at fellowship examinations, and it is the hope that in the process of acquiring the necessary knowledge required to become a functional consultant that the required professional attitudes and behaviors have been instilled as well. The expectation is that this transformation should occur over a period of approximately 5 years. While structural frameworks are relatively easy to establish and codify, how these goals are realized by the trainee are often nonlinear in their progression and are realized at different points along the course of the training program.

Junior radiology resident and senior radiology resident needs and learning objectives are fairly similar; however, their emphasis differs depending on where the trainee is on the learning continuum. In the early years of radiology training, the principal objectives of the junior trainee are to (1) develop the detection skills to distinguish the normal from the abnormal findings in a given imaging study; (2) to collate and reconcile imaging observations into a hypothesis of what is happening to a given patient in light of these findings and other relevant clinical information; and (3) to develop the required communication skills needed to express these findings in the appropriate radiologic discourse and lexicon, or radiologic "episteme" to borrow from Foucault (1980). An example of where this discourse is seen most clearly in the substance of the radiologic report where the wording, tenor, and focus of the report often depend on the target audience, i.e., the nature of the clinical service. For example, in recommending subsequent radiologic follow-up, the report will be more prescriptive if the audience is a generalist physician, whereas the recommendation to the specialist surgical service will be more veiled. This is often done since the relative knowledge of the needed follow-up examinations will be invariably different between generalist and specialist services.

As it currently stands, the radiology training program at the University of Western Ontario sees training at the junior levels being focused on the acquisition of the knowledge and professional skills needed to assume independent on-call duties. On-call duties are a vital and fundamental component of radiology training. These activities help lay the foundation of the consultancy skills that are expected as the majority of interactions between residents and referring clinical services occur during these call activities. It is here where the trainee is presented with a clinical scenario and hypothesis that the subsequent imaging examination will serve to provide evidence either for or against that hypothesis and the trainee is expected to synthesize these findings and to communicate them to a referring service with a recommendation for follow-up if appropriate. A common example is provided by the clinical scenario of right-lower-quadrant pain and an elevated white blood cell count and imaging findings either on ultrasound or computed tomography suggestive of appendicitis and the importance of an urgent surgical referral.

Unfortunately, this knowledge and professional skill acquisition does not occur in a linear fashion. Often it occurs rather stochastically. This is common in radiology training and marks a rapid departure from the conventional progressive stepwise learning the trainee was accustomed to prior to beginning formal radiology training. A period of adjustment is required and a possible role for transitional curriculum such that these skills may be introduced in a more stepwise fashion. This suggests a role for education departments to become involved in the development of such curricula with the academic radiology department and national boards if appropriate.

The progression of the trainee to more senior levels sees a shift in focus from foundation laying in the context of knowledge acquisition and basic consultancy skills to a greater depth of knowledge and a refinement of these consultancy skills. The focus of the trainee also shifts in the final years towards fellowship examinations and the ultimate goal of independent practice. These evolving needs of the senior trainee need to be addressed by several interrelated groups: the trainee, the training program, and the academic radiology department.

Current schemes to realize these needs can include a dedicated senior resident curriculum that can include an examination preparation curriculum, radiology practice management, interprofessional relations and conflict resolution, and continuous quality improvement initiatives. These latter components are all areas that governing bodies have highlighted as essential components of training and would seem to be most appropriate if introduced at the senior levels of training.

The current format and structure of radiology training programs need to recognize these different trainee goals and needs. As described, knowledge acquisition and professional skill development occur in a nonlinear fashion. Recognizing that residency training is an apprenticeship with progressive independence granted as seniority and competence develops, training programs and governing bodies should consider a formalized curriculum that caters to the needs of trainees at different levels. This curriculum should be pedagogically based on the adult learner model of self-direction and needs-based knowledge acquisition. A balance must be struck, however, to ensure that the necessary learning is delivered and that self-direction does not lead the learner to focus on irrelevant issues. The ultimate goal of radiology training is to transform the trainee from a rather undifferentiated general physician to a professional radiologic expert. Training programs, academic departments, trainees, and governing bodies should consider a formalized evidence-based curriculum that covers the goals and objective of licensing bodies, recognizing the unique level-specific needs of the trainee.

3.9
The Ideal Academic Environment for Postgraduate Radiology Residents

Gunderman and Huynh (2007) posed the question, "Is radiology presented to students as a fulfilling career?" An examination of the extrinsic and intrinsic factors at play in radiology presented a sobering picture: Exclusive attention to extrinsic factors ("workplace policy and administration, supervision, work conditions, compensation, and relationship with peers") could not compensate for a lack of attention to the intrinsic factors ("a sense of achievement in work, recognition for the quality of work we do, the nature of the work itself, the degree of responsibility we have in our work, and their sense that we are growing personally and professionally in the work we do"). Extrinsic factors in radiology have put great pressure on residency programs and their RTPDs to balance the clinical, teaching, administrative, and research needs of the department with those of the residents. As clinical workload increases, it is not uncommon for faculty to complain that they are "too busy to teach". How can this be addressed?

3

The most important concept in maintaining and enhancing a residency program is shared responsibility. The majority of teaching cannot be done by a few exceptional, dedicated radiologists. Instead, every member of the faculty needs to contribute to the academic mission of the department, including resident supervision and education. But how much is enough? To answer this question, a program needs to know how much teaching is required to achieve its academic mission. In our program, we decided that all residents should receive 1 h of rounds each day and an additional session of in-depth teaching once a week. We also wanted each resident attending a rounds session to be given the opportunity to "take a case." Since it takes, on average, each resident about 10 min to discuss a case, the number of attendees at rounds should be no greater than six. With up to 18 residents in our program spread among three hospital sites we could achieve our goal if each teaching site gave rounds once a day. Each hospital is staffed by slightly more than ten radiologists, meaning that we could achieve our teaching goal if each radiologist gave rounds every other week. Since all three sites already had various teaching rounds in place, we determined that we could still meet our teaching goal if each radiologist personally supervised a rounds session for the residents once a month. Thus, we had developed our first teaching standard for our radiology faculty – each radiologist was expected to supervise a rounds session for residents at his/her site at least once a month. This was embraced by the radiology faculty, as our expectation from them for supervising rounds was now clear and easily achievable.

Our department, until this point, did not have written expectations of either residents or faculty radiologists. A similar process as described above was used to develop an expectation by faculty for giving weekly in-depth radiology teaching sessions – one session per year. We are currently working on similar expectations for undergraduate radiology teaching, resident supervision of research, and administrative assistance. Similarly, expectations of residents for teaching and research were developed. Our residents play an integral part in teaching undergraduate radiology education in the hospitals for clinical clerks (medical students doing clinical rotations). By establishing expectations for teaching, we expect all of our residents to teach and they now benefit from the learning which comes from the preparation and presentation of these sessions.

Administration of a radiology residency program is becoming an increasingly complex task. There is a constant need to update and refine the residency program to accommodate rapid advances in imaging technology. The requirements of programs to teach residents a greater volume of more complex material have led to increased expectations and stricter standards. It is not possible for a RTPD to keep abreast of the advances in all of the subspecialty fields of radiology. To assist the RTPD in this regard, we are developing a committee of subspecialty directors. The role of the subspecialty director is to act as a contact person and resource for the RTPD for issues pertaining to that subspecialty area of radiology. We have proposed the following subspecialty directors:

Abdominal imaging (including woman's imaging)
Thoracic imaging
Musculoskeletal
Cardiac imaging
Vascular imaging and image-guided therapy

Breast imaging
Neuroradiology
Pediatric radiology
Ultrasound
Magnetic resonance imaging
Nuclear medicine

The role of the subspecialty director would be to oversee training in the subspecialty area, including the following:

1. Incorporate standards of residency training into rotation-specific goals and objectives
2. Develop a teaching curriculum
3. Liaise with his/her subspecialty faculty peers throughout the academic radiology department to optimize resident rotations and education
4. Develop evaluation tools, including an oral examination and a practice objective structured clinical examination
5. Oversee requests for training in the subspecialty area from other departments and co-ordinate these commitments to prevent interference with radiology resident education

In summary, we recommend that a strong radiology program requires:

1. Financial/time support for RTPD to do the role.
2. A committee of subspecialty directors to

   › Assist/advise the RTPD
   › Optimize teaching
   › Coordinate rotations
   › Take optimal advantage of local radiologists/equipment/service resources

3. Financial/time support for an undergraduate director to coordinate radiology teaching at the undergraduate level and encourage medical students to consider radiology as a career in collaboration with the RTPD.
4. Close collaboration with nuclear medicine department to optimally train specialists from both branches of diagnostic imaging. There will be an increasing blur in the distinction between these two specialties as hybrid imaging (positron-emission tomography/computed tomography, single photon emission scintigraphy/computed tomography, positron-emission tomography/magnetic resonance imaging) becomes more commonplace.
5. Leadership at the chair and chief level that mandates reasonable staff radiologist participation in the academic mission, and recognition of the importance of the postgraduate role.
6. Financial support for the administrator to perform required roles for undergraduate and resident education.

3

References

1. Anonymous (2008) Slacker stories and how you can get away with more than you think. Med School Hell [http://medschoolhell.com/2008/01/24/slacker-stories-and-how-you-can-get-away-with-more-than-you-think/] Accessed 28 Feb 2008
2. Dixon AK (2008) Current thoughts about academic radiology. Clin Radiol 63:115–117
3. Foucault M (1980) Power/knowledge. Hetfordshire, Harvester, Wheatsheaf
4. Gunderman RB, Huynh J (2007) Is radiology presented to medical students as a fulfilling career? J Am Coll Radiol 4:704–710
5. Howell RE (2004) Resident duty hours: The rest of the story. J Am Coll Radiol 1:104–7
6. Khasgiwala VC, Boiselle P, Levine D, Lee KS, Barbaras BS, Kressel HY (2007) Resident as a teacher: Assessing the benefits. Acad Radiol 14:1422–1428
7. Musick DJ, Gunderman RB (2004) The cultural dimension of radiology residency. Acad Radiol 15:265–267
8. Ten Cate O, Snell L, Mann K, Vermunt J (2004) Orienting teaching toward the learning process. Acad Med 79:219–28
9. Thind R, Barter S (2008) The Service Review Committee: Royal College of Radiologists. Philosophy, role and lessons to be learned. Clin Radiol 63:118–124
10. Toms AP (2008) The decline and fall of academic radiology. Clin Radiol 63:113–114

Teaching and Learning: Defining the Scholarship of Teaching

4

T. Van Deven, K. Hibbert, H.C. Ellinor

The ultimate goal of radiology and therefore, radiology education…is to help patients.
(Nyce, Steele, Gunderman, 2006, p 629)

In professional education, it is insufficient to learn for the sake of knowledge and understanding alone; one learns in order to engage in practice.
(Shulman 2005, p 18)

4.1
Narrative

Prior to joining the Centre for Education, the full extent of my knowledge of hospitals came from the television series Scrubs. As I began my work, there were so many aspects of radiology education that I had never heard of before: objective structured clinical examination, CanMEDS, Royal College of Physicians and Surgeons of Canada (RCPSC). I initially found it to be overwhelming, but I developed some useful tools: first I developed an acronym dictionary to help me with the acronyms involved in my day-to-day work; I designed a comparative curriculum map that positioned our department's radiology curriculum alongside the Royal College's expectations and the curricula of other radiology departments across Canada. This gave me a better understanding of what radiology programs entail.

One of my earliest tasks was to look for funding to help sustain the mission of the Centre. I began by searching our university's database and the Canadian Institutes of Health Research's Web site and came to the realization that there is little funding specifically for a venture such as ours. Similarly, it appeared as though we were entering comparatively uncharted waters when I began searching the literature for research that had been done in the area of scholarship in radiology education.

T. Van Deven (✉)
Centre for Education in Medical Imaging, Schulich School
of Medicine and Dentistry, University of Western Ontario, London, ON, Canada N6A 5C1
E-mail: tvandev@uwo.ca

Radiology Education. R.K. Chhem et al. (Eds.)
DOI: 10.1007/978-3-540-68989-8, © Springer-Verlag Berlin Heidelberg 2009

4

I attended a course that introduced me to PubMed and My NCBI where I learned about medical subject headings (MeSH) and how to best use the search methods of PubMed. In the summer of 2007, I presented what I had learned to the education research assistants hired by the Centre.

I have been involved in creating annotative bibliographies and summaries to locate key references in the field. These activities have made me feel a valued and respected part of the team and have also made the goals of the Centre more explicit to me as I have begun to understand the issues that radiology education is facing today.

This information has also contributed to the development of a new Web site that I have helped design and maintain, and helped me understand what information would be useful for potential residents, current residents, faculty, and staff.

In the summer of 2007, I worked with the team to organize the First Annual International Conference on Expanding Scholarship in Radiology Education. This involved managing the Conference's Web site, searching educational radiology journals and university and hospital Web sites for potential invitees and speakers, arranging for and scheduling speakers for scientific sessions, organizing travel and accommodation for keynote speakers, and securing a facility and preparing a program for the conference. This was a wonderfully rewarding experience personally, as it brought together many individuals who shared the Centre's goals. I have grown passionate about the direction of the Centre as it seeks to bring scholarship to our radiology department. The team I am working with have encouraged the expansion of my knowledge and have made me feel very much a part of the Centre's goals.

Holly Ellinor

4.2
Introduction: What do We Mean by "Scholarship of Teaching"?

Education in any learning domain can only be determined by the way in which scholarship is defined and also how it is ultimately rewarded. The intellectual activity we know as "scholarship of teaching" has been taken up by various scholars over the past few decades in an attempt to name and describe a complex term (Cross and Harris Steadman 1996; Glassik et al. 1998; Bender and Gray 1999). Nearly two decades ago, Ernest Boyer focused on the futility of even beginning discussions about improving the quality of teaching if faculty are not given the same recognition for time spent teaching, tutoring, or mentoring as that accorded to research pursuits (Boyer 1990). Recognizing, acknowledging, and rewarding a scholarship of teaching must be attended to, as ultimately, with many of the intrinsic awards of academia diminishing, "medical schools are in serious danger of losing their academic vision" (see p. 2 in Gunderman and Cohen 2002).

Today, the conditions appear to be shifting more favorably toward such recognition. The reasons for the shift are unclear, but may have something to do with the emergence of a more competitive global market for higher education, increased scrutiny and accountability by governing bodies, the changes in our students' learning styles and the access to information that they have at their fingertips, and the constant pressures of a booming knowledge economy and the requisite demands to keep up. The *need* for "excellence" in teaching is apparent. The *scholarship of teaching*, according to Hutchings and Shulman "is the mechanism through which the profession of teaching itself advances, through which teaching can be something other than a seat-of-the-pants operation" (1999, p 14). For us, understanding the scholarship of teaching in this way served as a catalyst that drives our vision for what we collectively want to accomplish in radiology education and stimulates the kind of dialogue, debates, and exchange of ideas that we believe will inform our practice, and ultimately result in improved learning.

We agree with Hutchings and Shulman (1999, p. 13) that "*all* faculty have an obligation to teach well, to engage students, and to foster important forms of student learning". In our experience working with the radiology faculty and residents, it became clear that they shared this goal and were seeking assistance to improve their practice, their techniques, and their overall planning and curriculum development – all within a context in which they generally felt enormous time pressures, a lack of confidence in their pedagogical knowledge, and a lack of compensation or acknowledgement that their teaching contributed to the department.

4.3
Creating the Conditions to Foster "Scholarship in Teaching"

We should remind the reader that our involvement with the Department of Radiology and Nuclear Medicine resulted from a desire to optimize the role and function of education in radiology. Early on, we decided that we would form a center – a deliberate attempt to create a space and a place to invite dialogue and an exchange of ideas. As we immersed ourselves in the *existing practice* by attending rounds, classes, meetings, etc. we began to consider how we might work toward what Shulman refers to as a *wisdom of practice*, "the full range of practical arguments engaged by practitioners as they reason about and ultimately make judgments and decisions about situations they confront and actions they must take" (2007, p 560). As educators, we brought 25 years of teaching experience each, and a degree of comfort with what Shulman calls pedagogical content knowledge (i.e., the synthesis of subject matter knowledge, knowledge of pedagogy and knowledge of context) in our own teaching (1986). This, however, was new territory. We did not have any of the subject matter knowledge and were only beginning to get a sense of the context. Our colleagues in radiology indisputably had wide-ranging clinical knowledge, but lacked understanding of even the general principles of teaching, or the role that context may play to create pedagogically powerful learning opportunities (Miller 1980; see pp. 1–113 in Lowry 1993). We were thrust into a relationship in which we both stood to learn a great deal as we learned to negotiate shared understandings from which we might launch new ways of thinking about, talking about, and practicing education within the Department of Radiology.

4.3.1
The "Series"

In one of our earliest conversations, radiology faculty suggested that perhaps we might begin by offering a 1-h workshop in which we gave participants the "tools" of teaching. We smiled; theirs was a familiar request often sought by novice teachers. We responded that we would be delighted to do so, if they might first spend an hour with us to give us the "tools" to become radiologists so that we could put our session in an appropriate context. Our point was well taken, and what emerged instead was a decision to run an educational series designed to provide the opportunity to bring the knowledge we each had together in a way that would lead to richer understandings of existing practice in a way that would help us map strategies to achieve a wisdom of practice.

We took, as our starting point, the issues that emerged from our needs assessment to create the "Educational Series: Part 1." It was composed of

a. Anatomy of curriculum
b. Theories of teaching and learning
c. Assessment and evaluation
d. Building a culture that supports mentorship

According to Shulman, *scholarship* has three defining features; it is visible and public, it is subject to critical review by one's peer group (in this case, radiologists), and members of the department begin to use and build upon what they have learned in ways that advance the scholarship of radiology education.

4.3.1.1
"Anatomy of the Curriculum"

These features are certainly not new. Gunderman (2006, p. xv) reminds us of Socrates claim "that an unexamined life is hardly worth living. Likewise, medical education can achieve its potential only if we reflect carefully on it". We approached the *anatomy of the curriculum* as a way to encourage our new colleagues to look at their existing and past practice and begin to identify and name the theoretical underpinnings that were informing their decision-making, and what the implications of those choices (even when subconscious) might be to both the teaching and the learning scenarios. In many cases we learned that it was necessary to also introduce the language of "critique" in order to engage in the kind of dialogue that could serve to advance our understanding of the ideas. Since radiology and nuclear medicine is a profession dealing primarily with the interpretation of images, we created a presentation that used simple images to stimulate a dialogue around "theories-in-use" (Schon 1987).

To give you an example, we show a photograph depicting a simple pitcher pouring liquid into a bowl. We pose the questions, "What teaching scenario is reflected in this image? Where are the teacher and student positioned? What are the implications for the curriculum?" We have presented this session a number of times locally and in other parts of the world. The responses never cease to intrigue us. The image not only provokes antic-ipated discussions about transmission models and concern about the capacity to "hold" more knowledge, but interestingly, it often raised questions about the directionality of the flow of knowledge, and the similar materials that were used in the construction of the *pitcher* and the *bowl*. Indeed, in one presentation, participants suggested that the reality of practice was more akin to what they call "teh tarik," or pulled tea. They explained that to make teh tarik, the tea must be poured back and forth in order to mix it with milk and create a thick froth, and suggested that it was this reciprocal exchange of information with their students that they found to be the richest learning experience. Insights such as the teh tarik example often led participants to make subsequent connections with current practices as they are viewed through a new lens, inevitably leading to realizations and ideas about what might be done differently.

4.3.1.2
Theories of Teaching and Learning

> ...the basic purpose is not to destroy. Rather it is to strengthen pedagogy already good, to salvage techniques which could serve more usefully, to point out principles and practices that have not yet found their way widely into medical schools.
>
> (Miller et al. 1961)

As noted a few times in this book, the goal for our educational series was not to present a recipe book of "how to" or to provide a formula for effective teaching pedagogy. Rather, we aim to provoke reflective practice and inspire new approaches that improve both efficiency and effectiveness within the radiology teaching program. Ultimately, we aim to develop an educational program that will help radiologists generate self-efficacy along with the dispositions necessary to participate in the profession as lifelong learners.

Our implicit theories of learning shape our educational practices. As noted educator Debra Britzman observes, "Teaching is one of the few professions where newcomers [can] feel the force of their own history of learning as if it telegraphs relevancy to their work..." (2003). In any teaching environment, whether it is recognized or not, theories of learning are in play. Drawing on the principles of adult learners, we began this presentation by exploring participants' existing knowledge of teaching theories. We stress that the purpose of discussing teaching theories is not to suggest that one must be chosen and others elimi-nated, but that each theory encompasses different goals, different ways of constructing learners, different aims, and ultimately different forms of evaluation and assessment. By activating their existing or prior knowledge of teaching and learning theories, we have found that once faculty begin talking about their teaching strategies, they quickly realize that they actually employ a variety of theories throughout their teaching.

Most, however, begin by talking about their didactic teaching. Recall our earlier image of the pitcher and the bowl. While various names have been applied to this particular teaching theory, we describe it as a "crude learning" theory. It has many other names – the "federal express" theory, the "dip-stick" theory – but most often the label applied is a pejorative one associated with "the empty vessel." The educator (presumably full) pours

4

information into the empty vessel (presumably the learner). In this scenario, the goal of the educator is to pour as much information as possible into the learner; the goal of the learner is to retain as much information as can be held. Evaluation would be measured by opening up the learner and measuring what spills out – what can be reproduced, what can be recalled. Virtually all of us have experienced this scenario as students and participated in it as teachers as some time in our lives. It is important to recognize that while this theory has its limitations, it certainly has a place within a continuum of strategies and approaches, and indeed didactic teaching itself can include participatory strategies. For example, many faculty employ questioning techniques such as prompting recall, prompting explanation, and counterexamples that serve to engage the learners in an active role. We repeat this process, working through some of the more commonly used theories such as gestalt and cognitive theories, behaviorism, and constructivism. We also examine notions of problem-based learning and evidence-based practice typically found in medical education practices. Working together has provided a forum to introduce the various discourses that we each employ to each other which ultimately, we hope, will enable us as a collective to refine our understanding of the "scholarship of teaching" and move us toward a purposeful "wisdom" in practice.

4.3.1.3
Assessment and Evaluation

Assessment and evaluation have proven to be two of the more contested and challenging areas to work through. We have discovered these two components to be understood in a very narrow sense, limiting the potential that more comprehensive understandings of assessment and evaluation can offer to both the teacher and the learner. The power and legitimacy afforded to the end-of-training RCPSC certification examination and the prerequisite assessment overshadow all other processes. Our department, like many others, attempts to prepare students for the final examination by creating numerous opportunities, for example, for students to write practice examinations, participate in mock oral examinations, and present regularly during rounds. This is currently a necessary process given the gate-keeping function of the RCPSC examination.

Our focus in this presentation then is to work on expanding our understanding of the role and function of assessment and evaluation, and how limited understandings may rob us of opportunities for employing meaningful practices. For example, we have observed the prevalence of PowerPoint presentations in the didactic lecture (predominantly in the large undergraduate classes). Students have demanded (and faculty have complied with their request) that the slides for each lecture be posted on a Web site to allow them to download and print them for study reference. This practice has left both students and faculty frustrated: students are frustrated if faculty talk about anything other than what is on the slides (since they have agreed that only what is on the slides will ever be in a test), and faculty are frustrated because the slides create a very technical rational approach to teaching – reminiscent of the crude learning theory we have already discussed. In other words, their teaching conforms to the limitations of the medium.

When students move into their postgraduate years, they bring the same set of expectations into a very different learning environment. In a specialty such as radiology, the classes are much smaller, and opportunities for direct interaction between residents and faculty increases exponentially. What often get lost, however, are clear guidelines around what is being assessed, how the assessment is undertaken, and how assessment can inform the instructional "next steps." It has become a part of our mandate therefore, to focus on moving assessment and evaluation beyond accountability and toward a method for improvement. Jolly and Peyton argue that at the end of the day it is not enough that learning has occurred; "rather it is important that new behaviours are of practical significance in the normal working environment and … have some effect on the community, for instance, by improving patient outcomes" (1998, p. 108). Viewed broadly, assessment and evaluation go beyond functioning solely as an instrument to measure learners' abilities toward becoming a means of evaluating the program and processes, and then as a means to guide the future direction of the department. By gauging the impact of certain learning/teaching strategies, faculty can begin to use that evidence to modify their learning and teaching practices.

In this way, faculty begin to understand those forms of assessment and evaluation that they do have control over, and the implications of making even subtle changes. Our presentation therefore includes an introduction into the many forms and purposes of assessment, the requisite time involved in ongoing assessment as compared with that for information that is gathered in "snapshot," one-dimensional processes; the difference in data that are gathered to understand a learners' progress as well as data that reveal information about the suitability of the teaching strategies used; and the different function of formative and summative assessment in an effort to move beyond what has been termed "feedback sandwich" (Milan et al. 2006).

We do not limit our discussion to assessment of students. A critical component of assessment is learning how to self-assess, and this is true for students and faculty. Teaching portfolios are increasingly being used as tools to contribute to the development and growth of individual teachers (Bird 1990). A teaching portfolio is a way of documenting your teaching activities, tracking your evaluations (i.e., your strengths and weaknesses), compiling resources, and stimulating reflection. Similarly, residents can begin to build professional portfolios to document areas such where improvement is needed and strategies to address any weaknesses, feedback received, continuing medical education courses, innovative educational experiences, etc.

The portfolio can play a key role in what we have found to be a difficult, yet important component of the assessment and evaluation component: giving and receiving feedback. In our discussions with radiology colleagues in our own department and in the literature, it seems that a focus on the pitfalls of feedback dominates the discussions. Frequently, feedback is viewed only as an opportunity to identify mistakes for the purpose of correcting those mistakes. For example, Cowan's study (2001) showed trainees often feel they do not get enough feedback, while Gibson and Campbell's study (2000) reveals that teachers often think they give more feedback than learners claim to receive.

Giving feedback is not an end in itself; it needs to be constructed as a part of the learning process. The overall goal of feedback is to produce professionals who are self-reflective, thereby continually striving to improve themselves. To accomplish this, feedback has to go beyond the two questions that are usually asked: What went well and what could be

4

improved? Certainly reinforcing the positive aspects while attending to deficient aspects of performance is part of the feedback process; however, many situations are far more complex than this suggests, often involving a complicated interaction between the person giving the feedback and the individual receiving it (Milan et al., 2006). The exchange ideally should occur in an environment built upon an established rapport founded on trust. Using the transtheoretical model (Prochaska et al. 1992), Milan identifies three stages in feedback: the precontemplative stage; the contemplative stage; and the preparation stage. If a learner is situated in the precontemplative stage, he/she is often unaware of any problems; when the learner is faced with constructive feedback aimed at improvement, he/she either denies they exist or blames them on external forces. In the contemplative stage, the learner may be aware of problems, but when given constructive feedback is ambivalent about making changes. If, however, the learner has reached the preparation stage, we see a shift; the learner is committed to change and can receive the constructive feedback and make a plan for change that can then be generated into action.

Recognizing these subtle differences in where the receiver may be located allows the sender to tailor his/her feedback in a way that is more likely to scaffold the receiver into subsequent stages, making it more likely that the feedback can function as it is intended, until the receiver reaches a level of professionalism in which he/she sactively seeks feedback to improve practice, and ultimately to develop an effective process of continual self assessment. Indeed, Ende (1983) suggests that the

> ...trainee's reaction to the feedback would also be a valid indicator of the program's success. Like giving feedback, receiving it properly is not always a simple passive act. It requires maturity, honesty and a selfless commitment to the goal of improving clinical skills—traits that are certainly worth cultivating in our future physicians (p. 781).

4.3.1.4 Creating a Culture that Supports Mentorship

The final component in our first Educational Series focuses on creating a culture that supports mentorship. Elsewhere in this book, Bob Garvey writes extensively on mentoring programs that have been introduced into medical education in the UK. Similarly, we recognized early on that mentorship is a critical component of teaching, and even in the absence of a formalized mentoring process mentoring will occur. What is sometimes not fully appreciated is that our residents are watching us and learning from us, even when we do not think we are teaching. What are they learning then?

I our daily role-modeling and conversations are purely of a professional and academic nature, then we are serving our students well. If however, they include disparaging and disrespectful remarks made about colleagues, other residents, or patients, then we are contributing to a toxic environment for learning, and run the risk that such behavior will be reproduced by our residents when they enter their own work environment.

When professionals collaborate in a culture of inquiry, it is important to recognize that different perspectives, background assumptions, and underlying experiences will be brought to bear. Differences can be more pronounced when they involve cross-cultural discussions. Viewing cultural differences as a rich site for learning and exploring them up front, before they are linked to performance, can alleviate future misunderstandings. Such conversations require time and opportunities to build relationships between colleagues and residents – something that is often cited as a barrier to mentoring in a busy clinical setting such as radiology. However, doing so contributes to the creation of a professional culture that becomes more personally relevant to our working lives, leading us to perform our roles better and rekindling the passion that brought us into our chosen profession.

4.4
The Centre for Education in Medical Imaging: A Collaborative Effort

When we began the Centre, our mandate was to optimize the role and function of education within the Department of Medical Imaging through three main avenues:

1. Strengthen curriculum design and implementation in response to educational needs
2. Support and guide the "art of teaching" for faculty and residents at both the practical and theoretical level
3. Advance educational scholarship in medical imaging education

We understood early on that achieving our mandate would require the following conditions for success:

1. Staunch institutional support from the Dean of Education and the Dean of Medicine
2. Vision: A clearly communicated vision led by the Chair of the Department
3. Expertise: Curricular and pedagogic expertise developed through an interdisciplinary relationship with professional educators
4. Support staff: the inclusion of all members of the department to realize the educational mission and vision

Over the past 2 years, we have seen the need for an educational component to be included as a vital, planned, and integral component that permeates the radiology department. The aim of our series and individual consultations was at stimulating new conversations that we believe will contribute to cultivating a culture in which scholarship will take root and thrive. We see our role as participating in sustained faculty development in ways that will allow faculty to continually revisit, review, and reassess their own teaching. We fully acknowledge that this is only part of the equation; to build a culture that supports scholarship, there must be a willingness to find creative ways to protect radiologists' time and income for academic pursuits.

Changing a culture begins by first changing expectations, communicating them clearly, and supporting the development of activities to meet those expectations. Creating the Centre for Education has been one step toward changing that culture. We have benefited greatly from the areas of expertise from each member of our team. Much as our series has

4

been written and rewritten, our roles within our Centre have expanded and shifted. We have depended upon Rethy Chhem's unique combination of medical and educational expertise; we have drawn heavily upon our own educational background; and we have depended upon the superb administrative support offered by all members of the department. Working alongside the radiologists and scientists in the completion of this book has allowed us all to come to appreciate what we each have to offer the other, and possibilities for further scholarship endeavors as faculty begin to explore and challenge their notions of teaching. *Our work, like that of many others (Schön 1983; Van Manen 1995), underscores the power and institutional value afforded by integrating reflection in a community of practice founded upon respect.* Holly's narrative, presented at the opening of this chapter, captures the shift that we have all experienced, and illustrates that when we are new to something we begin with the practical and gradually move toward understanding our practice in more complex ways. We included her narrative in this chapter as it highlights the notion that change is the most important component for creating a different culture. Holly's narrative, which speaks to the shifts and changes in her role within the Centre, highlights not only her personal growth but also the endless possibilities when we embrace and accept new challenges.

References

Bird T (1990) The school teachers's portfolio: An essay on possibilities. In: Millman J, Darling-Hammond LE (eds) The new handbook of teacher evaluation: Assessing elementary and secondary schoolteachers. Corwin Press, Newbury Park

Boyer EL (1990) Scholarship reconsidered: Priorities of the professoriate. Jossey-Bass, San Francisco

Britzman DP (2003) Practice makes practice: A critical study of learning to teach. State of New York Press, New York

Cohen MD, Gunderman RB (2002) Academic radiology: Sustaining the mission. Radiology 224:1–4

Cowan G (2001) Assessment and appraisal of doctors in training: Principles and practice. Royal College of Physicians of London, Salisbury

Cross KP, and Steadman MH (1996) Classroom research: Implementing the scholarship of teaching. San Francisco, California: Jossey-Bass Inc., Publishers.

Ende J (1983) Feedback in clinical medical education. J Am Med Assoc 250:777–781

Gibson DR, Campbell RM (2000) Promoting effective teaching and learning: Hospital consultants identify their needs. Med Educ 34:126–130

Gunderman RB (2006) Achieving excellence in medical education. Springer, London

Hutchings P, Shulman L (1999) The scholarship of teaching: New elaborations, new developments. Change 31(5):10–15

Jolly B, Peyton R (1998) Evaluation. In: Rodney JW, Peyton R (eds) Teaching and learning in medical practice. Manticore Europe, Rickmansworth, UK

Lowry S (1993) Teaching the teachers to teach. Br Med J 306:127–130

Milan FB, Parish SJ, Reichgott MJ (2006) A model for educational feedback based on clinical communication skills strategies: Beyond the "feedback sandwich". Teach Learn Med 18:42–47

Miller GE (1980) Educating medical teachers. Harvard University Press, Cambridge

Miller GE, Abrahamson S, Cohen IS, Grasser HP, Harnack RS, Land, A (1961) Teaching and learning in medical school. Harvard University Press, Cambridge

Nyce JM, Steele JS, and Gunderman RB (2006) Bridging the knowledge divide in radiology education. Radiology 239:629–631

Prochaska JO, DiClemente CC, Norcross JC (1992) In search of how people change: Applications to addictive behaviours. Am Psychol 47:1102–1114

Schön D (1983) The reflective practitioner. Basic Books, New York

Schon D (1987) Educating the reflective practitioner. Toward a new design for teaching and learning in the professions. Jossey-Bass, San Francisco

Shulman L (1986) Those who understand: Knowledge growth in teaching. Educ Res 15(2):4–14

Shulman L (2005) Pedagogies of uncertainty. Liberal Educ 91(2):18–25

Shulman L (2007) Practical wisdom in the service of professional practice. Educ Res 36(9):560

VanManen M (1995) On the epistemology of reflective practice. Teachers Teach Theor Pract 1(1):33–50

Interdisciplinary Learning: A Stimulant for Reflective Practice

5

S.J. Rich

It soon became clear that the problems were going to be intractable. They were shaggy, they stank. In committee they would not keep quiet. (see p. 40 in Leonard 2003)

Such problems are encountered by professionals every day. One of the reasons that the problems often seem intractable is that we tend to try to solve them from the limitations of our own professional knowledge. Many of today's professional and practical problems cannot be solved in isolation. Knowledge has become so specialized that we need alternative perspectives and we need to be able to listen to the expertise of others in order to sometimes even understand the nature of the problem. Interdisciplinary learning and teaching begins to orient teachers and learners to the complexity of the problems that we must face daily and calls for us to listen to the wisdom of the other as we interrogate our own certainties.

As various levels and forms of disciplinary collaboration are being tested across the country, it has become clear that the trend, supported by granting agencies and by higher education institutions, is the establishment of centers that bring together a range of disciplines to explore problems that are of significance in today's complex world. Yet one of the challenges faced by those assessing such proposals is that all too often while many of the grant applications have the rhetoric of interdisciplinarity and suggest ways in which individual disciplines might work together, the reality of the proposals is that each discipline continues to work in isolation, drawing on the scientific methods and knowledge from individual disciplines without recognizing the potential of true collaboration.

At other times, proposals that are truly interdisciplinary are not recognized because they seem messy and unable to meet the rigorous scientific standards of traditional disciplines. They are viewed as "softer" than those from traditional disciplines and "lacking" the same scientific rigor that was assumed during the nineteenth century, a time when scientific method and objectivity became codified and seen as providing an epistemological outline for disciplinary research. Thus, those in the position of evaluating proposals often have the dilemma of evaluating two, one which may appear to have the identifiable rigor with minimal or superficial attention paid to interdisciplinarity, and a second which may not

S.J. Rich
Faculty of Education, University of New Brunswick, Fredericton, Canada
E-mail: srich@unb.ca

Radiology Education. R.K. Chhem et al. (Eds.)
DOI: 10.1007/978-3-540-68989-8, © Springer-Verlag Berlin Heidelberg 2009

5

demonstrate recognizable scientific hallmarks of rigor but reveals the potential to explore a significant human problem in an innovative way. This dilemma is one that confronts all of us who work within the traditional academy where the disciplines still hold sway. Even in areas like gender and cultural studies, where interdisciplinarity was one of the reasons for their establishment, the economic and political pressures present in the academy have led them, to some extent, to become more like traditional disciplines where the objects of knowledge have become reified and the disciplinary boundaries are fixed. Yet unlike claims by some, interdisciplinary programs were not solely the result of political pressures brought forward by various interest groups during the turbulent 1960s (Katz 2001). The call for interdisciplinarity existed long before the 1960s, although perhaps the 1960s enabled a serious consideration of such approaches. There had been recognition many years before that using the power of multiple forms of knowledge could help explore complex human issues. In this chapter, I explore interdisciplinarity. I outline its history and its potential and then demonstrate some of the ways in which it might become an effective part of programming for those in the health sciences and beyond.

5.1
Interdisciplinary Learning: A Century of Growth

John Dewey, an educational philosopher and advocate for democratic citizenship, believed that students need to be able to relate to the material that they were being taught and that they had to become active participants in learning. For Dewey, one of the best ways to engage students in learning was to ensure opportunities to explore questions of interest. In their explorations they were to draw from all disciplines as they investigated potential solutions. This educational process enabled the learner to learn how to learn and ensured that schools were not about preparing solely for a life that would happen after school (see p. 63 in Dewey 1916 and p. 292 in 1929). Indeed since democratic engagement was necessary for citizens, schools in their learning environments had to model learning experiences that reflected active social participation. Dewey's ideas, articulated in the early part of the twentieth century, advocated inquiry-based learning and have to some degree been reflected in educational curricula since that time. These notions of inquiry-based learning were taken up in public schools in Canada and the USA during the 1960s and perhaps reflected a combination of some of the political turmoil of the time and Vygotsky's (1978) notions of the social construction of knowledge. Conceivably, it may have been that at this particular juncture public schools and institutions of higher learning were more open to new ideas to help deal with the increasing diversity on campus and the influx of young women who had just been freed from their biology through the advent of the birth control pill. Whatever the reason, during this decade open classrooms became a feature of schools and educators were encouraged to plan and work together to capitalize on the expertise that various individuals brought to the classroom. The method selected demanded collaboration.

Although many educators found this to be an exciting time in their careers, what had been forgotten was that more than an open space was necessary for interdisciplinary teaching and learning. By the 1970s there was a backlash in public schools as many who attempted to use interdisciplinary, project-based learning did not have the requisite background or skills to collaborate successfully or to capitalize on the subject knowledge brought to the table by each partner. The backlash was further exacerbated by a shift in focus from authentic, individualized assessment toward more standardized assessments that theoretically removed subjectivity from evaluation. Interdisciplinary learning gave way to standards-based education, although in many pockets teachers still developed integrated units and talked with each other as they planned behind closed doors to keep interdisciplinarity alive.

By the 1980s educators had moved into camps with some, often those from traditional universities, championing the discipline or field-based learning, while others, often from some of the newer universities and professional schools, continued to favor interdisciplinary learning. Those who favored disciplinary or subject-based learning argued that learners could never master a field if they had to attend to the content of other disciplines, while the interdisciplinary camp argued that the ways in which subjects intersected provided learners with greater understanding of their field. However, by the end of the 1980s, the camps began to converge, with each group beginning to see what the other had to offer. A partial resolution to the situation came about when educators began to focus on higher-order thinking skills rather than discrete subject matter knowledge. Those who worked in the field of curriculum began to suggest that what was needed was a new approach to curriculum design, an approach that focused on the big ideas and the essence of what it was to know. Inquiry-based-learning came into favor once again as a way to look toward outcomes of an education program rather than focusing on discrete skills.

In higher education, two publications from the Carnegie Foundation assisted interdisciplinary learning to enter the mainstream of the universities. These publications, *Scholarship Reconsidered: A Mandate for the Professoriate* and *Ready to Learn: A Mandate for the Nation* (Boyer 1990, 1991), argued that traditional practices and traditional disciplines were not meeting the needs of the youth of the day. Not surprisingly, both of these reports focused on preparing learners not for the past but for a future that could only be imagined. The subject borders had been crossed and educators were encouraged to seek ways in which their disciplines could enrich each other. That is not to suggest that interdisciplinary learning has been an easy sell.

5.2
The Context Today

In today's academy, a number of converging trends have supported the increased interest in interdisciplinarity. One of the key reasons for the interest may be the complex issues that face today's communities. Homelessness, environmental illness, and poverty place an increasing strain on the ability of a single professional approach to tackle any problem. The physician, for example, may be able to treat a symptom of an environmental illness by prescribing asthma medication, but the underlying problem of pollution created by overindustrialization or of a contaminated water supply is not within that realm of that professional. The decision of whether to place a roadway through an environmentally sensitive area demands input from a number of separate knowledge bases. Complex problems give rise to emerging disciplines such as environmental studies and neurosciences where students and established scholars are drawn to the field because of the issues in which they are interested. Interdisciplinarity enables scholars and practitioners to work together to investigate such problems.

Changes in workforce expectations have also contributed to the current interest in interdisciplinarity. Employers often expect that their professional employees are familiar with working in teams in which individuals contribute their strength and knowledge to work on an issue. In schools, teachers are expected to be able to work as a part of a school team on which several professional disciplines (social workers, counselors, psychologists, and teachers) address the issues surrounding a particular child. In medicine, often many practitioners, nurses, physicians, and social workers must communicate to determine the nature of a medical problem and determine the most appropriate treatment course. In order to work within these emerging, complex environments, individuals must be able to solve problems collaboratively and develop a set of shared goals that appreciate and respect disciplinary roles. Effective communication skills and the recognition that no one discipline possesses the best solution are keys to working successfully in an interdisciplinary environment.

Yet interdisciplinary learning and interdisciplinary programs continue to be seen as transgressive, existing in a liminal space because learners and the material do not seem to really belong to any particular discipline even though some universities have introduced interdisciplinary programs at both graduate and undergraduate levels. Such programs can be found at times in undergraduate general education, where they augment traditional programs and enable students to specialize but then also look for connections to other disciplines. In other instances, programs may be conceptualized around the notion that solving any problem requires certain skills and knowledge, but that finding solutions is not defined nor experienced as the application of a discrete skill set or discrete disciplinary knowledge. Students may, for example, explore aspects of leadership from the perspective of a number of disciplines, then, in their culminating projects, frame the issues in a substantive piece of reflective researched work. However, because they do not have a disciplinary "home," these students and their faculty colleagues may be forgotten on campuses that remain structured along disciplinary lines. However, these programs can also suffer from the failure of the academy to support those faculty members who wish to interact with each other and their students to research these concerns. In short, although programs may exist, the traditional structures of the academy do not foster the types of interaction necessary at the borders of the disciplines. Even with a beginning acceptance, the space both physically and cognitively allocated is given grudgingly, especially when resources are limited and traditional programs are experiencing a lack of resources.

5.3
Interdisciplinary Learning and Learner Engagement

One issue that should, however, make anyone interested in higher education pay attention is the power of interdisciplinary learning to engage students. Since interdisciplinary learning is a form of experience that is complex, context-dependent, value-laden, and ethically bound, the actions of those involved are characterized by intuitive and tacitly engaged practices. This means that members of different disciplines have to learn to come together in ways that cross borders and engage with each other. In such a context, those who have been disciplined differently enter into conversations with each other in an attempt to understand alternative perspectives.

Dewey wrote of engagement in his initial work and his notions of engagement have been reflected in many quarters in higher education, including the National Survey of Student Engagement (NSSE 2007). For Dewey and for today's learners, engagement occurs when students believe they have the capacity for learning and when the demonstration of learning is relevant to their lives. Engagement theory suggests that for learners to be involved with their learning there must be meaningful interaction with others around a task that matters. In the interdisciplinary context, engagement theory holds as learners are involved in an activity that demands application of skills, communication about the task is essential, and the outcomes of the tasks can be shared with a larger community. In contrast to academic rationalism, interdisciplinary learning focuses on the wholistic learning process and, as noted by Shulman and Fenstermacher (see p. xvi in 2008), learning that involves teaching for practical reasoning leads to a more informed and responsible engagement. Interdisciplinary learning, because it goes beyond the mere acquisition of information and technical skills, adds a social disposition to the learning process. At its best, interdisciplinary learning demands practical reasoning and an application that requires reflection and criticism not just for its own sake, but for the consideration of what matters in society as a whole. When students are required to think about the ways in which their actions have an impact on others, engagement follows. It is no longer sufficient to learn skills in isolation or apply them in a limited context without thinking about the ways in which all actions have implications for both the self and the other. The next section outlines interdisciplinary learning.

5.4
Interdisciplinary Learning: It Is and It Is Not

There are many forms of interdisciplinary learning although in various disciplines it has assumed many pseudonyms and variations. For example, educators speak of problem-based learning, project-based learning, or integrated studies – all of which are variations on the basic theme articulated by Dewey at the turn of the twentieth century. Each discipline that has adopted some form of interdisciplinarity has adapted a "method" that fits with a particular world view. In business schools, students apply their interdisciplinary knowledge as they consider business cases from each perspective within business so that cases are considered from the perspective of marketing, finance, and so forth. In medical schools, clinical problems will be posed and medical students invited to consider the problems from multiple perspectives within the medical profession. In education, particularly social studies, complex social and environmental problems will be raised for groups of students to consider. In each of the aforementioned cases, students collaboratively solve problems and reflect on their experiences, but to some extent their experiences are limited by the boundaries of the discipline and subdisciplines. However, learners are challenged to listen to each other, and together unravel the complexity of the problem or case. The challenge for today's academy is giving appropriate recognition and space to those who recognize that such limited cases would be enriched by perspectives from outside the immediate discipline.

True interdisciplinary learning helps learners to develop meaningful links across the disciplines. These links provide both teachers and learners with a purpose that goes beyond the evaluation and memorization of facts and pushes learners to think about the ways in which information can be applied in new ways to old subject matters. Often interdisciplinary learning focuses on a complex problem that requires knowledge from several disciplines to be solved. Klein (1990) defines interdisciplinary learning as the synthesis of two or core disciplines, establishing a new level of discourse and an integration of knowledge. Klein goes on to suggest that interdisciplinary initiatives are often described by the form they take, as in team teaching, or by the motivation for them, such as serving societal needs. Yet for interdisciplinary studies to evolve, those participating must go beyond simply adding the knowledge of one discipline to another but must begin to integrate knowledge to create a new way of understanding. In the sciences especially, as knowledge advances, scientists who study biology must understand biochemistry and biophysics in order to truly examine the ways in which an organism adapts or fails to adapt to its environment. Interdisciplinary learning accepts and respects that different disciplines have knowledge to contribute to the solution of the complex problems that face everyday modern life.

When interdisciplinary curricula are created, the disciplines are bridged and at the same time the students' needs for content knowledge are met. The content informs the student and the student in turn informs the content. As each student discovers what is needed in order to complete a task, the learning become more meaningful and students have to apply practical reasoning. In settings where interdisciplinary learning is featured, students often find that content becomes more relevant and exciting especially if teachers can link the learning to aspects of the students' lives. For example, medical students who want to become family practitioners may well find that their understanding of anatomy and chemistry is enhanced if the information required is linked to a real patient. Their understanding of family medicine is enriched when they learn the perspective of the nurse or the social worker who works with the whole family. Those who work from an interdisciplinary perspective understand the interconnectedness and interdependence of the human condition. Treating information in the abstract does not foster learning as effectively as making the learning meaningful and enabling the learners to discovers the connections across the disciplines.

Interdisciplinary learning perhaps could be best developed in professional schools where learners, because of the nature of professions, have to engage with the messy reality of humanity. In professional schools, learners often have already developed some sense of what the disciplines look like and have some mastery of the knowledge bases of several disciplines. Learners are challenged to bring this knowledge together in order to solve the complex problems of professional practice. Such activities involve developing an identity as a professional. In the development of the identity, the practitioner has to become aware of conceptual knowledge, the "what" of practice, at the same time as he/she becomes familiar with the techniques of the profession, the "how" of practice. Finally, both the what and the how have to be used appropriately in particular situations and the what and the how of a particular profession may be juxtaposed with the what and the how of another profession. The juxtaposition of the two conceptualizations and sets of practices may transform both. Interdisciplinarity may ultimately speak to issues of identity because in the interaction with professions and disciplines other than one's own, the practitioner may become more attuned to what it is to be a good practitioner. That is, to understand the core values, beliefs, and deep commitments of a professional. Interdisciplinary practice then seems to have three key characteristics. It is inquiry-based, as Dewey outlined inquiry. It is field-oriented, that is, oriented to the life world and its problems. And, finally, it is learner-focused because there are always opportunities for the learner to work collaboratively, independently, and finally reflectively. Those involved in interdisciplinary learning engage in studying independently in order to review the disciplinary knowledge and collaborate across inquiries with peers, learning to respect difference as they do so. Ethical relationships and consideration of the perspective of the other play an important role in facilitating interdisciplinary learning. Central to the development of understanding in interdisciplinary learning is the art of reflection and perhaps the art of understanding through storying.

5.5
Interdisciplinary Teaching and Learning as Meaning Making and an Entrée to Reflective Practice

Aboriginal writer Thomas King writes "The truth about story is that's all we are"(King 2003, p. 2). Laurel Richardson suggests that the act of writing, of exploring who we are, frees us from "the intellectual myopia of hyper-determined research projects and their formulaic write ups…" (see p. 14 Richardson 1997). It seems only appropriate that the challenge of interdisciplinary work should turn to story as a way to articulate the problems and solutions investigated. Interdisciplinary projects are by their very nature ambiguous and uncertain. Since the problems border-cross, the way into the investigation demands that the practitioner discover the self in the problem. The process of self-discovery means that language is considered and each word is selected thoughtfully. Such consideration of the ethics of framing problems and their solutions means that we move from the certainty of false scientific language into the world of tentative and formative understandings that permit shades and areas yet to be explored. In interdisciplinary studies, practitioners come to terms with language and how it is used to shape disciplines and establish borders. As Gadamer (1989) noted, language is a vehicle for interpretation and thus for shaping understanding:

> A person who believes he is free of prejudices, relying on the objectivity of his procedures and denying that he himself is conditioned by historical circumstances, experiences the power of the prejudices that unconsciously dominate him (see p. 360)

In short, without knowing who we are, we cannot educate. The educator involved with interdisciplinary learning must be engaged in a reflective interaction with his or her own pedagogical practices and prejudices and may use the act of writing as a way in to

5

understand and shape them. It is through the interaction with disciplines other than one's own that one comes to see the world of practice through a different lens. The act of writing, because it forces the writer to engage with words, language, and self, can assist the would-be interdisciplinary scholar to unpack the prejudices and see them for what they are. Once this happens, there is an admission that what was once seen as certainty is tentative, and those participating in the shaping and solution of a problem can reframe the issues and free those involved from the tyranny of technical rational discourse.

5.6
Interdisciplinary Learning and Reflective Practice

Reflective practice has been a part of a dominant conversation in the professions since Schon's seminal work (1983), *The Reflective Practitioner*, and has been adopted in the education programs of a wide range of professional groups to the extent that it is now a part of the quality assurance programs of many accreditation bodies in the health professions and beyond. Reflective practice, if it includes the act of writing, of conceptualizing our approach to the world as story, enables us to recognize our prejudices and the history of our disciplines from the manner with which we engage the world around us. The challenge of interdisciplinary practice is to uncover or create a common language through which the various disciplines can interact. It also means that at times there must be a tolerance for ambiguity. In any profession, the entry to practice is characterized by shock at the messiness of practice and the problems encountered. No matter what profession, individuals do not behave as theories would suggest that they behave. There seems little direct applicability of the esoteric knowledge of their discipline to the real world of messy people, so reflective practice has been seen as a way to enable practitioners to think about the complex problems encountered in practice.

Yet, as Schon acknowledges, in reflective practice, the perspective of the individual practitioner can become very powerful and exclude the client, especially since the practitioner as expert is already in a position of power. What a focus on interdisciplinary reflective practice does is limit the dominance of a single expert group. Since multiple disciplines are called on to interact with and attempt to understand a common problem, the reflection becomes multilateral and no single perspective dominates. There must be give and take to make meaning of the situation. Interdisciplinary reflective practice then calls into question monolithic approaches to the solution of professional problems.

One of the challenges of interdisciplinary interaction is to consider how to engage in reflective practices that are not formulaic but that attend to collaboration. It is relatively easy to suggest that in interdisciplinary learning contexts individuals do not work in isolation or plan on their own but collaborate with colleagues to learn from each other. In this way interdisciplinary learning takes up the notion of the educator as a learner who communicates with respect for the knowledge that each person brings to the planning and teaching context. Those who have tried to develop programs that are interdisciplinary in nature have found that collegiality and respect for the knowledge of others is a natural outgrowth of the collaboration but the collegiality cannot be contrived. True collaboration and interdisciplinarity arise when real problems that matter to practitioners are involved. If this collaboration arises naturally from the identified needs of the group, then some might say that interdisciplinary learning has been a way to create professional growth or learning communities among educators. Yet all too often the practice itself becomes a process of going thorough the motions and not engaging in an in-depth reflection on the *what* and the *how* of the action.

Some suggest that interdisciplinary educators begin by thinking about the learner population. Next, they identify the disciplinary fields that are involved in practice. Finally, they develop a visual tool to help to determine the essential questions and the disciplines that students will need to explore. Dewey (1929) suggested the following sequence as a way to think about planning for interdisciplinary, inquiry-based learning:

1. Recognize a situation in our experience of the world
2. Think about the situation as a problem that can be investigated using inquiry
3. Hypothesize potential solutions that might solve the problem and what disciplines might have something to offer toward a solution
4. Think about the meaning of these solutions in relation to both the problem and the world experience
5. Apply the results of the inquiry to the situation and evaluate the results
6. Accept a scientific or commonsense explanation of the problem situation that reduces but does not necessarily resolve the original indeterminacy

For practitioners to understand what these steps mean however, they need to be able to write the self into each step. In medicine, for example, the current situation with respect to organ donations raises a number of moral and ethical problems. Before introducing the issue, the educator needs to think about (and write about) the nature of organ donation. What are the concerns involved? Who has the responsibility to make the decisions? On what basis might these decisions be made? A focus on the relatively simple act of harvesting the organ for transplantation to another person allows a consideration of the technical aspects of the issue but does not raise the sociological and psychological issues surrounding the act. Once a case has been developed, it is relatively easy to organize an interdisciplinary student group to discuss a clinical problem. When only one discipline is involved, the problem can be discussed in an abstract manner and the self is never really invested in the learning process. The problem solution becomes one of demonstrating what is known about the facts of the case and then being able to translate those facts into a diagnosis. What is missing is a step that engages the clinical practitioner and the students from other disciplines in a discussion of what the act might mean for the family of the donor or the recipient. In order to really consider such issues, learners have to be able to think about and reflect on who they are as people living in the world. What is their story and how does it intersect with the lives of others?

As the concept of interdisciplinarity has entered the university, professors from across various disciplines have found that they need to work together to establish the outcomes that are desired in various programs and then to determine what problematic situations might help students acquire these outcomes. In many professional schools, true interdisciplinary learning has not yet arrived since all too often these schools are still struggling for acceptance within the traditional boundaries of the university. The scholarship of discovery, long accepted as the norm in the university, is valued but too often the scholarship of application, the scholarship the professional schools know and do well, does not yet have the status it deserves. Yet there seems to be some hope.

5.7
Interprofessional Education and Interdisciplinarity

Interprofessional education, a concept that is emerging in many Canadian schools, focuses on the ways in which the traditional departments in the university are organized then systemically works toward breaking down those barriers. In order to connect people in these contexts across boundaries, successful techniques have included:

1. Taking advantage of informal as well as formal conversations
2. Using metaphors to describe student learning and teaching
3. Making implicit knowledge of each profession visible

It is the last point – making tacit knowledge visible – that is critical for interdisciplinary learning to succeed, especially in professional schools and in the university as a whole. The wisdom of practice that Schon speaks about is all too often tacit and can only be surfaced in problematic situations. In most professional schools the articulation of tacit knowledge is not featured but is left for learners to discover. It is perhaps only by bringing together different disciplines within the professional school that tacit knowledge can be made explicit.

For example, some professional schools attempt interdisciplinarity by mandating that occupational therapy nursing, medicine, vocational therapy, and dentistry are linked in one school but housed in separate buildings. However, in order for an effective interdisciplinary atmosphere to develop, those involved should be located near to each other so that they can engage in the types of informal conversations that build trust and enable asking the difficult questions. When disciplines and professions are isolated, the borders between them are reinforced and not crossed. Proximity makes it easier to learn about others, their stance, and their relationship to the subject.

Too often in these professional school "arranged marriages" the curricula are left as separate entities and researchers in these contexts are valued not for the work they do that is applied but for their contribution to "pure" research. For the interdisciplinary school or program to become truly effective (or for the marriage to work), the curriculum itself needs to be examined and critical questions asked. What do nurses need to know, what do physicians need to know, and so forth? The next critical question is at what place do these types of knowledge intersect and where might they have the potential to enhance each other. This type of discussion is rarely taken up within the academy, yet it must be if the power of interdisciplinary is to be unleashed. Sullivan and Rosin (2008) suggest a new model for undergraduate teaching, one which takes as a given that professional education needs the insights of a liberal education. In their book, they outline the experience of a research seminar that brought together educators from six professional fields as well as liberal arts colleagues. What happened in the seminar exemplified the engagement of teachers and learners in learning through interdisciplinarity, a process that caused them to inform judgment with knowledge. A key issue in the courses discussed in the book was that "…good citizenship and good work require that technical considerations be brought into proper balance with the sense of the kind of person one desires to be and that doing this successfully depends on achieving a good understanding of the consequences of one's actions" (see p. 20 in Sullivan and Rosin 2008). Although they do not label them as such, the courses they describe are interdisciplinary and to ensure their success they engaged people who had:

1. A reputation for academic rigor and excellence
2. An open-minded approach to learning and a passion for inquiry
3. The ability to ask good questions
4. An ability and a willingness to teach and to learn

Interdisciplinarity offers hope for all disciplines to be better and stronger together. What might be possible if you initiate a discussion with someone from outside of your profession, outside your discipline, and tackle a problem that interests both of you? What new insights might you both learn? It may be the beginning of your own interdisciplinary learning community.

References

Boyer EL (1990) Scholarship reconsidered: The priorities of the professoriate. Jossey-Bass, San Francisco

Boyer EL (1991) Ready to learn: A mandate for the nation. Jossey-Bass, San Francisco

Dewey J (1916) Democracy and education. Macmillan, New York

Dewey J (1929) My pedagogic creed. J Nat Educ Assoc 18:292

Gadamer HG (1989) Truth and method, 2nd rev edn. Weinsheimer J, Marshal D (transl) Continuum, New York

Katz C (2001) Disciplining interdisciplinarity. Fem Stud. Retrieved from http://www.accessmylibray.com. Accessed 08 March 2008

King T (2003) The truth about stories: A native narrative. Anansi Press, Toronto, ON

Klein JT (1990) Interdisciplinarity: History, theory and practice. Wayne State University Press, Detroit

Leonard J (2003) Jesus in Kashmir: Poems. Proensa, Woden, Australia

National Survey of Student Engagement (2007). Bloomington, IN. Experiences that matter: Enhancing student learning & success Annual Report: Indiana University Press.

Richardson L (1997) Fields of play: Constructing an academic life. Rutgers University Press, New Brunswick

Schon D (1983) The reflective practitioner. Basic Books, New York

Shulman LS, Fenstermacher GD (2008) Foreward. In: Sullivan WM, Rosin MS (eds) A new agenda for higher education: Shaping a life of the mind for practice. Jossey-Bass, San Francisco

Sullivan WM, Rosin MS (2008) A new agenda for higher education: Shaping a life of the mind for practice. Jossey-Bass, San Francisco

Vygotsky L (1978) Mind in society: The development of higher psychological processes. Harvard University Press, Cambridge

Feedback in Radiologic Education

6

R.B. Gunderman, K.B. Williamson

There is no such thing as a "self-made" man or woman. We are each made up of thousands of others. Everyone who has ever done a kind deed for us, or spoken one word of encouragement to us, has entered into the make-up of our character and thoughts.

George Matthew Adams

Feedback influences everyone's sense of whether they have been successful or not, and so influences how they will think and act in the future. In education, it is a critical component in how learners monitor and evaluate their own performance (Bransford et al. 2000). The absence of a clear program for assessing learner performance and providing feedback is a strong mark against any educational program (Quattlebaum 1996). Whether we realize it or not, feedback constitutes an important teaching strategy. Yet many radiologic educators do not employ feedback as effectively as they could, and some misuse it altogether. Improving the quality of feedback that learners receive is a crucial element in improving educational programs in radiology.

Despite the fact that all residency programs are required to provide regular feedback to residents, the nature and quality of that feedback vary. Most medical educators receive little or no training in how to provide effective feedback (Gallagher et al. 1977). Moreover, as clinical demands have grown, providing high-quality feedback has become a more difficult and, clinically speaking, more expensive proposition (Gunderman 2001). Overburdened with other responsibilities, faculty members may simply circle a few numbers on routine evaluation forms and write a comment such as "Doing fine" or "Needs to work harder," which provides very little guidance. Some may view the requirement to provide feedback as an unwelcome burden.

Despite these difficulties, the influence of feedback pervades our lives as educators. It should not be regarded merely as a means of keeping score or patting a learner on the back,

R.B. Gunderman (✉)
Education Division, Department of Radiology, Indiana University School of Medicine,
702 Barnhill Dr, RI 1053, Indianapolis, IN 46202-5200, USA
E-mail: rbgunder@iupui.edu

Radiology Education. R.K. Chhem et al. (Eds.)
DOI: 10.1007/978-3-540-68989-8, © Springer-Verlag Berlin Heidelberg 2009

but as one of the most important teaching opportunities educators enjoy (Curtis et al. 1988). When applied well, feedback encourages learners to improve and thus enhances educators' satisfaction with teaching (Cuttino and Scatliff 1987). When feedback is poorly applied and negative, however, learners tend to avoid it, and the quality of the teaching program suffers (Reynolds and Ende 2000). The purpose of this article is to review some of the key principles underlying high-quality feedback with the hope of raising the profile of this important strategic component of radiologic education.

6.1
Lack of Feedback

Resident: I have been working hard and learning a lot in this residency program, but nobody ever gives me any feedback on how we're doing. Could you give me some idea of how you see my strengths and weaknesses? Faculty member: Do you have any idea how much harder I am working now than I did 5 years ago? I am far too busy trying to get the clinical work done to take time out for that. If there is a problem, believe me, we'll tell you. Otherwise, you can assume you're doing okay. Resident: But I really want to improve. Any feedback at all would be greatly appreciated. Isn't that partly what residency programs are for? Faculty member: Here's some feedback for you: If you don't stop talking and focus on getting this work done, we'll be here all night.

This "No news is good news" scenario provides an important lesson about feedback, namely, the danger of failing to provide it. Many medical students and residents feel as though they are operating in a vacuum. In fact, one study of residents in another specialty revealed that only 8% of respondents felt "very satisfied" with the quality of feedback they received, while 80% reported rarely or never receiving useful feedback (Isaacson et al. 1995).

In the scenario above, a resident makes a reasonable request for some appraisal of his or her performance in the residency program. The way the question is phrased suggests that the resident is not fishing for praise but genuinely wants help identifying specific strengths and weaknesses. Instead of responding to the resident's request, however, the faculty member views the request as an intrusion and tells the resident to drop it. Clinical work must be completed, but failing to provide a high-quality education to the next generation of physicians and radiologists is too high a price to pay.

An alternative to the resident's request for feedback in this scenario would be the following:

Faculty member: We get pretty busy around here this time of day. That's just how it works. So what we need to focus on right now is completing this clinical work. One thing I can tell you is that no one has complained about your performance. That is good. Once we fulfill our clinical commitments, let's set aside some time to talk in more depth about the quality of your work. Is that okay?

6.2
Disparagement versus Feedback

Faculty member: What is the difference between compressive atelectasis and passive atelectasis? Resident: Compressive atelectasis means the lung is being compressed by something, but passive atelectasis means it is just collapsing on its own, for some other reason. Faculty member: No, that's wrong. Try again! Resident: Compressive atelectasis means the lung is being compressed by a mass, while passive atelectasis has to do with elastic recoil. Faculty member: Wrong again! Come on! Resident: Compressive atelectasis...it means that the lung...I mean....Faculty member: Yes, well, what do you mean? I can't believe you don't know this! Resident: I guess I don't know the difference. Faculty member: I guess not! [Turning to other residents]You know, this is a classic example of how NOT to succeed in residency. Let's move on to the next case.

We tend to suppose that learning failure involves an inability to recall something, but it can just as easily reflect a misunderstanding. Some educators prefer not to correct or contradict learners, fearing that they will give offense or diminish their own popularity. Yet failing to correct a misunderstood concept or relationship tends to perpetuate misinformation that may undermine the resident's performance, even jeopardizing a patient (Coulson et al. 1989). Pointing out mistakes is an integral component of every educator's mission.

Yet there are effective and ineffective ways of pointing out mistakes. There is a big difference between merely telling people that they are off course and providing them with guidance. Effective feedback provides real insight. In the case of the distinction between compressive and passive atelectasis, the faculty member might draw the resident's attention to the locus from which the mass effect on the lung arises, whether from within or from outside the visceral pleura.

Such guidance frequently works best when accompanied by an affirmation, such as "Well, you're on the right track about mass effect, but does it make a difference where the pressure on the lung is exerted from?" Above all, learners should be provided with opportunities to revise their thinking as they work on a problem.

While feedback may need to be negative or critical, it need not be malicious. There is rarely any benefit in humiliating people. In a profession such a medicine, where most members are accustomed to performing at a high level, providing feedback in a way that puts learners down may prove counterproductive. It can damage learners' self-esteem and produce a level of anxiety that actually interferes with learning. Sometimes learners' pulses may pound so loudly for fear of humiliation that they cannot hear themselves think. Furthermore, it may incite resentment or outright anger that can have adverse consequences for faculty members, for example, through poor educational performance evaluations. Malicious feedback undermines the camaraderie between educators and learners and represents neither professional nor humane conduct.

6.3
The Never-Satisfied Educator

Faculty member: What do you make of this image? Resident: It shows a poorly marginated, lytic lesion in the tibial diaphysis with a permeative pattern of bone destruction; aggressive-looking, onion-skin periosteal reaction; and Codman's triangles. The open growth plates indicate that this is a pediatric patient, and I would favor a Ewing sarcoma. Faculty member: What is the histopathology of Ewing sarcoma? Resident: It is one of the small, round blue cell tumors, like lymphoma and primitive neuroectodermal tumors. Histochemical and immunologic studies can be important in telling the difference. Faculty member: What is the prognosis? Resident: If the tumor hasn't metastasized at the time of presentation, it can be relatively good—70% 5-year survival or better. Faculty member: Who was Ewing sarcoma named after? Resident: I believe his name was James Ewing, and he was a pathologist at Cornell University. Faculty member: And where did he attend college? Resident: I don't know that. Faculty member: Oh you don't, do you? I didn't think you would. Well, as a matter of fact, Dr. Ewing was a graduate of Amherst College. You think you're pretty smart, don't you, but you just remember that you clearly have a great deal to learn.

In this case, the resident is clearly performing at an outstanding level, basically scoring direct hits with every response. One could hardly imagine a clearer, more succinct description of a bone tumor, and the resident responds equally well in addressing the tumor's histopathologic characteristics, prognosis, and even the derivation of its eponym. One gets the feeling, however, that this faculty member is determined to keep posing more and more difficult questions until the resident is forced to admit failure, resorting to trivia that no reasonable person should ever feel guilty about not knowing. At no point along the way does the faculty member provide any encouragement or praise for the outstanding job the resident is doing. Instead of leaving the resident feeling good about a first-rate performance, the faculty member concludes by putting the resident down.

Although this is an extreme example, many practicing radiologists may be able to think of an educator they encountered in the course of their own careers who seemed disappointed when a resident knew the answer to every question. The best educators are not so insecure about their own knowledge that they must seek satisfaction in exposing the ignorance of others. The faculty member's goal should be to form an educational alliance with residents and medical students, helping them to understand what they need to know for their level of training, helping them to identify where deficiencies exist, and providing praise where praise is deserved. Residents who really "know their stuff" deserve a pat on the back once in a while, and any resentment faculty members may feel about the fact that they rarely receive any praise is no excuse for not providing it to students and residents.

There is a distinct danger in radiology residency programs that the only feedback residents receive is corrective or negative feedback. How often do faculty members go out of their way to tell residents that they have done a good job, or to thank the residents for their help? Yet positive feedback can offer tremendous encouragement, increasing learners' dedication to learning and their will to excel. Such encouragement may be especially important for students and residents who seem disheartened or lacking in confidence, but even those who seem to be excelling are likely to benefit from sincere words of praise. Providing positive feedback is good for faculty members, as well. Most people, including medical students and residents, tend to like educators who make them feel good about themselves, and a faculty member who helps to build legitimate self-esteem among learners is more likely to be highly regarded.

6.4
Teachable Moments

> *Faculty member: You know, your performance in that last procedure clearly shows me that you don't understand the proper technique. Resident: What did I do wrong? Faculty member: Did you finish the assigned reading before you started this rotation? Resident: Well, I finished most of it, but we have been working here till late in the evening every night, and I just haven't had time to finish everything. Faculty member: Did you sleep last night? Resident: Well, yes.... Faculty member: Then you had time! Resident: In fairness, I really don't think there has been enough time to do all the reading you assigned. Faculty member: Really? If you feel that way, I'd be happy to help you find another position. There are plenty of other applicants who want to be in this program.*

In this case, the faculty member has identified a deficiency in how the resident performed a procedure, a crucial first step in improving performance, but failed to exploit the opportunity to provide focused, constructive feedback. If learners are not informed of deficiencies, they may never recognize their opportunity to improve. As a result, they become increasingly entrenched in bad habits. However, the best feedback to provide in such a situation is a precise diagnosis of the problem and a prescription for treatment; that is, point out what is wrong and show how to fix it. By shifting the discussion from procedural technique to the global issue of whether the resident has done all of the assigned reading, a teachable moment has been lost. In other circumstances, there would be nothing wrong with chiding a resident for failing to complete assigned readings, but the opportunity to redress a specific deficiency should be seized wherever possible.

The task in this case is not the recall of information or the solving of a cognitive problem, but the performance of a procedure. This renders the faculty member's questions about reading particularly unhelpful, because procedural skills typically prove difficult to learn solely from a book (Romiszowski 1999). Although procedure manuals are useful, procedural learning comes from doing and becomes far more effective with guided practice.

Sometimes it is the expectations themselves, and not the failure to meet them, that is the real problem. There is little to be gained by expecting learners to sacrifice sleep and other components of self-care in order to complete voluminous learning requirements. This approach may bring results when employed on an occasional basis, but if such expectations become the norm, they are likely to produce residents who are simply tired and discouraged. While occasional threats may spur some learners to improve their performance,

6

intimidation as a motivational technique eventually produces a defensive attitude toward knowledge that is antithetical to curiosity. Repeated threats engender a sense of distrust that can damage a program's morale and esprit de corps.

In the ideal, the educator might respond to the resident's query "What did I do wrong?" by describing or even demonstrating the problem, highlighting the difference between what the resident did and the proper technique. Another useful strategy in such a situation is to provide a second chance to get the procedure right. After the learner has had an opportunity to think through and mentally rehearse the task, repetition can help to solidify the proper technique.

6.5
The Spirit of Inquiry

Resident: I'm having some trouble understanding the difference between cytotoxic and vasogenic edema. Could you help me out? Faculty member: You mean you haven't read that yet? What's the matter with you residents today? You seem to think everything should be spoon-fed to you.

Learners need to become adept at recognizing what they do not understand. One way to encourage self-assessment is to respond helpfully to requests for explanation or clarification. When faculty members react indignantly to requests for clarification, blaming the resident for failing to know, residents learn to fear admitting their ignorance and lose opportunities to improve. In the worst-case scenario, an entire program becomes permeated by an attitude of intolerance for uncertainty. Faculty members and residents alike begin to behave as though their survival depends on never getting caught not knowing something.

Such attitudes undermine the spirit of open inquiry that characterizes an academic institution. They quell the appetite for investigation on which clinical and scientific advancements depend. Good questions are more important to the future of radiology than right answers, because they are the impetus to new discoveries that will build the future of the field. Moreover, good questions can enrich the understanding of faculty members, who may discover that they do not understand matters quite so well as they supposed and may learn something themselves as a result.

When a learner poses a question, an educator can respond helpfully without "spoon-feeding" the answer. When time permits, a good strategy is to probe the resident's understanding, answering a question with a question. The purpose of such an approach is not to embarrass or intimidate, but to help the learner better appreciate what it means to understand something and to ask the key questions that real understanding requires. Helpful questions might include the following: What do the terms "cytotoxic" and "vasogenic" mean to you? What are their underlying cellular mechanisms, and what different types of processes tend to produce them? What are their characteristic imaging appearances?

Asking questions helps learners to think problems through for themselves rather than merely memorizing what someone tells them. In many cases, faculty members could encourage students and residents to call on their peers for help (Barron et al. 1998). This encourages future radiologists to regard their knowledge base as a work in progress and to become comfortable consulting with others.

6.6
Conclusion

Feedback helps learners pay attention to what they are learning and to strive to improve the quality of their work. Feedback can help a medical student or resident who is not studying enough, or who approaches studying in an ineffective way, to identify that a problem exists and take steps to correct it. Not only does feedback help learners see their performance from the point of view of their instructors, it also helps them become more self-reflective and thus better able to monitor and adjust their learning approaches on their own. The mark of well-educated people is not merely how much they know but how well they learn, and the ability to monitor one's own learning is an essential skill that good educational programs cultivate.

A radiology educator who becomes better at providing feedback to medical students and residents is likely to realize additional benefits in other domains of professional life. In dealing with fellow radiologists and other physicians, it is important to be able to deliver criticism without giving offense and to find effective ways of saying "Well done!" Non-physician health professionals and support personnel such as nurses, technologists, and secretaries also benefit from good advice and words of encouragement.

Formal systems of feedback, such as annual reports, should be taken seriously by everyone involved as an opportunity to improve performance and make professional life more enjoyable and fulfilling. It is equally important, however, to remain alert for informal opportunities to help people perform better and to provide praise and encouragement for good work. Such opportunities are especially important in the case of medical students and residents, who are at a highly formative stage of professional development and for whom the right feedback at the right moment can make a big difference.

References

Bransford JD, Brown AL, Cocking RR. How people learn: brain, mind, experience, and school. Washington: National Academy Press, 2000

Quattlebaum TG. Techniques for evaluation of residents and residency programs. Pediatrics 1996; 98:1277–1283

Gallagher R, Donnelly M, Scalzi PM, Deighton M. Toward a comprehensive methodology of resident evaluation. Annu Conf Res Med Educ 1977; 16:6–12

Gunderman RB. The fight for education. AJR Am J Roentgenol 2001; 175:23–26

Curtis DJ, Riordan DD, Brower AC, Amis ES. Testing as a teaching tool. Invest Radiol 1988; 23:151–153

Cuttino JT, Scatliff JH. Resident performance evaluation. Invest Radiol 1987; 22:986–989

Reynolds EE, Ende J. Feedback in medical education. In: Distlehorst LH, Dunnington GL, Folse JR, eds. Teaching and learning in medical and surgical education: lessons learned for the 21st century. Mahwah: Lawrence Erlbaum Associates, 2000

Isaacson JH, Posk LK, Liaker DG, Halperin AK. Resident perceptions of the evaluation process. J Gen Intern Med 1995; 10:89

Coulson RL, Feltovich PJ, Spiro RJ. Foundations of a misunderstanding of the ultrastructural basis of myocardial failure: a reciprocation network of oversimplifications. J Med Philos 1989; 14:109–146

Romiszowski A. The development of physical skills: instruction in the psychomotor domain. In: Reigeluth CM, ed. Instructional-design theories and models. Vol II. Mahwah: Lawrence Earlbaum Associates, 1999

Barron BJ, Schwartz DL, Vye NJ, Moore A, Petrosino A, Bransford JD. Doing with understanding: lessons from research on problem and project-based learning. J Learn Sci 1998; 7:271–312

The Role of Mentoring in Professional Education

R. Garvey

7.1
Introduction: A Glimpse into the UK Health Service Story

Consider these four vignettes:

The Northern Deanery Mentoring and Professional Development Programme provides a benchmark mentor development programme for the UK National Health Service (NHS). The programme, led by Nancy Redfern from the Northern Deanery, provides multidisciplinary training and development programmes for health care staff in the northeast of the UK as well as other areas around the country – particularly, Yorkshire, Oxford, Portsmouth and Northampton. Nancy believes that building a network of well-trained mentors is essential to creating a "critical mass" of people to contribute to cultural change within the NHS.

Participants appreciate being able to learn with colleagues from different areas of the NHS. For the most part, they attend because they want to make a positive difference to patient care. Others come to "test" the programme out with a view to establishing a scheme in their own Hospital Trusts.

The programme is voluntary and focuses on mentor skills development. It does not focus on specific organizational issues and consequently it is essentially about personal professional development. This approach holds appeal to NHS staff. (see pp. 52–55 in Garrett-Harris and Garvey 2005)

R. Garvey
The Coaching and Mentoring Research Unit, Sheffield Hallam University, Howard Street, Sheffield, UK
E-mail: r.garvey@shu.ac.uk

Radiology Education. R.K. Chhem et al. (Eds.)
DOI: 10.1007/978-3-540-68989-8, © Springer-Verlag Berlin Heidelberg 2009

7

Mentoring in the National Blood Service

The National Blood Service (NBS) is committed to providing support for colleagues that meets their individual development needs. Developing mentoring skills is seen as essential for individuals within the Training Department to assist them in accomplishing this aim. However, it is not limited to those in the Training Department to meet their evolving roles but is also available to others within the organization, who are dealing with the changing nature of the NBS. Mentor development supports NBS' key objectives, specifically:

> Through learning and development opportunities motivating and supporting people to deliver their best
> Making the NBS an organization people want to join, work for and stay with

Three main lessons learned to date are:

1. Create time to learn and develop mentors and mentees
2. Strive to make mentoring multidisciplinary and across all levels of staff rather than *being used in a hierarchical way for development*
3. Place importance on developing both mentors and mentees (see pp. 55–61 in Garrett-Harris and Garvey 2005,)

Oxford Radcliffe Hospitals Coach/Mentor Scheme

Between 1999 and 2004, Oxford Radcliffe Hospitals have been involved in coaching and mentoring. During this time, prospective coaches/mentors enrolled in a 9-month diploma in professional coaching and mentoring programme to gain both theoretical and practical competence in the areas of professional coaching/mentoring. The main lessons learned are summed up as follows:

> Measure success
> Develop a marketing plan for coach/mentoring
> Promote the scheme
> Be specific about the service offered
> Develop a target market
> Be clear that this is an experiential process not a classroom-based one
> Allocate appropriate financial resources
> Develop networks and events for continuous professional development (CPD) purposes
> Share responsibility with all stakeholders
> Work with an external provider to accelerate the learning needed
> Hold on to the dream (see pp. 61–70 in Garrett-Harris and Garvey 2005,)

The Expert Patients Mentoring Programme

The UK has about 17.5 million people with at least one chronic condition. These conditions account for about 78% of health care spending and occupy 80% of general practitioner time. Therefore, chronic disease is a major issue in the UK and one which affects us all. Given these statistics, the health care, social and economic arguments for tackling this issue are overwhelming.

The NHS has run the Expert Patients Programme since 2002. The programme supports people with chronic illnesses by helping them to self-manage. The "expert patient" is someone with a chronic illness trained to help others with similar conditions.

In 2006, The NHS Expert Patients Mentoring Programme started in the East Midlands and the southeast of England. The idea was to draw on and develop the skills of trained expert patient facilitators to mentor health care staff from Primary Care Trusts to:

> Release expert patients' knowledge and skills for the benefit of staff
> Offer mentoring and development opportunities to patients who had completed the Expert Patients Programme
> Offer mentoring and development opportunities to health and social care staff working in patient self-management
> Promote a wider understanding amongst Primary Care Trust staff of the Expert Patients Programme
> Promote wider understanding and take-up of the emerging strategy for patient self-management
> Support the patient engagement process by modelling staff and patients as equal partners in the planning and delivery of healthcare
> Supporting multidisciplinary teams working in the NHS

Comments from participants were as follows:

"Find all the means you can to keep this programme going, as getting volunteer mentors is such an untapped resource, and as our early experiences of mentoring are so positive in promoting knowledge that helps improve people's lives, this surely must have a place in the NHS's future".

"The mentees have said that they have learned so much, they understand more, and they have put some of the new skills into practice and they have worked".

"You have given me a great insight into how a patient is able to take back control of their illness, without being dependant on the nursing/medical profession".

"I think I have also become more empathetic to the frustrations that patients with long term conditions endure on a daily basis". (Based on Garrett 2006)

Mentoring in the UK health service is significant in size and varied in its applications. The 2004 NHS Staff Survey (2005) across the UK health sector noted that at least 17% of staff had been involved in some form of mentoring in the previous year. With a workforce of 1.2 million people, this is substantial number. The contexts of the four vignettes relating to mentoring in the UK health service are decidedly similar as they relate to:

> Change and transition
> Multidisciplinary working
> Enhancing performance
> Patient involvement and self-management
> Developing service quality
> Knowledge and experience sharing
> CPD of health care professionals

At Oxford Radcliffe Hospitals, a distinction is made between mentoring and coaching. Essentially both involve the same skills and processes but with subtly different purposes. Both mentoring and coaching have their roots in education. Both are associated with learning, development and performance enhancement. This distinction will be discuss further later in this chapter.

7.2
What Is Mentoring?

In the world of mentoring, a single definition is difficult to grasp. Generally this is because definitions attempt to position a concept within a tight framework. Whilst there is some merit to this approach in some contexts (e.g. cause and effect methods), mentoring deals primarily with social and human activities – activities which defy simplification through definition. It is therefore more appropriate to offer a description in the tradition of Geertzian philosophy (Geertz 1971).

7.3
Descriptions of Mentoring Through History

Mentoring has a long and illustrious history in education. The first mentor was reportedly the goddess Athena, who worked with Telemachus, the son of King Odysseus. Athena assumed the role of Mentor, as the trusted friend and adviser to Odysseus. This is believed to be the first account of this type of learning dyad. As a Mentor, Athena helped Telemachus to learn how to become a king.

In his seminal work *Les Aventures de Télémaque,* Fénélon (1651–1715), Archbishop of Cambrai (and later tutor to Louis XIV's heir), further developed the mentoring theme of Homer's *Odyssey*. Fénélon's work offers a case history of human development depicting the ways that life's events may provide potential learning experiences (see Sheehy 1974 for further comment on this point). Fénélon shows us that the activity of observing others provides both positive and negative learning opportunities. He suggests that prearranged or chance happenings, if fully explored with the support and guidance of a mentor, may provide opportunities for the learner to acquire a high level understanding of "the ways of the world" very quickly. This concept relates to the American researcher Kathy Kram's (1983) idea that mentoring performs a "psychosocial" function.

At the time, Fénélon's work was viewed as a political manifesto presenting an ideal political system based on the concept of the paradox of a monarchy-led republic. There was a clear focus on the development and education of leaders – something with which mentoring is associated today. Fénélon implied that leadership could be developed through guided experience. Louis XIV viewed this as a challenge to the divine right of kings and consequently banished Fénélon to Cambrai and cancelled his pension.

Les Aventures de Télémaque appeared again in France in Rousseau's educational treatise Emile (first published in 1762). Rousseau, considered by many as the founder of "experiential learning", was profoundly influenced by Fénélon's ideas on development. Rousseau focused on dialogue as an important element in learning and gave clear guidance on the ideal class size for effective education – one to one! In Emile, Telemachus becomes a model, perhaps even a metaphor for learning, growth and social development. The central character, Emile, is given a copy of Les Aventures de Télémaque as a guide to his own developmental journey.

Further early writings on mentoring can be found in the work of Louis Antonine de Caraccioli (1723–1803). As Engstrom (2005) noted, de Caraccioli wrote Veritable le Mentor ou l'Education de la Noblesse in 1759 and it was translated into English in 1760 to become The True Mentor, or, an Essay on the Education of Young People in Fashion. This work describes mentoring mainly from the perspective of the mentor. De Caraccioli acknowledges the influence of Fénélon's work on his own. In The True Mentor (1760) de Caraccioli writes, "…we stand in need of academics to form the heart at the same time that they enrich the mind" (p. vii). This is a direct invitation to what we now understand as holistic learning found in current discourses in mentoring and could be regarded as the precursor to the idea of emotional intelligence.

At about the same time, according to the Oxford English Dictionary, in 1750 Lord Chesterfield used the term "mentor" in a letter to his son to describe a developmental process – "the friendly care and assistance of your mentor". Later, Lord Byron (1788–1824) used the term "mentor" in his poems The Curse of Minerva and Childe Harold's Pilgrimage "Stern Mentor urg'd from high to yonder tide" and in The Island Byron refers to the sea as "the only mentor of his youth". Given the classical educational background of these writers (Ancient Greek literature was a part of their curriculum), it is likely that they derived the concept from Homer. It is also interesting to note the dual description of "mentor" as either "friendly and caring" or "stern".

Two volumes of the publication The Female Mentor emerge in the English language in 1793, with a third volume in 1796. These works are recordings of conversations about topics of interest among a group of women referred to as "the society". The author, Honoria, identifies and describes the characteristics of the female mentor, not as the substance of the

7

book, but rather as a commentary and series of asides made throughout the volumes. The introduction to volume 1 provides the purpose of the books:

> If the following conversations should afford you some amusement, and if you should think them calculated to lead the youthful and unbiased mind in the ways of virtue, I shall feel highly gratified (Vol. 1, p. i).

The mentor, Amanda, was aware of Fénélon and his approach to education and life and appeared to have served as a role model for *the society*.

The philosophical underpinnings of the discussions in the books are broad and draw on, for example, the philosophy of ancient Egypt, Christianity, Greek civilization and ideas on nature. There are also a number of discussions about famous women as positive role models, for example "Anne Bolen, Queen Consort of Henry Eighth" and "On Learned Ladies". Indeed, there are many examples throughout history that document famous mentoring relationships:

> › Moses and Joshua
> › Lord Cecil and Queen Elizabeth I
> › Annie Sullivan and Helen Keller
> › Mentor (Athena) and Telemachus

Today, many have come to recognize and appreciate the function and purpose of successful mentoring relationships as vital to an organization's growth and sustainability. Modern-day descriptions of mentoring contain links to the historical roots:

> In mentoring, the relationship between mentor and mentee is all-important. There is a high degree of trust and mutual regard. The mentor helps the mentee become what that person aspires to be. The mentee is helped to realise his or her potential. The mentor learns and develops also, through being a mentor and developing mentoring skills. (see p. 18 in Alred et al. 2007)

In *Transformational Mentoring: Creating Developmental Alliances for Changing Organizational Cultures* Julie Hay (1999) describes mentoring essentially as:

> › Showing people the ropes – and helping them climb them
> › Passing on knowledge and/or skills, formally or informally
> › Looking after people
> › Acting as a sounding board
> › Helping people put learning into practice
> › Being a role model
> › Being a guide
> › Being a champion
> › Talking to people about their careers
> › Coaching
> › A guide not a guru

A simple definition which seems to capture the essence of these descriptions is "Off-line help by one person to another in making significant transitions in knowledge, work or thinking" (see p. 4 in Megginson et al. 2005).

Pulling these threads together, mentoring can best be described as learning relationships between two people that requires a range of human qualities such as trust, commitment and emotional engagement to be effective. Mentoring also involves a range of skills, including listening, questioning, challenge and support. Relationships have a time scale. In some contexts they may become lifelong, while others may last for a predetermined time.

7.4
Why Is Mentoring Powerful?

Mentoring is a powerful approach to CPD and learning because it relates so well to many different theories of learning. For example, many forms of mentoring relate well to the "person-centred" view of learning put forward by Carl Rogers in his core conditions of learning:

> › Learning is a social activity
> › Individual authority, responsibility, control
> › Security and empathy
> › Extensive open information exchange
> › Climate of trust based on mutual respect and genuineness
> › Unconditional positive regard for other people
> › An ability to communicate all these to others (after Rogers 1969, p. 281)

Similarly, it can be argued that mentoring is central to Levinson's (1978) work on adult development. In this work, Levinson presents the concept of age-related transitions in adults and notes that the average age transition is typically about 7 years – a number that can be reduced to 3 with the inclusion of a mentor. Levinson's work became the foundation of the modern mentoring movement in the USA, as a psychosocial function aimed at accelerated development. Indeed, according to Daloz (1986), mentoring relates well to the developmental theories of no less than nine researchers: Dewey (1916); Jung (1958); Perry (1968); Kohlbergh (1969); Freire (1970); Knowles (1970); Gilligan (1977), Levinson (1978) and Kegan (1982).

As a human dialogic learning process, mentoring also relates well to Erikson's (1950) generativity concept and as such it is an essential process for human progress – we learn by, with and through other people. Mentoring is therefore a fundamentally human development process, it is centuries old, and it links to major theoretical frameworks on learning. It makes sense therefore to ensure that mentoring forms an essential part of CPD in any profession.

7.5
CPD and Mentoring

According to Megginson and Whitaker:

Continuous Professional Development is a process by which individuals take control of their own learning and development, by engaging in an on-going process of reflection and action. This process is empowering and exciting and can stimulate people to achieve their aspirations and move towards their dreams (2003, p. 5).

As we consider this description in relation to the four vignettes offered at the beginning of the chapter, it can be observed that reflection, autonomy and empowerment are central features in any mentoring programme. Indeed, Levinson's (1978) work on male development points out that mentoring is in fact about the mentee's dream.

Curuso (1996) takes Levinson's idea further, noting that

> …traditional mentoring and most structured programs assume top down mentor to protégé and frequently give no or inadequate consideration to the protégé's dream. Quite often the protégé's dream is replaced by either a mentor objective or an organizational goal.

Here, Curuso suggests that the starting place for mentoring is necessarily with the mentee's aspirations and while organizational issues are important (for the organization at least), they are rarely the main motivation for the individual. When we think about our vignettes, we see this reflected in the level of voluntarism inherent in the programmes we described. So, although mentoring serves an organizational need and purpose for CPD, the main drivers of mentoring and CPD lie with the individuals' needs and requirements within the organizational setting. This seems an important philosophy for both CPD activities and mentoring. As Kessels (2002) reminds us, "you cannot be smart against your will", so autonomy and self-direction remain important ingredients. Since learning is a social activity, an organizational context can make it more or less possible for people to learn and develop (Rogers 1969; Habermas 1974; Vygotsky 1978; Bruner 1990; Lave and Wenger 1991). Therefore, organizational structures and practices play an important role in creating and developing learning environments conducive to forming positive mentoring relationships.

Curuso (1996) argues for a theory of mentoring, in which the qualities of learning (as conceptualized, for instance, in Lave and Wenger's 1991 theory of situated learning) and the potential benefits of mentoring move away from the traditional one-to-one mentoring relationship, to characterize relational activities in the organization as a whole. In practice, this means that mentoring can be afforded by a "variety of individuals and/or institutions who provide help to a protégé" (Caruso 1996). It then becomes appropriate to talk about a "mentoring organization". A mentoring organization can be characterized by:

> - The compatibility of individual and organizational aspirations
> - High employee commitment
> - A focus on collaboration and team development
> - A complex web of practices and relationships that are supportive and developmental of the individual and the organization

Above all, it is important to understand that people who have a developed an enthusiastic sense of themselves as learners inhabit a "mentoring organization". This concept resonates well with Higgins and Kram's (2001) notion of "multiple mentoring relationships" where any one individual may have a range of developers. Therefore, the links between CPD, mentoring and organizational development are natural and powerful, and this is perhaps why so many UK NHS organizations engage with it.

7.6
Connections with Practice

Medical work is not just about scientific facts. It requires practitioners to apply scientific knowledge in the context of individual lives and complex human systems. It crosses many domains of knowledge, including the social and interpersonal. Doctors are exposed constantly to risks, including stress, alienation, over-involvement, automatic behaviour and burnout. Other professions have rightly recognised that they need organized support as professional oxygen in order to sustain reflective practice in the face of such risks. The medical profession has until now been in the paradoxical position of needing as much of this oxygen as any other group of clinicians (if not more) but generally getting less (see p. 24 in Launer 2006).

In this statement, Launer, a passionate supporter of mentoring in the UK health service, advocates for mentoring support for physicians. Although he emphasizes the psychological support mentoring offers, research suggests that mentoring has a great deal to offer many working in the health sector. For example, mentoring promotes the growth and development of nurses, some of whom will become the future leaders in their profession. In their 2001 study, Smith et al. (2001) identify the benefits for mentored nurses as:

> › Enhanced thinking, risk taking and self-esteem
> › Job enrichment and professional development
> › Improved wisdom, commitment, growth, power, political awareness and job performance

Similarly, in a UK Department of Health (2004) study *Mentoring for Doctors* the benefits cited for physicians participating as *mentees* are described as:

> › Improved reflection skills
> › Support for dealing with specific problems
> › Developing strategies for dealing with and resolving
>   › Major crises in professional life
>   › Major change in ways of thinking and acting
>   › Significant changes in direction
> › Confidence building in decision making
> › Improved self-worth and job satisfaction

And as *mentors*:

> › Increased motivation and job satisfaction
> › Satisfaction for playing a role in developing talent
> › Improved relationships with patients, colleagues and family members
> › Improved problem solving abilities

7

Indeed, some mentoring physicians suggested that the concepts, principles and skills of mentoring provide them with a generic approach to practice which pervades all that they do.

7.7
Making the Transition

If mentoring has appeal as a personalized and effective approach to CPD, much can be learned from Kram's (1985) framework for developing mentoring. It is adapted here as follows:

1. Defining the purpose and the scope of mentoring
2. Diagnosing the elements that will support mentoring and those that will hinder it
3. Implementation
4. Evaluation

7.7.1
Defining the Purpose and Scope

It is important for each organization to decide what mentoring is for and who it is for. In doing this, it becomes possible to focus on specific groups and target recruitment to the scheme.

7.7.2
Diagnosis

Before developing mentoring, it is also important to have good knowledge of the organizational context and its cultural issues. This is particularly true in attitudes towards learning and development.

Much has been written (Megginson et al. 2005) about the importance of voluntarism in mentoring. An organizational culture may be developed in order to make it possible for people to volunteer to become mentors and mentees. Developing capacity within the organization requires attention to and support for the capacity and abilities of the mentors themselves. As Alred et al. (1996) noted, individuals may be concerned about their ability to serve as a mentor. Concerns generally relate to issues such as:

> Do I have the experience and the qualities required?
> What am I supposed to do?
> What is involved?
> How will my manager or colleagues view this?
> How does mentoring fit with organizational policies?

Organizations must therefore understand the skills, attitudes and behaviours required to achieve successful mentoring practices, and whether there is a need for training or professional development to ensure that those skills are acquired. An organizational "assessment" can help them identify their level of readiness. First, they need to consider the level of experience that staff could bring to a mentoring relationship. A staff with a wide range of experience can more easily sustain the demands of a mentoring programme and allow for meaningful mentor/mentee pairing or grouping. It is also important for organizational leaders and administrators to recognize that in times of change, there is often a greater need for mentor support.

Similarly, mentors also need to have an awareness of their work environment, its opportunities, challenges and values. This is necessary because it relates to Kram's (1983) concept of mentoring performing a "psychosocial" function. In essence, a potential mentor who is aware of the politics of an organization can help others to adapt and learn. However, while political awareness is important, it is also important that a mentor is committed to the organization's vision of its future and wishes to contribute to its progress and development. This means that in addition to having a genuine desire to serve in the role, a potential mentor needs a "thinking" approach to work and is prepared to see concerns of colleagues as opportunities for discussion and development. Mentoring can assist people to develop resilience and the capability to prepare for the unexpected and make appropriate judgements in the heat of action.

Mentors therefore need an appreciation of the skills and abilities that may be required to navigate challenging situations and a willingness to develop these skills and abilities in others through modelling and dialogue. It is also necessary to understand where resistance to mentoring exists within an organization, what form this might take and a way of working with this resistance.

7.7.3
Implementation

As with the introduction of most programmes, when implementing a mentoring programme, institutions may face some potential challenges. These challenges include, for example:

> Elitism
> Excluding the socially different
> Replicating management behaviour rather than changing it
> Maintaining the "status quo" based on "accumulation of advantage"
> Replicating and sustaining exploitative hierarchical systems
> Manipulation and social engineering
> A power and control relationship
> Mentee dependency

Some research suggests that these challenges are more likely to manifest themselves under certain conditions and in certain types of organization. For example, in "fast-track, career-oriented schemes" some of these negative effects are more likely.

Within the context of the health sector, other issues may affect the implementation of a mentoring programme. These relate to the conflicting roles of coaching and supervision. Outwardly, coaching is a very similar activity to mentoring. Research (Willis 2005) suggests that both coaching and mentoring activity share the same skills and processes. Differences may be found in the contexts in which the activity takes place and the intent of the coach or mentor. Mentoring is fundamentally a voluntary activity. It works best in a cross-functional, off-line context where the intent is the holistic development of an individual. As such, the process of mentoring develops the capacity of both the mentor and the mentee.

Coaching, as derived from Oxford and Cambridge universities in the UK in the mid-nineteenth century, was initially associated with improving academic attainment. Around the same time, coaching activity migrated to sport, particularly rowing and cricket. Coaching today, in some contexts, can be a paid activity, but in organizations it is often done within the line structure. The power and authority which comes with the line relationship creates a strong short-term, performance orientation where specific knowledge and skills are developed. Coaching can be very effective; however, both mentoring and coaching work best in developmental, learner-centred environments with willing participation and with the learner establishing the agenda. The introduction of power differentials always has the potential to distort the relationship.

Supervision, in the health context, often relates to governance. However, the various health professionals view supervision differently. For example, those engaged in therapeutic work understand supervision as working with an experienced colleague with a view to developing and improving practice. Supervision in this context can also have a quality assurance agenda. In the more general health context, it may be tempting to conflate mentoring with supervision, but this has the potential to create confusion about roles and function and ultimately lead to the ineffective application of both. By keeping supervision separate from mentoring, one maximizes the advantages of both. In broad terms, mentoring works best in a developmental climate, free from the problems introduced by a need for evaluation or judgement.

Other variable conditions that offer potential for difficulties may be found in the social context (culture, climate, type of business, values, etc.). Garvey and Alred (2001, p. 552) quoting Antal (1996), for instance, note that "unfortunately, many companies foster highly competitive behaviour and stress bottom-line results in a way that discourages supportive behaviour between members of the organisation". Arguably, there is the potential for the same kinds of behaviour in a heavily target driven organization like the UK NHS. Within some environments mentoring may be viewed either as an activity for "high-flyers" (those on their way to leadership positions) or alternatively as a "remedial" activity. Neither characterization is helpful or constructive. Mentoring is effective when viewed as a normal developmental activity for all who engage in it.

One of the most common challenges raised when attempting to implement an initiative such as a mentoring programme is the concern that it will require extra time. This need not be the case. It would be hard to think of a functioning organization where colleagues did not talk to each other as part of their normal daily interaction. Mentoring interactions generate a purposeful kind of dialogue which focuses on the learner and the learning. It is not limited to giving advice or instruction, but rather it involves listening, supporting, questioning and challenging. Mentoring works best when the relationship between the two parties is paramount and issues of power and authority are minimized. The "chemistry" in mentoring between people creates a positive learning environment. A challenge of implementation is to recognize mentoring as a legitimate work activity, and one that enhances the culture of the organization to become a rich learning environment for everyone.

Finally, feedback is an important part of mentoring. However, it is also important to remember, as Einstein pointed out, that not everything that can be counted counts and not everything that counts can be counted. Feedback needs to start at the beginning of a mentoring arrangement and continue as a regular component of the process over time. It is also important to consider the combinations of all the above-mentioned issues in any research or evaluation as well as to consider Rogers's (1969) core conditions raised earlier in this chapter.

7.8
Expanded Understanding of the Mentoring Role

7.8.1
Conditions for Success in Mentoring

In addition, a survey of the literature produces a number of suggestions that may guide institutions as they aim to create the conditions that will lead to the implementation of a successful mentoring programme.

Voluntarism – Mentoring is essentially a voluntary activity. The degree of voluntarism will depend on the situation and the circumstances. In some cases, putting people together and asking them to contract for a specific number of meetings (i.e. three) before they review the relationship can be helpful. It can also assist the process if both parties agree on a "no fault divorce clause" so that they can end the relationship by mutual agreement and with clarity. Institutions in which members of the senior administration get involved and serve as positive role models in the programme often meet with great success and "buy in".

Training – All the vignettes presented previously in this chapter focus on skills development for mentors, but it is also important that there is some orientation towards mentoring for mentees. This may involve skills training for both parties together in the same programme. For example, while mentors need to develop skills in offering constructive feedback, mentees may require some orientation in how to receive constructive feedback. Both groups often need some parameters delineated for them to identify how to engage in a conversation that allows them to focus on the issues in a way that ensures the dialogue is about the professional, and not the personal.

Ongoing support – Mentors often need support. This may take the form of a mentor support group or one-to-one mentoring supervision – a mentor to the mentor. There is also benefit in mentors from different sectors coming together to share practice and experiences. The purpose of bringing mentors together is to discuss mentoring process issues, debrief mentors and develop skills and to improve understanding.

Matching – It is important to have a clear matching process to which the participants subscribe. In some organizations, it works well to assign mentors within the pool of volunteers. In others, it may be best to create opportunities for potential matches to meet and get to know each other, their experiences and their interests.

Establishing reviewable ground rules – It is important to clarify the boundaries of the relationship at the start. Garvey's (1994) "dimensions framework" is helpful here. While mentors and mentees need to develop a capacity for empathy, it is equally important that the relationship does not deteriorate into "therapy sessions".

Ongoing review – Recent research from the USA (Nielson and Eisenbach 2003) has concluded that the most important factor in successful outcomes to mentoring is regular feedback and review within the relationship about the relationship. Establishing ground rules at the start can facilitate this process.

Whose agenda? – Mentoring is for the mentee. Attempts to impose the agenda on the mentee can often result in problems related to the mentee feeling manipulated. The benefits of mentoring to all stakeholders result from broadly following the mentee's agenda. The mentor can facilitate this process by working with the mentee to develop new goals to work towards at the end of each feedback cycle.

Evaluation and monitoring – Ongoing evaluation of an institution's mentoring programme from the start of the scheme is important. There is little point in evaluating the scheme after, say, 2 years to unearth problems which could have been resolved at the time.

Self-awareness and the ability to give and receive feedback – A mentor needs to be self-aware in order to help someone else, but it is also important that both mentee and mentor are able to give and receive feedback. Feedback can be a vital element in successful and accelerated CPD.

7.9
Conclusions

Mentoring has the potential to be a powerful process within a CPD framework. It is, in essence, two colleagues talking with a purpose. If developed with the above in mind, it offers benefits for the mentor, the mentee and the host organization. With mentoring it is important to start with those who show interest, but what is clear is that mentoring offers individualized learning and development within a supportive environment.

References

Alred G, Garvey B, Smith RD (1996) First person mentoring. Career Dev Int 1(5):10–14
Alred G, Garvey B, Smith R (2007) The mentoring pocket book. Management Pocket Books, Arlesford, Hants
Antal A (1996) Odysseus legacy to management development: Mentoring. Eur Manag J 11(4):448–54. In: Garvey B, Alred G (2002) Mentoring and the tolerance of complexity. Futures 33:519–530

Bruner J (1990) Acts of meaning. Harvard University Press, Cambridge

Caruso RE (1996) Who does mentoring? Paper presented at the third European Mentoring Conference, London, November 7–8

Daloz LA (1986) Effective teaching and mentoring. Jossey-Bass, USA

de Caraccioli LA (1760) The true mentor, or, an essay on the education of young people in fashion, J. Coote at the Kings Arms in Paternoster Row, London

Department of Health (2004) Mentoring for doctors: Signposts to current practice for career grade doctors. Crown Copyright, New Zealand

Dewey J (1916) Democracy and education. Macmillan, New York

Erikson E (1950, 1995) Childhood and society. Vintage, London

Engstrom TEJ (2005) Individual determinants of mentoring success. Dissertation, Northumbria University, Newcastle

Fénélon De La Mothe FS (1699) The adventures of telemachus, vols 1 and 2. Transl. Hawkesworth J. Union Printing Office, St. John's Square, London

Freire P (1970) Pedagogy of the oppressed. Herder and Herder, New York

Garrett R (2006) Expert patient mentoring project evaluation. Sheffield Hallam University, Sheffield

Garrett-Harris R, Garvey B (2005) Towards a framework for mentoring in the NHS. Sheffield Hallam University, Sheffield

Garvey B (1994) A dose of mentoring. Educ Train 36(4):18–26

Geertz C et al (1971) Myth, symbol and culture. WW Norton, New York

Gilligan C (1977) In a different voice: Women's conception of the self and of morality. Harvard Educ Rev 47:481–517

Habermas J (1974) Theory and practice. Heinemann, Portsmouth, NH, USA (first published in 1971 as Theorie und Praxis)

Hay J (1999) Transformational mentoring: Creating developmental alliances for changing organizational cultures. McGraw-Hill, UK

Higgins MC and Kram E (2001) Reconceptualizing mentoring at work: A developmental network perspective. Acad Manag Rev 26(2):264–288

Jung CJ (1958) Psyche and symbol. Doubleday, New York

Kegan R (1982) The evolving self: Problem and process in human development. Harvard University Press, Cambridge

Kessels J (2002) You cannot be smart against your will. In: Garvey B, Williamson B (eds) Beyond knowledge management: Dialogue, creativity and the corporate curriculum. Pearson Education, Harlow

Kram KE (1983) Phases of the mentor relationship. Acad Manag J 26(4):608–625

Kram KE (1985) Improving the mentoring process. Train Dev J 39(4):40–42

Kohlbergh L (1969) Stage and sequence: The cognitive-developmental approach to socialization. In: Goslin D (ed) Handbook of socialization theory and research. Rand McNally, Skokie

Knowles MS (1970) The modern practice of adult education: Andragogy versus pedagogy. Association Press, New York

Launer J (2006) Supervision, mentoring and coaching: One-to-one learning encounters in medical education. Association for the Study of Medical Education, ASME Office, Edinburgh

Lave J, Wenger E (1991) Situated learning: Legitimate peripheral participation. Cambridge University Press, New York

Levinson D (1978) The seasons of a man's life. Alfred Knopf, New York

Megginson D, Whitaker V (2003) Continuous professional development. CIPD, London, UK

Megginson D, Clutterbuck D, Garvey B, Stokes P, Garrett-Harris R (eds) (2005) Mentoring in action. Kogan Page, London

Nielson T, Eisenbach R (2003) Not all relationships are created equal: critical factors of high-quality mentoring relationships. Int J Mentor Coach 1(1):online article

NHS National Staff Survey (2005) Summary of key findings 2004. Health Care Commission, UK

Perry WG (1968) Forms of intellectual and ethical development in the college years: A scheme. Holt, Rinehart and Winston, Austin, TX

Rogers CR (1969) Freedom to learn. Charles E. Merrill, Columbus, OH

Sheehy G (1974) New passages: Predictable crises of adult life. E.P. Dotton, New York

Smith L, McAllister L, Crawford C (2001) Mentoring benefits and issues for public health nurses. Public Health Nurs 18(2):101–107

Vygotsky LS (1978) In: Cole M et al (eds) Mind in society: The development of higher psychological processes. Harvard University Press, Cambridge

Willis P (2005) European Mentoring and Coaching Council. Competency Research Project: Phase 2. June, EMCC, Watford

Radiological and Biomedical Knowledge Integration: The Ontological Way

8

R. Arp, C. Romagnoli, R.K. Chhem, J.A. Overton

8.1
Introduction

Imagine a scenario where a surgeon, oncologist, and radiologist at a research hospital work together to treat a cancer patient suffering from esophageal adenocarcinoma. After treatments of cisplatinum and fluorouracil administered by the oncologist, a round of teletherapy treatments from the radiologist, and a successful esophajectomy performed by the surgeon, the patient develops cauda equina syndrome (CES) weeks after the surgery which causes severely decreased mobility in his legs. The radiologist is perplexed by this and is interested in whether the megavoltage teletherapy treatments administered to the patient may have caused the CES. So, she sits down at her computer to do some research. She queries PubMed, MedNet, Dynamic MepPix, DynaMed, and MedlinePlus only to find a vast amount of disparate data from a variety of different sources. Not only is it difficult to find a set of relevant and precise terms, but she also has great difficulty discerning the connections between various seemingly related results. Further, regarding what little she does find, she must go to the journal's Web sites, or to her university's medical library, in order to piece together this disparate information for herself. She continues with a general Web search: there is something that looks *vaguely* relevant from a laboratory in Germany, but the researchers in that laboratory have not annotated any of their information for the benefit of other researchers on the Web; a laboratory in the Netherlands is composed of

This work is funded by the United States National Institutes of Health (NIH) Roadmap for Medical Research, Grant 1 U54 HG0040208.

R. Arp (✉)
National Center for Biomedical Ontology, University at Buffalo, New York, USA
E-mail: rarp@buffalo.edu

Radiology Education. R.K. Chhem et al. (Eds.)
DOI: 10.1007/978-3-540-68989-8, © Springer-Verlag Berlin Heidelberg 2009

8

researchers with impressive publications in journals such as *Radiology*, *Science*, and *Nature*, but they deliberately choose *not* to make their results available on the Web, as they are vying for million-dollar research grants; still another laboratory in Columbia has what appear to be relevant conclusions that are available to anyone on the Web, but the researchers there have annotated their information in such a way that only other members of the laboratory can decipher it. Owing to this informational quagmire, the radiologist gives up her research and moves on to other projects. The surgeon and oncologist encounter the same sea of confusion in their own searches, and move on to other projects as well. Although the cancer patient is treated for CES, no reliably certain cause of the syndrome is discovered and, in addition to the complications due to his esophajectomy – such as gastric dumping syndrome – the patient's right leg atrophies, becomes gangrenous, and must be amputated.

Now imagine the same scenario again where, this time, the radiologist sits down at her computer and, with a click of her mouse, is able to find several relevant results from research laboratories, all of which are clearly and coherently annotated so that anyone with medical training in radiology could utilize this information in his/her own research and treatment regimens. Our radiologist is able to devise a course of treatment for the CES which allows the patient to make a full recovery. The patient is ambulatory the rest of his life, and gastric dumping syndrome is the worst of his troubles.

This scenario with a more positive outcome should be how the story ends, every time, with physicians, researchers, and other interested persons being able to access relevant biomedical information from the Web that is classified, categorized, coded, curated, and, above all, *calibrated* so that it may be interoperable and reuseable for diagnoses, prognoses, and courses of treatment. After all, when reciting the Hippocratic oath, a physician swears that she or he will "impart a knowledge of the art of medicine to others." In today's world that revolves around the collection, storage, and retrieval of various forms of electronic information, databases and other computational tools are essential for "imparting a knowledge" of the biomedical sciences. Other than making phone calls, sending e-mails, attending conferences, and reading the latest journals, physicians and researchers use the Web to gather relevant biomedical information. However, as our first imagined scenario hints at, there are numerous *real-life* scenarios where information has been isolated in multiple research laboratory silos – creating a silo effect (see Fig. 1) – making it difficult or impossible to share and reuse potentially significant pain-easing and life-saving information.

So, how can we collect, categorize, manage, store, process, mine, query, and, especially, retrieve and disseminate all of this biomedical information appropriately and efficiently by computational means? Progress in biomedicine depends upon making use of the results of previous biomedical research, treatments, and clinical trials. Thus, it is crucial that the information contained in biomedical textbooks, journals, and clinical trial reports be efficiently accessible to, and usable by, individuals, physicians, and research groups other than its original authors, for purposes of performing research and treating the diseases of patients (among other things). The problem, then, is to chart the ever-growing sea of biomedical information – including information from radiology and nuclear medicine – in such a way that the various parts, portions, and depths of it can be efficiently accessed, used, navigated, and reasoned about by human individuals. This has been a central problem, along with the silo effect, that the burgeoning sciences of bioinformatics, medical informatics, and biomedical informatics are trying to solve (Baxevanis and Ouellette 2005; Polanski

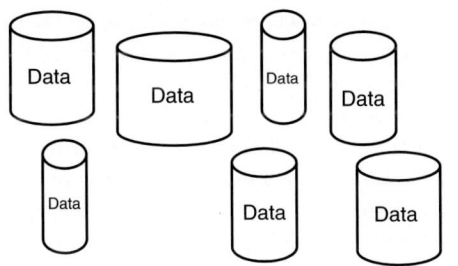

Fig. 1 The silo effect

and Kimmel 2007; Lesk 2005; Shortliffe and Cimino 2006; Berman 2006; Gruber 1993; Grenon and Smith 2004; Smith et al. 2006; Fielding and Marwede 2006).

8.2
Domain Ontology

The obvious solution to the problem of navigating the sea of biomedical information, as well as dispelling the silo effect, has been to make use of the superhuman memory and reasoning capacities of computers. Thus, the basic tool of the bioinformatician is the computer, principally because computers have three great virtues: first, computers are able to store a tremendous amount of information reliably; second, with human influence they are able to retrieve and reason about (to a certain extent) the information that they store automatically, efficiently, and reliably; third, information stored in a computerized format can be made instantly accessible to individuals in all parts of the globe via the Internet.

Medical practitioners from various fields are already seeing the benefits of new information systems in the administration of hospitals. Electronic health records, hospital information systems, radiology information systems, and databases of medical images such as picture archiving and communication systems all demonstrate the power of computers to improve medical practice. But these tools would not help the radiologist in our fictional example. What is needed is the application of similar methods and tools beyond administration and deeper into medical research and practice.

Now, computer programs are dumb beasts in that, at present, they do not understand the information present in their repositories, and they need to be programmed to reason with the information that we humans give them. Most importantly, substantial care needs to be taken, at the outset, to ensure that the terminology, definitions, relations, and the like that are entered into biomedical information databases (1) accurately reflect reality, to the best of our developing state of knowledge in the biomedical sciences, (2) are internally coherent, (3) are clearly defined, and (4) are interoperable with other databases. To ensure requirements 1–4, especially requirement 4, researchers over the past 20 years (or so) have worked with computer scientists and programmers to set up what are known as *domain ontologies* in their fields of study. What exactly is a domain ontology?

A *domain* is an area, sphere, aspect, or delineated portion of reality which humans seek to know, understand, and explain (also, predict, manipulate, and control) as fully as is possible through the development of a subject matter, field, science, or discipline (as well as sub-disciplines) concerning that area, sphere, or aspect of reality. Examples include all of the various subjects investigated at a typical university, such as medicine, engineering, mathematics, law, computer science, economics, philosophy, psychology, and the like, complete with their respective, subsumed subject matters such as radiology and nuclear medicine.

An *ontology* is a little more complicated to define. The word "ontology" can refer to a branch of Western philosophy – having its origins in ancient Greece with philosophers such as Parmenides (fifth century BCE), Heraclitus (sixth century BCE), Plato (427–347 BCE), and Aristotle (384–322 BCE) – the concern of which is the study of what is, of the kinds and structures of objects, properties, events, processes, and relations in every area of reality. From this philosophical perspective, ontology seeks to provide a definitive and exhaustive classification of entities in all spheres or domains of being. As a theoretical discipline concerned with accurately describing the taxonomy of all things that exist, ontology is synonymous with classical metaphysics. This philosophical sense of the term is what Rudolf Göckel (1547–1628) and Jacob Lorhard (1561–1609) had in mind when they independently coined the term "ontology" (*ontologia*). Ontology derives from the Greek words *ontos* (meaning "existence" or "being") and *logos* (meaning "rational account" or "knowledge"), so it makes sense that Nathan Bailey's 1721 *Oxford English Dictionary* defined ontology as "an Account of being in the Abstract" (Smith 2003). In fact, people are naturally philosophical ontologists of one sort or another since all of us form systems of classification as we try to understand, navigate, control, and predict the complex workings of this universe. For example, we sort things into genus/species hierarchical relationships of greater and lesser degrees of complexity. Consider, too, all of the models, illustrations, schematizations, flow charts, and other pictorial renditions – such as Linnean cladistics in biology and the periodic table of the elements in chemistry – that utilize a philosophically ontological categorization in order to capture the classification of entities and their relationships to one another.

Related to this philosophical sense, since the emergence of the information age "ontology" also has come to be understood as a structured, taxonomical representation of the entities and relations existing within a particular domain of reality such as geography, ecology, law, genomics, or radiology. Domain ontologies, thus, are contrasted with ontology in the philosophical sense, which has all of reality as its subject matter (Arp (2008); Smith 2003).

A domain ontology usually evolves in several steps. First of all, the terminology used in the ontology should be laid down in a lexicon. A *lexicon* is a structured vocabulary of terms and their definitions, and its key benefit is better communication through shared language. The definitions in a good lexicon will contain many instances of the phrase "is a," and the form "A is a B which has C." The "is a" relation gives the lexicon a structure, and by using this relation we can transform the lexicon into a taxonomy (more will be said about this evolution later, when we lay out steps one can follow in constructing a radiology domain ontology). A *taxonomy* is a tree-form, graph-theoretic, representational artifact that is organized into subsumed hierarchical relations with nodes (representing universals or classes) and edges (representing "is a" or subset relations). Ideally, a *domain ontology* is a taxonomy that provides a controlled, structured vocabulary and framework to annotate data within a particular domain, in order to make the data more easily searchable by human beings and processable by computers.

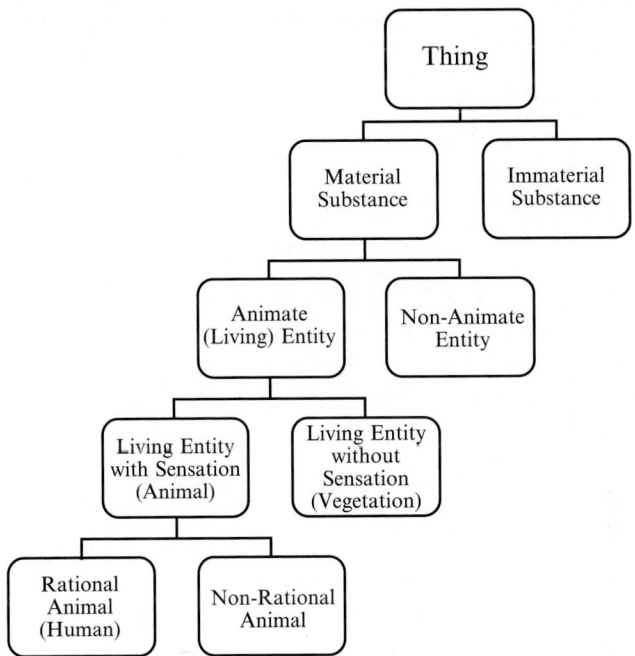

Fig. 2 The Porphyrian tree

Figure 2 represents a section from one of the first taxonomies created in Western history by the famous Greek philosopher Porphyry (ca. 234–305), called the Porphyrian tree. Notice that, in the tree, there is a kind of hierarchical classification of entities as well as a basic "is a" or "is a subtype of" relationship found between lower and higher entities. Material substance "is a" or "is a subtype of" thing, whereas animate (living) entity is a material substance, living entity with sensation is a living entity, rational animal is a living entity with sensation, and human is a rational animal, an example of which is Plato. Thus, Plato is a human, is a rational animal, etc. and, ultimately, is a thing.

Also consider Fig. 3. This is a simplified classification of one of the parts of the processes associated with the production of glutathione, which is a coenzyme and antioxidant. Once again, we can see the value in a taxonomic classification as it becomes evident that the construction of glutathione involves biosynthetic processes which are types of a metabolic process, itself a type of biological process. Of course, there are myriad other biological processes, e.g., cellular process, as well as many other metabolic processes that are not represented here. Further, there are many other processes and factors that are associated with the production of glutathione which have not been schematized in this one "branch" of the process.

Thus, the radiologist in our positive scenario described above likely would have queried something called "A Lexicon for Uniform Indexing and Retrieval of Radiology Information

8

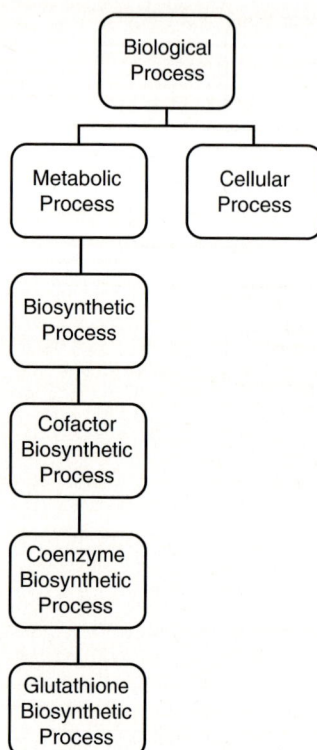

Fig. 3 A classification of part of the processes associated with glutathione production

Resources" (RadLex, http://www.rsna.org/Radlex/), a product of the Radiological Society of North America which uses a domain ontology to organize and retrieve all of the "images, imaging reports, and medical records" that have "moved online," to quote from the Web site. Echoing the information and concerns already expressed in this chapter, the researchers at RadLex note:

> Radiologists currently use a variety of terminologies and standards, but no single lexicon serves all of their needs. RadLex is a single unified source of radiology terms that is designed to fill this need... Terminology is increasingly vital to the practice of medicine. Many of the benefits of clinical information technology cannot be realized unless information is stored using standard terms in a structured format. Unfortunately, almost all radiology reports are stored as text narratives rather than in a structured format, thereby hampering radiologists' ability to participate in the ong oing changes in our health care system, which are increasingly driven by information technology (http://www.rsna. org/RadLex/index.cfm).

Now, RadLex is one database among many others that utilize domain ontologies to classify, categorize, code, and curate biomedical information, and researchers such as Kahn et al. (2006), Fielding and Marwede (2006), and Bertaud et al. (2007) have illustrated the benefits of RadLex to the domain of radiology in terms of interoperability of radiology and nuclear medicine databases, as well as improved accuracy of queried searches (Rubin

2007; Rubin et al. 2006; Marwede and Fielding 2005; do Amaral et al. 2000; Pommert et al. 2001). Other biomedical domain ontologies include the Gene Ontology (GO), the Foundational Model of Anatomy (FMA), the Cell Ontology (CL), the Disease Ontology (DO), and many more (see, for example, http://obo foundry.org/).

RadLex also demonstrates the relation between a lexicon and a taxonomy. The set of terms and definitions is the lexicon, while the additional structure of the "is a" relations make it into a taxonomy. Other than the "is a" relation, taxonomies sometimes use the "part of" relation, but a good taxonomy should stick to just one of these two relations to avoid conceptual confusion. Other examples of useful relations for some domains include "participates in," "adjacent to," "contains," or "transformation of," and the advantage of an ontology over a taxonomy is that an ontology can contain multiple relations. The edges which connect nodes in an ontology will be labeled to indicate the relation that holds between the nodes, and a particular node may be related to many others using several different relations. The richness of these additional relations makes ontologies much more powerful than taxonomies. A computer that is properly programmed can take advantage of these relations to do much more powerful reasoning than is possible with just the "is a" relation. Ongoing work with RadLex aims to add such a rich structure of relations between terms.

By utilizing domain ontologies, researchers are taking the first step toward "de-siloing" their information and allowing for the sea of biomedical information to be trolled effectively. The following is a list of the several benefits gained from utilizing an ontology:

(1) Formation of a controlled vocabulary of terms
(2) Clearly defined terms and relations between terms in a structured taxonomy
(3) Normalization of terms used among practitioners
(4) Interoperability of databases ("de-siloing")
(5) Improvement of searches
(6) Improvement of basic computer reasoning on collected data
(7) Easier revisions and improvements of the annotation system over time
(8) A committee or organization which controls the evolution of the ontology

Note that a lexicon alone could provide benefits 1, 3, 7, and 8, and to some extent benefit 5, but the additional structure of relations between terms is required to get all of these benefits. These benefits accrue to the whole community of participants, and the more widely the ontology is used the greater the benefits become. This results in a *network effect*, a positive-feedback loop, where new participants benefit from joining the community, and the community benefits from new participants.

However, problems still remain. There is a whole new set of problems associated with the construction of domain ontologies that is analogous to the silo and sea of information problems just mentioned. Now, it is the *domain ontologists* who are categorizing the information in their respective domains in such a way that the information is not interoperable, even concerning research from the same laboratories! Poor conceptualizations abound in these ontologies that are rooted in error, myth-making, faulty linguistics, antiquated information, and, most significantly, poor logical reasoning (Ceusters et al. 2004; Vizenor et al. 2004; Smith et al. 2006). RadLex is not immune from similar problems (Fielding and Marwede 2006; Rubin 2007).

8.3
Formal Ontology

To remedy these problems of conceptualization, reasoning, coding, mining, and querying pertaining to domain ontologies, a third kind of ontology – a *formal* ontology – has emerged. Insofar as it concerns bioinformatics, the ultimate goal of formal ontology is the calibration of all biomedical domain ontologies into one single, organized, interconnected, and interoperable computer repository, accessible in real time to anyone anywhere in the world. It aims to accomplish this goal, principally, by giving an articulate internal structure to electronic biomedical information repositories, and making possible the interoperability or intertranslatability of different repositories containing different information, in such a way that the information in these repositories can be understood in terms of a common formal framework for the categorization of entities and the reasoning about those entities.

The term "formal ontology" was coined by Edmund Husserl (1859–1938) in his *Logical Investigations* and was further developed by Roman Ingarden (1893–1970) in the middle of the twentieth century. Here, as Barry Smith and David Woodruff Smith note, "formal" means applicable to "all domains of objects whatsoever… independent of the peculiarities of any given field of knowledge" (See p. 28 Smith and Smith 1995). In our own day, through the work of researchers such as Tom Gruber, Michael Ashburner, Cornelius Rosse, Werner Ceusters, Pierre Grenon, and Barry Smith, formal ontology is increasingly being applied in bioinformatics, intelligence analysis, management science, and in other fields, where it serves as a basis for the improvement of classification, information organization and retrieval, and automatic reasoning (Gruber 1993; Smith et al. 2007; Grenon and Smith 2004; Smith and Grenon 2004).

Many people use the word "formal" as interchangeable with "upper-level," "top-level," or "higher-level" and, indeed, this is appropriate since "formal ontology" refers to a discipline which assists in making communication between and among domain ontologies (envisioned as bottom or lower-level ontologies) possible by providing a common formal framework or ontological "backbone" (illustrated in Fig. 4b). Some examples of extant, upper-level or formal ontologies include the Standard Upper Ontology (SUO, http://suo.ieee.org/) of the Institute of Electrical and Electronics Engineers, the Descriptive Ontology for Linguistic and Cognitive Engineering (DOLCE, http://www.loa-cnr.it/DOLCE.html), and Basic Formal Ontology (BFO, http://www.ifomis.org/bfo).

The fact of the matter is that, until a formal ontology such as BFO arrived on the scene, domain ontologies such as the ones concerning genetics, diseases, ecology, evolution, primatology, cardiology, and radiology were much more insulated, and the shareability, reusability, and interoperability of information between and among these domains was limited (as illustrated in Fig. 4a). This insulation is understandable given the varied perspectives, ideologies, terminologies, experiments, and the like of researchers in these domains. In other words, given the varied perspectives and terminologies used by different researchers in different scientific domains, one major problem is that data are isolated in multiple, incompatible silos. Because bodies of data are insulated from each other in this way, shareability and reusability is greatly limited. The result is that experimentally and clinically derived information does not cumulate.

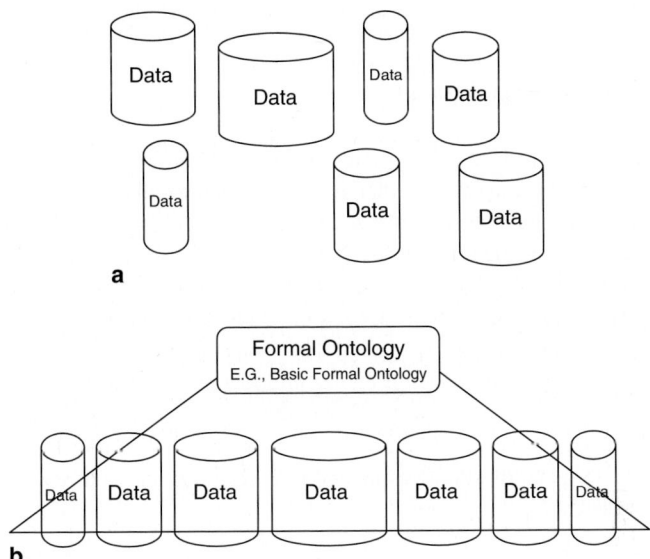

Fig. 4 a The silo effect (again). **b** Formal ontology as a backbone facilitating interoperability among domains

In fact, in a very real, concrete, and practical fashion, formal ontology enables semantic interoperability between heterogeneous databases, as well as terminology control of domain ontologies, which foster accurate document retrieval, knowledge extraction and management, natural language processing, and formal reasoning about knowledge structures in computational systems. By enforcing certain axioms and principles within a domain ontology database, formal ontology has made it easier to annotate, code, query, retrieve, share, reuse, and integrate data across multiple levels of granularity in various disciplines. Thus, in the logical sense of the word, a formal ontology such as BFO truly is an upper-leveled, *formal* ontological approach applied to any and all lower-leveled, *domain* ontologies (as illustrated in Fig. 4b, in comparison with Fig. 4a).

So, ideally and analogously, whereas a domain ontology assists in organizing the data of a particular domain to make those data understandable and accessible to the interested parties of that domain, a formal ontology *assists in organizing the data of multiple domain ontologies* to make all of those data from the domain ontologies understandable and accessible to interested parties. Stated simply: *interoperability of domain ontologies is virtually guaranteed, because researchers are all using the exact same upper-level ontological categories and relations*. The work involved in formal ontology and best ontology-building practices is especially important for researchers doing work in radiology and nuclear medicine since radiologists will, in fact, be interacting with oncologists, thoracic surgeons, and others from a variety of disciplines (as was emphasized in our fictional scenario). It is of vital importance, then, that domain ontologies are calibrated so that data in one biomedical domain can be interoperable, intertranslatable, and interinterpretable with data in any other biomedical domain.

8.4
Constructing a Radiology Ontology

Researchers doing work in radiology and nuclear medicine can, and *should*, classify, categorize, code, curate, and calibrate their data so that they may be shareable and reusable in their communities and others. They can do this (1) by setting up a radiology ontology (RadO) in an accurate and logically consistent fashion so that other members of the radiology and nuclear medicine community may benefit from this information and (2) by making sure that the categories and relations used in the RadO will be compatible with a high-quality formal ontology so that *any* researcher, in *any* laboratory, group, consortium, department, or wherever may benefit from this information. In what follows, we will first offer a general step-by-step procedure one can utilize in constructing a RadO. Then, we will suggest utilizing a well-known, working formal ontology called Basic Formal Ontology (BFO) in order to make the RadO calibrated and interoperable with any other domain ontology in the sciences.

8.4.1
Steps in Constructing a RadO

Much of what we say below will be found, implicitly and explicitly, in Rubin (2007), ANP Fielding and Marwede (2006). Also, members of the Qualitative Spatiotemporal Reasoning Unit of the Ontology Research Group (Buffalo, NY, USA, http://org. buffalo.edu/) at the University at Buffalo are providing a new avenue for the representation of canonical anatomy – and the processing of X-ray, MRI, EEGs, and other forms of image data – by applying ontological methods from geographic information systems and qualitative spatiotemporal reasoning. Ideas and information from that group may be helpful in the construction of a RadO (see http:// org.buffalo.edu/rarp/QSRUnit%20Page.html; Donnelly et al. 2006).

For easy reference, the steps themselves can be found in Fig. 5. Although following these steps will *guarantee* neither a "perfect" domain ontology nor interoperability between or among domain ontologies, they will be useful to those researchers interested in setting up a RadO or *any* domain ontology. And, we believe that they will make a perfect domain ontology, as well as interoperability between or among domain ontologies, *more likely*.

8.4.1.1
Step 1: Determine the Purpose of the RadO

As rational beings, before engaging in any activity whatsoever e.g., making a decision, embarking on a journey, choosing a career, writing a book, or building a domain ontology, we naturally want to establish the ultimate objective, goal, or purpose of the activity. Constructing a RadO is analogous to building a tool in that the tool's intended usage needs to be established first, before one can fashion it the correct way in order to get the job done most efficiently utilizing it. Thus, when building a RadO, it is essential at the very beginning

Step #1: Determine the purpose of the RadO

Step #2: Provide an explicit statement of the intended subject-matter of the RadO.

Step #3: Determine the most basic (a) **universal terms** *and (b)* **relations** *dealt with in the RadO.*

Step #4: Construct a list for the RadO, starting with the most basic terms.

Step #5: Put the terms in a taxonomic hierarchy complete with appropriate relationships.

Step #6: Regiment the information in order to ensure logical and scientific coherence.

Step #7: Regiment the information in order to ensure compatibility with other relevant ontologies.

Step #8: Concertize this information in a computer tractable language, like Protege.

Step #9: Implement the RadO in some specific computing context.

Fig. 5 Steps in constructing a radiology ontology

to ask the question "What is the ultimate purpose of this RadO?" This will include considering whether it is primarily intended to be a comprehensive representation of scientific information in a given domain for *reference* or general educational purposes (referred to as a *reference ontology*), or whether it is intended to be *applied* in order to accomplish certain very specific goals, such as the data mining of electronic health records and clinical trials, or medical treatments (referred to as a *task, use,* or *application ontology*).

8.4.1.2
Step 2: Provide an Explicit Statement of the Intended Subject Matter of the RadO

An explicit statement of the intended subject matter of a domain indicates what information and principles should and should not be included in the RadO. For example, the documentation for the FMA reads "The FMA…is strictly constrained to "pure" anatomy, i.e., the structural organization of the body" (http://sig.biostr.washington.edu/projects/fm/AboutFM. html). This statement makes it relatively clear what information is and is not properly a candidate for inclusion in the FMA and, thus, also what terms, ontological categories, and relationships might need to be included.

8.4.1.3
Step 3: Determine the Most Basic Universal Terms and Relations Dealt with in the RadO

In the jargon of ontologies, we can distinguish between instances and universals. An *instance* is a particular entity in the world, such a particular frog, the Louvre, or a particular

8

performance of "Eleanor Rigby." On the other hand, a *universal* is an abstraction, such as *frog*, *museum*, or *performance*. Universals have instances, and it is universals which we are interested in when building ontologies. Although any experiment, diagnosis, or treatment deals with instances (e.g., particular patients, particular pills), the goal of science is to make true statements about *universals*.

Determining what the universals of the RadO (such as *radiation, medical image, electromagnetic energy, X-ray machine,* and others) and the relations among these universals (such as "is a," "is a part of," " participates in," "is adjacent to," "develops from," and others) is a matter of analyzing the subject matter itself – with locating the various entities with which it deals in the context of a more general taxonomy or partonomy, much like the Porphyrian tree or periodic table of the elements mentioned earlier. The most basic universals will be related to one another in, at least, basic "is a," genus/species-type fashions: recall living entity with sensation is a living entity, rational animal is a living entity with sensation, and human is a rational animal, etc. for the Porphyrian tree, as well as biosynthetic process is a metabolic process is a biological process, for glutathione production.

Obviously, this requires the expertise of the researchers, professors, clinicians, and other thinkers associated with radiology and nuclear medicine. Here, relevant questions include: What are the most important, general, basic universals and relations dealt with in radiology and nuclear medicine? How do the universals and relations function in scientific theories pertaining to radiology and nuclear medicine? Are the universals and relations that have been collected an adequate reflection of what is most crucial for understanding the truth about radiology and nuclear medicine as reflected in current scientific knowledge?

8.4.1.4
Step 4: Construct a List of Terms for the RadO, Starting with the Most Basic Terms

Once a determination of universals and relations has been made, then one can compile these into an initial list of terms – on paper, chalk boards, dry erase boards, or using word processors – preferably with some definition and organization into tentative categories. This likely will entail answering: What are the essential or defining features of radiology and nuclear medicine as a whole, as well as of the particular entities and relations that have been selected as crucial?

Such a terminology may be acquired from existing dictionaries, thesauri, or radiology and nuclear medicine handbooks, or by consulting the literature and the opinions of experts. The initial RadO terminology should include, for each term, a listing of common synonyms or alternative expressions; and a clear, concise natural language definition of the term; an initial statement of the most likely ontological category to which the entities referred to by the term belong (object, quality, function, process, etc.). The following is important: *The terms and definitions in the initial terminology are basic, commonly accepted, and already clearly defined and, hence, do not necessarily represent the final state of the terms and definitions that will be included in the RadO.* Rather, they are a first draft, or gloss, for the sake of getting the relevant information organized and assembled in a single place.

8.4.1.5
Step 5: Put the Terms in a Taxonomic Hierarchy Complete with Appropriate Relationships

A system of well-defined terms regarding a specific domain should, in normal cases, form a hierarchically structured taxonomy. More specifically, if all or most of the terms being defined refer to universals on the side of reality, then the hierarchy among universals from more general (e.g., animal, plant, bacteria) to more specific (e.g., mammal, arthropod, sponge) should be reflected in the definitions of the terms that refer to these universals. Terms lower down in a taxonomic hierarchy should inherit all properties and characteristics from their "parents" (the genus–species relationship, oftentimes, is called the parent–child relationship), ensuring logical consistency in the definition of terms, clear demarcations among levels of abstractness within the ontology, and the possibility of automated reasoning. And each term in the taxonomy should have *only one* parent, in order to ensure that the best computational properties of the taxonomy are preserved. Once the taxonomy has been established using the "is a" relations between terms, other relations can be added in. While each term should have only one parent according to the "is a" relation, other relations may not include this requirement.

8.4.1.6
Step 6: Regiment the Information in Order To Ensure Logical and Scientific Coherence

This is probably the most important step, as the goal of this regimentation is to develop a RadO that is as logically coherent, unambiguous, and true to the facts of reality as possible. Importantly, if the goal is to use this RadO for purposes of representation in a computer-based ontology (as it should be), then a more rigorous formalization of this terminology is needed (because, like we said, computers are dumb beasts). In general, the syntax of the terminology selected for inclusion in *any* domain ontology should be formulated in terms of clear and explicitly stated conventions (whatever those may be), and should be such as to be familiar to, and easily recognizable by, potential users of the ontology – especially, but in some cases not limited to, domain experts. Regimenting a terminology, thus, involves both the explicit statement of – as well as *ruthlessly* consistent adherence to – syntactic conventions for the writing of terms and explicit consideration of the intended audience or user-base for the ontology.

Make sure to check the universals, relations, and domain-specific terminology contained in the RadO for logical, philosophical, and empirical adequacy, including consistency and human intelligibility. More specifically, in the RadO avoid the problems of (1) simply getting the facts wrong, (2) perception/reality confusions, (3) using examples instead of definitions, (4) circular definitions, (5) equivocation, (6) use/mention confusions, and (7) unclear or incoherent definitions. In fact, coherent definitions are essential to constructing any domain ontology, and a lot of the effort in domain ontology building – just like with the building of any regimented taxonomy or partonomy – consists in putting forward clearly defined terms. Anytime a definition of a term is presented, a critically thinking individual automatically tries to think of counterexamples that would make the term's definition inconsistent. So, if we tried to define "table" strictly as a "raised platform having four legs on which one can place food," the critical thinker would immediately consider counter-examples such as platforms having four legs *other* than tables on which one can place food (a construction worker eating on the floor of an unfinished second-story building having four leglike beams supporting it?), or tables with three legs, or tables on which one is not meant to place food, etc. When building a RadO, it is of paramount logical importance to ask: Are these terms consistent and free from counterexamples? Are the terms defined precisely within the confines of necessary and sufficient conditions?

Further, a defined term in the RadO should be *intersubstitutable* with its definition in such a way that the result is both (1) grammatically correct and (2) truth-preserving. The basic idea behind this principle is that wherever a term refers to a thing, the definition of that term should also successfully refer to that thing. Thus, for example, in the FMA the extension of the term "heart" should be identical with the extension of its definition "organ with cavitated organ parts, which is continuous with the systemic and pulmonary arterial and venous trees" (see http://sig.biostr. washington.edu/projects/fm/AboutFM.html). This will yield a claim like this:

"The (*heart*) pumps blood."

This means the exact same thing as, is as grammatically correct as, and is as equally true as this claim:

"The (organ with cavitated organ parts, which is continuous with the systemic and pulmonary arterial and venous trees) pumps blood."

The intersubstitutability of a term, and its definition with regard to the truth-value of sentences in which it occurs, is important both for preserving truth across inference in automated reasoning contexts *and* for ensuring intelligibility for human users of ontologies.

8.4.1.7
Step 7: Regiment the Information To Ensure Compatibility with Other Relevant Ontologies

The RadO should not only consist of representations of reality which are correct according to our current understanding, but the application of the RadO in a database should also be structured for the purpose of managing and manipulating that data, supporting (1) inter-connection, (2) calibration, and ultimately (3) interoperability of various computational resources. Is there coherence within the ontology as a whole, as well as coherence with other relevant domain ontologies? Is there a discernible taxonomy, especially one containing "is a" hierarchies? Is there human understandability? As will be made clear in the next section, BFO will be of direct assistance in this regard, by giving an articulate internal structure to electronic biomedical information repositories, and making possible the inter-operability or intertranslatability of different repositories containing different information, in such a way that the information in these repositories can be understood in terms of a common formal framework for the categorization of entities and the reasoning about those entities. Thus, when building any domain ontology, it is important to consider what formal ontological categories and relations – such as "entity" and "is a" – might apply to the domain at hand, and to select a formal ontology with sufficiently clear categories and relations to handle the basic kinds of entities to be found in the domain in question. This is why several groups in the Open Biomedical Ontology Foundry – including the GO Project, the FMA, FlyBase, and WormBase, to name just a few – utilize the categories and relations found in BFO to assist in the structuring of their respective domain ontologies, so as to achieve interoperability of terms they have in common (see http://obo foundry.org/).

8.4.1.8
Step 8: Concretize This Information in a Computer-Tractable Format, Such As Protégé

This step of regimenting the RadO is essentially a *syntactical* one, and involves translating the terminology, relations, etc. contained in the ontology into a format that is computer-tractable, whether this be some fragment of first-order logic, a description logic, or something else. This is an obvious place where formal ontologists and the expert scientists of a particular domain need to be working together with computer programmers and informaticians. Protégé is a free, open-source knowledge-base framework and ontology editor (available through Stanford University at http://protege.stanford.edu/) that numerous researchers use to set up ontologies, but there are others that come and go (see, for example, http://en.wikipedia.org/wiki/Ontology_editor).

8.4.1.9
Step 9: Implement the RadO in Some Specific Computing Context

Finally, then, comes the process of implementing the formalized representational artifact in some actually functioning computing context, such as one's laboratory *and* the Internet. This step is essentially an *implementational* one. Concerning this step and the previous one, it is important to remember the fact that computers are dumb beasts, and that they will only be able to *output* accurately and efficiently what we *input* accurately and efficiently.

8.4.2
Basic Formal Ontology

As we have mentioned already, a formal ontology – such as BFO, developed by Grenon and Smith (2004) – assists domain ontologies by giving an articulate internal structure to electronic biomedical information repositories, and making possible the interoperability or inter-translatability of different repositories containing different information, in such a way that the information in these repositories can be understood in terms of a common formal framework for the categorization of entities and the reasoning about those entities (Smith et al. 2007; Arp et al. 2008); http://www.ifomis.uni-saarland.de/bfo/). It does this by dividing up those universal entities recognized by the scientific world into their most basic categories, starting with *continuants* (entities that *continue* or persist through time; for example, objects, qualities, and functions) and *occurrents* (entities which *occur* in time; for example, processes, events, and happenings). These categories are linked together

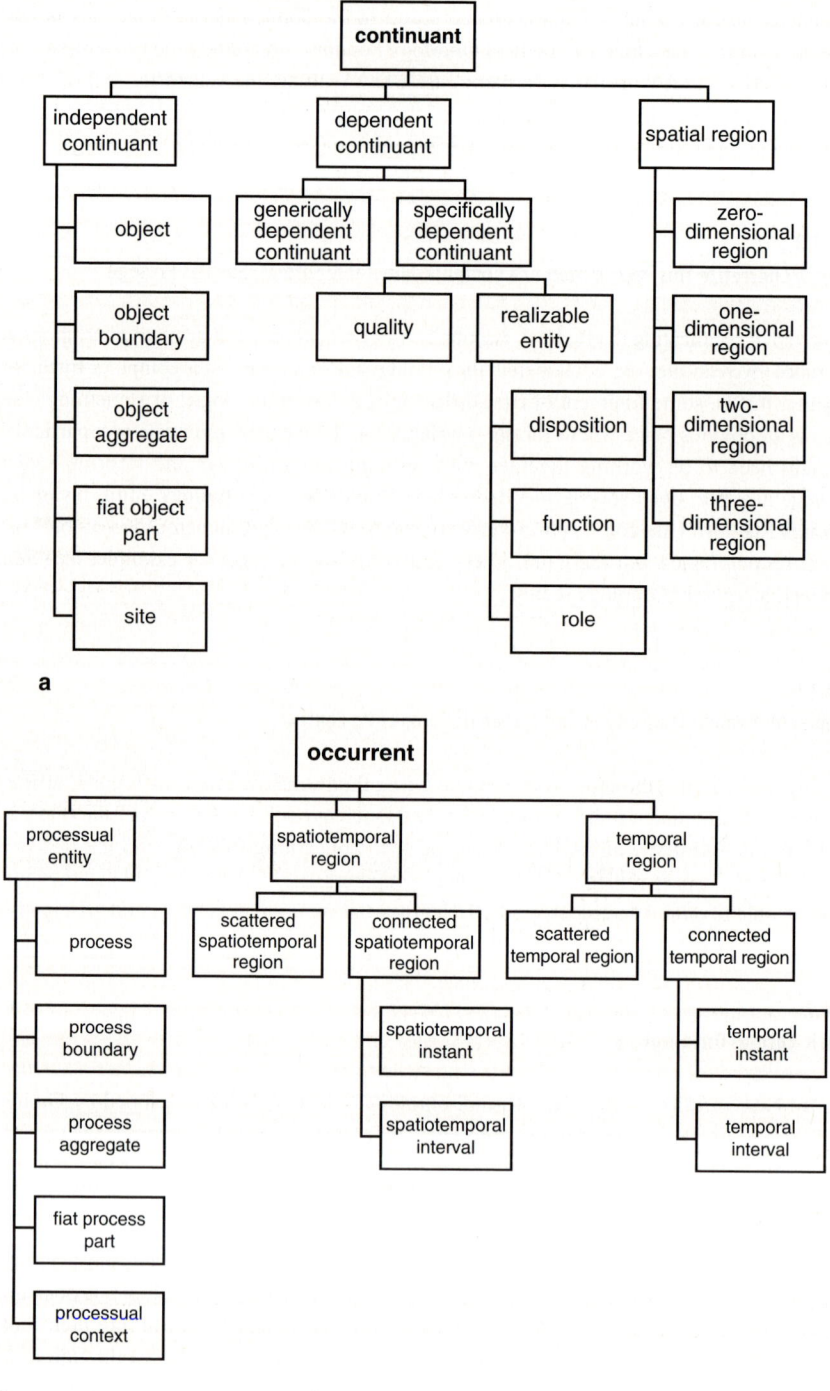

Fig. 6 a Continuant and its subtype children. **b** Occurrent and its subtype children

by means of various kinds of relationships, including "is a" (the taxonomical subtype relation), "part of," and "participates in." This way – and here is the crucial point already mentioned – *interoperability of domain ontologies is virtually guaranteed, because researchers are all using the exact same upper-level ontological categories and relations.* Illustrations of BFO categorizations can be found in Fig. 6, where, for example, object *is a* independent continuant and independent continuant *is a* continuant, while process *is a* processual entity, and processual entity *is a* occurrent.

BFO is increasingly being applied in bioinformatics – and in other areas such as the geospatial sciences, ecology, and social epistemology – and has been used to assist in the classification, categorization, calibration, annotation, recording, and coding of scientific phenomena accurately and efficiently (see http://ontology.buffalo.edu/smith/; Smith and Grenon 2004; Smith et al. 2006; Smith et al. 2007). The Open Biomedical Ontologies Consortium of researchers, in general, embraces BFO (see http://obofoundry.org/) and the various groups in the consortium (e.g., the GO Project, the FMA, FlyBase, WormBase, and others) utilize its basic tenets.

BFO appears to be working and standing the test of time. Thus, radiologists setting up a RadO would do well to consider not only the steps spoken about in the previous section, but also ultimately linking the entities in the RadO to the categories of BFO. This way, positive outcomes (like the one mentioned at the beginning of this chapter in our fictional scenario) might become a consistent reality in biomedical research and treatment.

References

do Amaral M, Roberts A, Rector A (2000) NLP techniques associated with the OpenGALEN ontology for semi-automatic textual extraction of medical knowledge: Abstracting and mapping equivalent linguistic and logical constructs. Proc AMIA Symp 2000:76–80

Arp R (2008) Domain ontology. Formal ontology. Philosophical ontology. In: Williamson J, Russo F (eds) Key terms in logic. Continuum Press, London (in press)

Baxevanis A, Ouellette B (2005) Bioinformatics: A practical guide to the analysis of genes and proteins. Wiley, Hoboken

Berman J (2006) Biomedical informatics. Jones and Bartlett, London

Bertaud V, Belhadj I, Dameron O, Garcelon N, Hendaoui L, Marin F, Duvauferrier R (2007) Computerizing the radiological sign. Radiology 88:27–37

Ceusters W, Smith B, Kumar A, Dhaen C (2004) Mistakes in medical ontologies: Where do they come from and how can they be detected? Stud Health Technol Inform 102:145–164

Donnelly M, Bittner T, Rosse C (2006) A formal theory for spatial representation and reasoning in biomedical ontologies. Artif Intell Med 36:1–27

Fielding J, Marwede D (2006) Four ontological models for radiological diagnostics. Stud Health Technol Inform 124:761–766

Grenon P, Smith B (2004) SNAP and SPAN: Towards dynamic spatial ontology. Spat Cognit Comput 1:1–10

Gruber T (1993) A translation approach to portable ontologies. Knowl Acquis 5:199–220

Kahn C, Channin D, Rubin D (2006) An ontology for PACS integration. J Dig Imag 19:316–327

Lesk A (2005) Introduction to bioinformatics. Oxford University Press, Oxford, UK

Marwede D, Fielding M (2005) The epistemological-ontological divide in clinical radiology. Stud Health Technol Inform 116:749–754

Polanski A, Kimmel M (2007) Bioinformatics. Springer, Berlin

Pommert A, Höhne K, Pflesser B, Richter E, Riemer M, Schiemann T, Schubert R, Schumacher U, Tiede U (2001) Creating a high-resolution spatial/symbolic model of the inner organs based on the visible human. Med Image Anal 5:221–228

Rubin D (2007) Creating and curating a terminology for radiology: Ontology modeling and analysis. J Dig Imag, Available at: http://www.springerlink.com/content/978708n776738132/fulltext.pdf. Accessed 28 April 2008

Rubin D, Dameron O, Bashir Y, Grossman D, Dev P, Musen M (2006) Using ontologies linked with geometric models to reason about penetrating injuries. Artif Intell Med 37:167–176

Shortliffe E, Cimino J (2006) Biomedical informatics: Computer applications in health care and biomedicine. Springer, Berlin

Smith B (2003) Ontology. In: Floridi L (ed) Blackwell guide to the philosophy of computing and information. Blackwell, Malden

Smith B, Grenon P (2004) The cornucopia of formal-ontological relations. Dialectica 58:279–296

Smith B, Smith D (1995) The Cambridge companion to Husserl. Cambridge University Press, Cambridge

Smith B, Kusnierczyk W, Schober D, Ceusters W (2006) Towards a reference terminology for ontology research and development in the biomedical domain. Proc KR-MED 1:7

Smith B, Ashburner M, Rosse C, Bard J, Bug W, Ceusters W, Goldberg LJ, Eilbeck K, Ireland A, et al. (2007) The OBO Foundry: Coordinated evolution of ontologies to support biomedical data integration. Nat Biotechnol 25:1251–1255

Vizenor L, Smith B, Ceusters W (2004) Foundation for the electronic health record: An ontological analysis of the HL7's reference information model. Available at: http://onto-logy.buffalo.edu/medo/HL7_2004.pdf. Accessed 28 April 2008

Educational Insights About Professional Ethics in Radiology

9

L. Brazeau-Lamontagne

9.1
Introduction

Twenty years ago when I started my M.A. in ethics, I recall a colleague asking, "How in the world is ethics relevant to you, a radiologist?" Today, the same question is asked. In this chapter therefore, I intend to focus on professional ethics as it is embedded in what the radiologist does as a physician, what professional ethics implies for his/her daily practice, what radiologists have to learn to maintain their professional commitment, now, and in the future. By professional ethics, I do not mean the fence separating ethics from nonethics. Here, professional ethics means demonstrating the necessary competencies to solve respectfully and carefully practical ethical dilemmas arising from grounded heath problems by way of addressing genuine radiologists' actions as physicians.

Daily radiology practice is fertile ground for genuine dilemmas. How can a resident be exposed to such a dilemma in the midst of his or her training? The following example, drawn from previous work (Brazeau-Lamontagne 2002), depicts one perspective of ethics: the duty to disclose. This example illustrates that ethical questioning can open meaningful communication that can be found embedded everywhere in the radiology service.

"Just before noon, I (a radiology resident) was completing an abdominal ultrasound examination on a woman self-aware of her cancer and well informed on what the present ultrasound examination was for. The diagnosis was obvious: numerous liver metastases. She asked for the result at once. As a resident, instead of answering, I referred to the attending physician, who, already late and in a hurry, disappeared before the patient could talk to him. Facing my "silence," the patient told me her conclusion: she was sick enough to leave me speechless."

L. Brazeau-Lamontagne
Department of Radiology, Centre Hospitalier Universitaire de Sherbrooke,
Sherbrooke, Canada QC J1G 2E8
E-mail: Lucie.brazeau@usherbrooke.ca

Radiology Education. R.K. Chhem et al. (Eds.)
DOI: 10.1007/978-3-540-68989-8, © Springer-Verlag Berlin Heidelberg 2009

9

9.2
Radiologists Are Physicians

Is it stating the obvious to say that radiologists are physicians? For the Royal College of Physicians and Surgeons of Canada (RCPSC) it certainly is. In Canada, the RCPSC sets standards for specialty, assesses and accredits residency programs, assesses residents' education and training, and certifies specialists, among which are radiologists (McKarthy and Smith 2007). The RCPSC embedded both ethics and professionalism within its framework, the CanMEDS roles (see Chap. 10 of this book). In doing so, the RCPSC targets all the specialties, including radiology, and emphasizes a common denominator to all physicians no matter what the specialties are. The common denominator could be summarized as the profession's moral endeavor it stands for. The RCPSC officially promotes radiologists as physicians but is far from being unique in that matter. The radiologists themselves do so as well. No matter what country they are working in, radiologists are getting the professional title of physician, and then get postgraduate specialty training. Therefore, from the accreditation/certification organizations' point of view or from the "working at the base" radiologists' view, it is the same. Radiologists are physicians.

That said, what of professional ethics pertains to radiologists? Robert Hattery challenged radiologists to think further about this in his presidential address at the 2006 Radiological Society of North America meeting. Hattery intended to provide "a wakeup call for radiologists to renew their commitment to ethical behavior." He proposed a few ideas aimed at bolstering professional behavior among radiologists:

> › *Read* the physician's Charter on Medical Professionalism (2002)
> › *Recognize* the sacredness of the physician-patient relationship
> › *Give back*: mentor, teach, and lead by example
> › *Have the fortitude* to identify and deal with unprofessional behavior
> › *Help* bolster public confidence

These five ideas provoke some interesting thoughts. The next step, however, was to find a way to progress from ideas to action in daily practice in order to realize a significant impact. The challenge here is to understand the ethical competencies well enough to translate them into day-to-day radiologists' actions. What does that mean?

From an "educational insights from experience in the field" point of view, I think that it means to escape the second-class physician status to which radiologists are sometimes relegated. What do I mean by *second-class physician*? Two illustrations drawn from the daily work come to my mind. First, let us go back to the example given above. For many years, radiologists were (and are still) "denied" by the referring physicians and among themselves deny the role of communicating results to patients. Such denial is not candid. It implicitly denies radiologists the basic roles that physicians hold with respect to interactions with patients. Second, the way radiological examinations are ordered by the referring physicians spans from receiving no information at all to receiving pertinent clinical signs and symptoms. It is important to remember that taking pictures in the absence of pertinent clinical information reduces the role of the radiologist to that of a "photographer," and further removes us from participating fully as part of a health care team working in the best interests of our patient.

What are the ethical competencies involved for *first-class* physicians? To me it means quite simply that "radiologist" is a synonym of "physician." In order to illustrate what this shift implies, I have rewritten the preamble of the physician's charter on medical professionalism, substituting *radiologist* for *physician*, and *radiology* for *profession*:

> Professional ethics *is the basis of radiology's contract with society*. It demands placing the interests of patients above those of the *radiologist*, setting and maintaining standards of competence and integrity, and providing expert advice to society on matters of health. The principles and responsibilities of the *radiologist's* professionalism must be clearly understood by both radiology and society. Essential to this contract is public trust in *radiologists*, which depends on the integrity of both individual *radiologists* and the whole radiology profession (Adaptation from Medical professionalism in the new millenium: a physician's charter, op. cit.).

Translating ethics competencies into daily practice reveals numerous ways in which radiologists participate as physicians within the health care delivery system, ranging from the one-on-one relationship with the patient, to continuous quality improvement through imaging, consulting, communicating, and so forth. Indeed, Oljeski et al. (2004) proposed no fewer than 16 topics pertaining to ethics education in radiology pointing to a wide range of radiologists' responsibilities. In order to fulfill these responsibilities effectively, we need to progress one step further.

There is a broad spectrum of how we radiologists think about ourselves and our roles. At one end of the spectrum, the radiologist views himself/herself as integral to the health care team, and linked to the care of the patient and family either directly or through the primary care provider. At the other end of the spectrum is the radiologist content to read and generate reports at the computer, with the patient seen as simply an object in the marketplace. Honoring the sacredness of the patient is neither spontaneous nor easy. It belongs to the historical endeavor of the entire medical profession. In the Middle Ages, Maimonide referred to this in his prayer:

> N'admets pas que la soif du gain et la recherche de la gloire m'influencent dans l'exercice de mon art, car les ennemis de la vérité et de l'amour des hommes pourraient facilement m'abuser et m'éloigner du noble devoir de faire du bien … toujours prêt à servir le pauvre et le riche, l'ami et l'ennemi, le bon et le mauvais.

Radiology is relatively "young" in this secular endeavor of the profession, but it is vital that radiologists do not forget to nurture the physician's commitment toward the patient. We need also to remember that the term "patient" here is a holistic word. The term "patient" means not only an individual but also a collective, applying to the patient in front of us as well as to those we will care for in the future. Professional ethics in radiology rests only at one side of the spectrum, where patient is situated at the heart of professional activities as their only goal. Therefore this chapter will not pay any attention or consideration to any radiological activities transforming the patient in a footstep for personal power or financial success of radiologists. Having discarded what cannot participate of radiological ethics, this chapter focuses on what it includes.

9

9.3
What Is Included in Radiology Ethics?

Armstrong (1999) described seven elements of the radiologist's responsibilities to the patient (Table 9.1).

Table 9.1 Armstrong's seven elements of radiologist's responsibilities to the patient

1. Assessing the *appropriateness of a patient's examination* ideally challenges us to listen to the patient's story; engage in discussion and perhaps argument with the referring physician; question the indications for the requested examination; reflect on the patient's circumstances; and analyze the possible consequences of each action, such as performing the examination, modifying [it] in some important way, delaying the study until more information is available, offering an alternative study, or not performing the requested examination
2. The *informed consent process* involves… disclosure of a core set of information to the patient including… the physician's recommendation and the purpose of seeking consent…; [the radiologist's] comprehension of pertinent information about the examination, alternative choices… and voluntariness of consent…; determining the patient's decisional capacity and securing an appropriate surrogate in the event that… a patient lacks the capacity for medical decision making…; and empowerment of a patient to consent or withhold consent, called "informed refusal"
3. The concept of *patient protection* includes considerations of patient safety and comfort, examination timeliness, preparedness for emergent resuscitative care, and patient follow-up; adequate management of pain and amelioration of suffering during interventional procedures using sufficient analgesia and conscious sedation…; and protection from inappropriate examinations, procedures, and impaired or incompetent care providers
4. *Image interpretation* is the process of monitoring image quality; monitoring individual and group performance with respect to errors of search, detection and recognition…; [deciding if/when] additional patient information should be sought; what specific question(s) are expected to be answered through the intended study…; and which specific wording should be used to spell out findings, their significance, and a recommendation for action
5. *Communication with patients and physicians* can include a dialogue focused on whether the requested examination is appropriate for a patient…; discussing the results of a patient's examination with a patient or family…; and the requirement the referring physicians receive information in a timely manner and understand the importance, relevance, urgency, and possible consequences of the findings, together with further requirements for patient evaluation and treatment. Communication is ideal in face-to-face consultation
6. *Continuous learning* requires critical thinking about the question "what [if anything] have I learned from this process?" [Continuous learning also can be] stimulated by examination of one's own mistakes… and how one responds to mistakes of any magnitude ([which] is in significant part determined by the institutional ethical milieu and the attitude's of one's colleagues in acknowledging errors…;) and particularly a willingness to be self-critical and acknowledge one's limits and the limits of one's methods
7. To *continually improve the quality of patient care*… [radiologists must] learn to… systematically examine the processes through which service is provided, requiring that key indicators of quality be identified and that the processes responsible for providing quality care be understood, measured, and systematically adapted. Moreover, changes initiated must measurably improve and sustain quality

In medical professional ethics, the central position of the patient is at stake. Do we need to have the patients physically in front of us in order to be dedicated to them? The answer is obviously no. The evolution in the medical health care delivery models has transformed yesterday's solo practice into today's medical team model, putting each member of that team alternately at the forefront during the care scenario. Each radiologist play an active role in this scenario, sometimes serving as a consultant to the consultant, sometimes in direct one-on-one relation to the patient (or family). No matter who initiates a referral, a patient coming to radiology comes to get a radiologist's expertise, with all the expectation that goes with it. First, let us consider imaging as an example. As Milton Guiberteau argued in his 2006 American College of Radiology presidential oration, "X-ray, CT or PET scan don't do show or tell. ...Medical images in themselves have no value until they are interpreted by qualified and experienced imagers" (Guiberteau 2007). Second, let us consider the "real-time presence," If the visit of the patient implies a direct interaction with a radiologist during that visit, then the patient personalizes his/her professional expectations and focuses them on the radiologist as a physician. The patient expects the radiologist to treat him or her with the regard and attention a physician normally pays to a patient. In both instances, the expectation is nothing less than professional care, with all the expertise and *doigté* it implies. Answering the patient's questions is part of it.

The focus on patients while they are actually in the radiology suite should not overshadow how strongly their care and treatment depends on image-based diagnoses. Radiology patients do not vanish from our professional attention when they walk out of the department, although as radiologists we do not pursue direct communication with the patients. Instead, we usually extend our commitment through our colleagues to whom we address our interpretation of imaging. Sometimes, all the relation we get with the patient is through our colleagues, as precious as precarious it can be. Therefore our interpretation of imaging ALWAYS remain our crucial commitment to the patients.

Our interpretation activities deserve a few more thoughts. Answering our colleagues' questions about patients is central to our daily work. The growing sophistication in radiology raises the need for the radiologists' expertise in the care system. A significant portion of the patient care plan is based upon evidence that is provided by the radiologist's interpretation. The patient/physician relation takes place in several ways. When we meet the patient in person directly, and when we relate to the patient through colleagues. In all instances, we have to keep seeing the actual patient behind the view box or the screen. This is central to radiology trainning. Remaining meaningfull to the patient implies a very wide spectrum of competences, much beyond the confinement of a "dark room" to expand into the full range of health care. The interpretation of imaging is an act of communication. Therefore we need to refrain from generating "one style fits all" reports. Instead, we must always keep in mind that we are answering a clinical question pertaining to a real patient. The message we communicate needs to be meaningful to the colleague who requested the radiology consultation. As in all other communication settings, we need to continue to learn about it, we need to cultivate mutual understandings, and we need to protect communication channels.

9.4
Learning Professional Ethics in Radiology

9.4.1
Learning Professional Ethics

During the last decade, calls for improved teaching of professionalism, from the undergraduate medical level to continuing professional development (Cruess and Cruess 1997), received wide attention. In a recent study Goold and Stern (2006) focused on specialty training. They reported that resident and nonresident informants identified consent, interprofessional relationships, family interactions, communication skills, and end-of-life care as essential components of training. Nonresidents also emphasized formal ethics instruction, resource allocation, and self-monitoring, whereas residents emphasized the learning environment and resident–attending physician interactions. The authors concluded that learning needs for ethics and professionalism include many topics relevant for most specialties. They underline the opportunities provided for shared curricula and resources.

If we keep in mind Hattery's 2006 presidential address, sharing curriculum resources could look very appealing. However, we have to be cautious. A "one size fits all" teaching strategy does not match with what is learned from the evidence-based education literature. The crux of the issue relies on the distinction between learning and teaching. Teaching emphases the explicit content of the curriculum whereas learning emphases on the process of "internalization" of competences. Learning can be compare to a cognitive metabolism needed to translate what is taught in what is done. There is no other way to monitor the process of learning than communication. It is ever more true of professional ethics. Therefore radiology teachers depend upon appropriate meaningful context to facilitate durable learning.

Learning professional ethics requires not only explicit teaching, but also the provision of opportunities where learning can flourish in an authentic context. As documented by Cruess and Cruess (2006), the past decade has seen development of new approaches to the teaching of professionalism. These approaches combine what is often referred to as the "hidden curriculum" in the medical academic community and the explicit teaching of what professionalism is all about, ethics background included. Therefore, as in any medical field, professional ethics in radiology is an integral part of radiology itself: it gives its sense and reason for action. Practically speaking, it implies that day-to-day exposure to genuine professional ethics questioning nurtures learning critical and reflective thinking, both of which are crucial to professional ethics learning. Action springs from critical reflection and critical reflection guides the action. Unless action is taken into account, teaching ethics remains ethereal:

> We need to bear in mind that ethics is not a subject that lends itself to memorization … Ethics matters are best addressed through example and conversation… Yet, ethical insight lies neither in lists of concrete rules nor in an ethereal realm of mere subjectivity and taste. It involves trying to understand who we are … and what we stand for or care about, personally, professionally, and as members of a community (Gunderman 2006).

Haccoun (1998) described four levels of efficacy a training program can reach:

> *When a training program is effective, trainees will be satisfied (level I), they will have learned the material (level II), they will behave differently on the job (level III), and the organization will be better after it (level IV) (...with) ultimate training question: Do trainees use the new knowledge, skills, abilities, and attitudes on the job?"*
>
> [Haccoun R. Training in the 21st century: some lessons from the last one. Canadian Psychology Feb-May 1998 from the WEB http://www.findarticles.com/p/articles/mi_qa3711/is_199802/ai_n87883]

9.4.2
Ethics in Daily Radiology Practice

One persistent concern addresses the ethics content itself in the daily radiology practice. Is there such a thing that relates to professional ethics in radiology? Does it really get dedicated attention in education? I recall my colleague's reaction 20 ago. In 2003, a qualitative study on academic radiologists evaluating the professional ethics of their residents was published. It used Armstrong's description of morality, ethics, and radiologists' responsibilities described earlier. It found that the US reference was shared by academic radiologists in France and in Quebec on the one hand, and found great similarities between France and Quebec academic radiologists in evaluating ethics among their residents on the other hand (Brazeau-Lamontagne et al. 2003). Not one of the eight academic radiologists interviewed was missing element on the matter. On the contrary, they shared the same preoccupations about professional ethics in radiology. Moreover, they all mentioned that they felt left alone by their academic institutions when they tried to focus on trainees' needs/deficiencies regarding professional ethics. That brings us back to the notion of a hidden curriculum Hafferty and Franks (1994) described, and how it interferes with the education process.

There is a strong belief that professional ethics is learned through role modeling. Originating from the old *exempla trahunt* of ancient Rome, the major trust in imitation for teaching sets the needs for professional behavior to look up to. But does imitation represent all that is needed to foster professional ethics learning in radiology, both in initial and in continuing education? We must realize that imitation does not suffice. Rather,

> *...professionalism is fundamental to the process of socialization during which individuals acquire the values, attitudes, interests, skills and knowledge – the culture – of [the radiology profession] which they seek to become a member [of].... If [radiologists] as rational human beings are to incorporate a set of values into their day-to-day life, they must be able to articulate them, along with the reasons for their existence* (Adapted from Cruess and Cruess 2006).

These values belong to and flow from the foundational ethics that the whole medical profession stands for. To illustrate the vital connections radiology makes with the professional medical ethics core, let us translate clinical ethics into the realm of our departments. In doing so, I will consider alternately consent, professional confidentiality, end-of-life matters, personal convictions and faith, resource allocation, and collegiality. Personal interactions

9

between certified radiologists themselves on the one hand and between certified radiologists with residents in radiology on the other hand are considered, representing the significant professional actors in the living context where radiological ethics is promoted. Therefore, it is deliberate that acquiring and persisting in radiological professional ethics are addressed together. It is considered a responsibility shared by educators and by trainees in the very theater where the action is, that is where achievement of professional excellence by all radiology physicians is fostered.

9.5
Consent in Radiology

Consent is an explicit or tacit manifestation of will by which a person approves an act to be undertaken by another. In recognizing the patient's right to consent, we necessarily and implicitly recognize the patient's right to refuse (Collège des médecins du Québec 2006). As radiologists we act no differently, as long as we strive daily to recognize our role in the clinical circuit in which the patient is scheduled to take part. In the stream of investigation or treatment, the radiologist is part of the care team. How do we learn that? The whole diagnostic or therapeutic "match plan" might not have been fully discussed with the radiologist in advance. Nevertheless, that does not authorize the radiologist to become a robot in her/his imaging contribution. We all must take over as attending physicians in the radiology suite, at least for the time the patient is under our care, and continue in that role until the imaging episode is over. We must address this particular issue with the residents and see with them how we all cooperate with the rest of the clinical team. This approach illustrates the "orchestrated," sequential responsibilities that positions the patient at the center of care in each of our departments. Practically speaking, that means we make room for reassessment if this particular patient is still willing to be examined and so forth, when we come to interact with her or him. Our residents will never learn about that if we do not explicitly agree as a group on this matter. The required agreement can be summarized as follows: Since the consent must be free and informed, it also implies validation that the patient understands what we propose to do in radiology. Therefore, we need to "translate in" what it means in the patient's clinical context. Freedom to decide goes hand in hand with being informed. This means that we explain in lay terms what the imaging procedure is for (the kind of diagnostic information it provides, for instance), how it will proceed, what the alternatives are, and the option of refusal. It also implies that we answer the patients' questions honestly. We ought to remember that the "I don't know" answer needs a high level of confidence both from the patient to believe it and from us to dare such honesty. In the case of a resident, the "I don't know" answer can be well accepted if the trainee status is disclosed. We all need to remember that "I don't know" could easily be misunderstood as a substitute for "I don't want to tell you the truth." In such an event, the patient usually mistrusts us, and allows his or her imagination to substitute possible outcomes to complete what we did not say. The resiliency during the rest of the investigation and treatment scenario is then easily jeopardized. We are then facing dilemmas about the quality of imaging and the appropriateness of our contribution.

A free and informed consent is much more than a simple signature on an authorization form. The written consent is nothing other than an aide for memory. It needs ongoing communication between the patient and the radiologist to monitor that the agreement is still in place. Therefore, no matter how official the consent form looks, we need to emphasize that it never takes over the consent process itself. The consent process takes time. We all depend on sharing protected radiological time in order to achieve genuine communication with patients in our department.

The patient is presumed to be capable of giving consent until there is evidence to the contrary. She or he cannot be considered incapable simply because her/his choice differs from the one we or the referring physician would make. In the case of an incapable patient, we call for a third party to provide substituted consent, with the additional provision to do so in the best interest of the patient. Depending on the country, legal procedures for the third-party designation vary. If there is an emergency and the consent cannot be obtained in due time either by the patient herself/himself or by her/his representative, the physician must act in the best interests of the patient. In an emergency situation, only the treatments immediately required by the emergency may be carried out. With the growing trust in imaging to provide diagnostic evidence for selecting many treatments, radiologists are increasingly involved in emergencies.

9.6
Professional Confidentiality

Our professional confidentiality originates in the Hippocratic oath. Does respect for private life, particularly in the context of radiology, still hold meaning today? The primary concern of professional radiological confidentiality is to safeguard the independence and private life of the person. The purpose of the physician's ethical duty to maintain patient confidentiality is to allow the patient to feel free to make a full and frank disclosure of information to the physician, with full knowledge that the physician will protect the confidential nature of this information (Johnson et al. 2005). What special understanding do we need to meet our commitment given the new technologies we now depend on? How can we gain public confidence in terms of radiological confidentiality? First of all, it is of paramount importance to realize that radiological reports and images are milestones in a patient's chart. Second, we need to treat the radiology information with due attention. Third, we need to educate our supporting staff that we care about radiological confidentiality, and demonstrate that care through our actions. Waiting areas and examination radiology suites must provide a discreet, welcoming, and calm atmosphere that preserves the private nature of conversations between radiologists and patients as well as with the radiological technicians. We need to remember that the more sensitive the content of the conversation, the greater is the obligation to observe discretion. Protecting conversations of a private nature between the radiologist and the patient extends to institutional administrators, who must support settings conducive to confidentiality. The same reserve and discretion applies to the discussion of cases with residents, with colleagues, or with other professionals. In these circumstances, we need to pay special attention to the place and manner in which the investigation of patients is discussed. Radiological notes and reports are part of the patient's chart. Moreover, the imaging documents themselves are part of the chart. Therefore, all our storage strategies must be congruent with preserving confidentiality. Discretion in radiology is a collegial matter. We need the efforts of all department members to secure patients' computerized data against informatics predators, which is part of security management of any radiology department or private office.

9.7
The End-of-Life Issues

Usually for physicians and the whole care team, the end-of-life issues raise the question touching on proportionate treatment as opposed to disproportionate treatment. These notions help us better evaluate the reasonable options, given the diagnosis, on the one hand, and the intensity of the treatment sought, on the other hand. Care is said to be proportionate or disproportionate according to the desired goal: Does one envisage a cure, maintenance, or relief for the patient? Answering these questions many times implies diagnostic accuracy, among which imaging has a significant part. Therefore, as radiologists, we often help to elucidate end-of-life issues in that respect. Hence, active questioning about cessation of treatment versus aggressive treatment can bring us to the corollary: cessation of imaging versus aggressive imaging. We have all experienced clinical colleagues "shopping" for services until someone in the department relents and provides a radiology procedure. Without active and explicit commitment from all of us, radiology residents will not build a responsible participation in end-of-life care with the clinical team nor will we. That implies that we show compassion not only to the implied patient but also to our clinical colleagues who have to cope with end-of-life agonizing processes.

The proportionate versus disproportionate care issues raise the question of futility. Treatment is generally considered "medically futile" or not beneficial to the patient if it offers the patient no reasonable hope of cure or improvement or any other kind of genuine benefit. Three questions should be asked in assessing the futility of treatment and its diagnostic counterpart:

1. Is the proposed procedure in keeping with the patient's expectations?
2. Does the proposed procedure have adverse effects that must be evaluated in relation to the expected beneficial ones?
3. Will the proposed procedure benefit the patient as a whole? The futility of medical treatment cannot be evaluated without taking into account the point of view of the patient himself/herself.

All the comments previously addressed in the Sect. 9.5 still apply here. We must not offer care not required by the state of a patient. All physicians, radiologists included, must agree to treatments compatible with a serene and dignified death. This includes refusal of ill-considered investigations/treatments by the patient or his/her family. In determining end-of-life care, we must favor free and informed consent – keeping in mind that information implies active listening and dialogue. Whenever imaging procedures are taken into consideration, we, together with the clinical team, must come to grips with death in order to reach a shared understanding as to the required supportive care the patient wishes to receive. If an imaging contribution is contemplated, it must point to a direct therapy option. If such direct impact from imaging is not the case, the imaging procedure will be unduly burdensome for the patient. We must share the patient's wishes. Practically this requires us to maintain an open mind since radiologists, as any other physicians, can also happen to be first-hand witnesses of those wishes sometimes.

End-of-life issue are all too often a taboo subject in the clinical settings – radiology departments included. Indeed, death is broadly a **cultural** taboo in many of our societies. Care systems are situated within such a culture. For all physicians, including us, the end-of-life issue is doubly taboo. On the one hand, Western society tends to avoid the subject of death to the point of altering the language and rites attached to it. On the other hand, it increasingly entrusts the care of the dying to hospital institutions, whom are themselves caught up in the dynamics of an all-out fight for life and an "efficiency" rationale. It is there that the ambiguous quest for evidence particularly targeting radiologists stands. Should radiologists not relearn how to provide support and solace in the same measure as they seek to heal? Without wanting to single-handedly change the culture of the society in which we live, as radiology physicians we can, through our professional commitment, play a decisive role in the approach to the care of the dying. Just as we do at other times in the lives of patients, we must contribute to provide supportive care and information to them and their family at the end of life and, in so doing, help patients and family conclude life in dignity.

9.8
Personal Convictions

Patients may refuse treatment on the basis of convictions. Religious conviction is recognized as a valid and accepted reason for a patient to refuse a treatment because freedom of faith is part of self-determination embedded within the consent solicitation process. Freedom of faith represents one way to respect the global autonomy and inviolability of the person. The freedom of conscience and belief means that one may choose freely to adhere to a faith and make its precepts one's own. However, respect of patients' convictions does not imply that we volunteer interventions for religious purposes. Refusal of a treatment by the patient does not have the counterpart of forcing a physician to do a procedure under pressure that would "protect" the patient's right of freedom of faith. The voluntary cessation of pregnancy provides an example of where our imaging expertise might come in conflict with our own personal convictions. This limited occurrence should not overshadow a much wider one: complying with "image" as requested under the pressure that "we have no choice" because a colleague asked for it does not upgrade any meaningless imaging demand to a meaningful one. We might be prone to shirk personal implication on that matter because we may find that we have insufficient skills (Armstrong 1999) or because we are much too insignificant in the greater hospital environment to justify what we believe to be a right. However, it is our personal and collective responsibility to keep our focus on the patient, including our commitment to proceed with meaningful imaging only.

9.9
Resource Allocation

I do not know any radiology department that is not the theater of gate-keeping scenarios. From the very beginning, we get involved in the radiation issue and the motto "As low dose as possible" is of utmost importance for all radiologists and residents. This opens the way to a broader topic: the appropriateness of the imaging examination.

> *Assessing the appropriateness of an examination ideally challenges us to listen to the patient's story; engage in discussion and perhaps argument with the referring physician; question the indications for the requested examination; reflect on the patient's circumstances; and analyze the possible consequences of each action, such as performing the examination, modifying the examination in some important way, delaying the study until more information is available, offering an alternative study, or not performing the requested examination* (Armstrong 1999).

It is stating the obvious to say that the resources in question are not financial means only. Resource allocation issues directly relate to fundamental justice well underlined in the charter on medical professionalism itself with a commitment to a just distribution of finite resources. Let us consider what happens if we substitute the word *radiology* for *profession* and *radiologists* for *physicians* and so forth it in terms of our commitment:

> *While meeting the needs of individual patient, radiologists are required to provide investigation/intervention that is based on a wise and cost-effective management of limited imaging resources. They should be committed to working with other radiologists, others physicians, hospitals, and payers to develop guidelines for cost-effective care. The radiologists' professional responsibility for appropriate allocation of resources requires scrupulous avoidance of superfluous tests and procedures. The provision of unnecessary imaging procedures not only exposes patients to avoidable harm and expense but also diminishes the imaging resources available for others* (adapted from Charter on Medical Professionalism, 2002).

What does distributive justice imply? Does it suggest that we provide the same thing to everyone? Or is it not rather that we respond to the patients' needs, no matter what their gender, socioeconomic status, ethnicity, religion, or any other social category is? When we speak of care, we must keep in mind that justice is responding to needs which "shape" the design of care, including allocation of time. Time catches us in two ways: how we schedule imaging appointments and how we utilize the time of our colleagues. As gatekeepers, we must remember both to take into account and to pay due attention to it in our daily work.

Care cannot be addressed in the way material goods are. Care cannot be but adapted to the patients' need. Therefore, we must discuss justice matters with respect to resource allocation with our residents. I suggest three reflective questions which, if combined, might help radiologists sort out justice issues: First, would I do the same if the patient were a renowned executive or a poor unknown person? Second, would I do the same if the patient were me? Third, would I do the same if I were "role modeling" before a journalist? A frank and sincere Yes to all three together is needed to meet our professional oak. In teaching, we must keep in mind that ethics requires authentic examples combined with dialogue that reflects our own professionalism and ethical approach to dilemmas in order to grow.

9.10
Collegiality

To consider our residents as colleagues means that we enter into dialogic relationships with them that can be mutually beneficial. For instance, dedicated small-group learning sessions, adapted from a clinical variant of problem-based learning sessions, may constitute "gifted opportunities" that allow open discussion and reflection on sensitive professional dilemmas the residents experience in real life (Brazeau-Lamontagne 2002). Considering residents as colleagues also calls for deeper understanding of what collegiality is all about. One way to introduce the meaning of collegiality is through the quality improvement approach.

> Teaching of evidence-based medicine addresses only one of the many challenges involved in raising the level of clinical performance. Most importantly, all care of individual patients by individual practitioners is embedded in a complex, nested set of human organizations; and because (as is often said) every system is perfectly designed to get exactly the results it gets, medicine's many shortcoming can be attributed as much to inadequate human organizations (dysfunctional systems) as to the deficiencies of individual clinician performance (Batalden and Davidoff 2007).

Organizations imply ways of acting together. What does collegiality mean? It means the interdependence of pairs, grounded on respect for professional expertise and nurtured by common engagement toward the ends and the values of the profession (Ihara 1988). Collegiality entails a certain way of acting together. How do we get to act together professionally?

9

The shared cooperative activity theory (Bratman 1992) allows us to distinguish three ways human beings act together:

(1) *Aggregation*: Individuals are juxtaposed and rely on their *mimetic skills* to accomplish common actions. Hence, their group action takes on the requested tasks by way of duplication of individual gestures by the others without reference to the motivating reasons for doing it. Therefore, aggregation lacks the reasons of action needed for discernment. It relies on imitation only.

(2) *Hierarchy*: It mobilizes the individuals in common actions, by way of the influence of the leader, who persuades the group by way of the reason she or he sees as right. The leadership puts in charge to make out for what reasons. Here the reasons of action are neither shared nor submitted for consensus. They are rather centralized by the leader, because she or he is the unique holder of the global vision. Therefore, the leadership is giving way to due commands and orders to persuade by means of coordination. Individual actors welcome the commands by persuasion; that implies without critical reflection, which would debate the reasons for the actions needed and would allow discernment in changing or doubtful context.

(3) *College* as in our professional group: Its mode of action toward the "we together" is again different from aggregation and hierarchy. The professional college builds a project of common actions, considers those actions significant by way of its own reasons of action according to its own *professional ethics* that the members endorse by conviction to assume the common responsibilities of the group. Here, the actors cooperate in sharing not only the actions they do but also in sharing the reasons why they are doing them. Therefore, even if they are no longer actually together, the individuals in a professional college can still modulate their actions without disrupting their group coherence, even in challenging moving context, because the group maintains its actions coherent by sharing ends and values (Agliette and Orléan 2000).

If we go back to the first example of the present topic, how might collegiality work? We could start by sharing the issue between the attending physician and the resident explicitly of course, but also by coming to a shared department approach to communicating bad news to the patient. In the example cited, the attending physician was in a rush. It would be unrealistic to ignore rushes. Instead, we need to learn how to cope with them. In fact we need to learn how to share workload really. That implies that we take it one step further and delineate what actually is considered in the workload by including answering patients' questions. The role of the residents in that particular aspect cannot be "taken for granted" nor dismissed as irrelevant.

Collegiality calls for our active sharing of ends and values. Since there is no arm-to-arm transfusion of values, we have to talk about them, both among ourselves and with our residents. "Once in a lifetime" is not enough. We need to keep talking about our reasons for action in order to validate the context adjustment we perform. If ethics fosters the achievement of professional excellence by every radiologist, collegiality fosters the expression of our professional commitment to the patients' care. If we come back to the charter on medical professionalism, several commitments stand out as collegially compulsorily: commitment to improving quality of care, commitment to improving access to care, commitment to scientific knowledge, commitment to maintaining trust by managing conflicts of interest, and commitment to professional responsibilities. That is not to discard the individual responsibilities we all have toward those commitments. But we cannot meet our individual responsibilities without holding on to our pairs. For instance, how can we improve access to care if we do not orchestrate our actions with our colleagues? How can we improve quality of care without conjugating our efforts with those of our pairs? Denying such evidence is the equivalent of pretending we ensure the full range of care by ourselves!

How to achieve collegiality? There are no quantitative data on the matter. Instead the literaure stresses the endeavor of collegiality, as with the charter of medical professionalism. In fact, collegiality is a long way to go. Radiologists, educators and trainees in radiology, need to be well aware that spontaneous collegiality does not exist. We continuously learn about it and need by way of active and explicit dedication. On a broader institutional standpoint, the Conférence internationale des doyens et facultés de médecine d'expression française (CIDMEF) came up with a charter of institutional ethics for the Faculties of Medicine (*Charte de l'éthique des Facultés de médecine* . Pédagogie médicale 2004; 5:213–17. English translation available at http://www.sante.univ-nantes.fr/med/ethique/ under the index "charte") That charter is aimed to continuously promote discussing and sharing ends and values towards social medical responsibilities and professional commitments during the whole process of medical education. Taking the hidden curriculum phenomenon into account, tadaptation of that institutional charter of ethics must occur in radiology. There is a real need for us all to join and explicitly depict the many aspects of professional excellence in radiology, including the dynamic environment in which we teach our residents.

9.11
Conclusions

This chapter has addressed key issues involved in pursuing excellence in medical education through professional ethics. It has emphasized the need to recognize radiologists as physicians in a shared professional endeavor. Translating the charter on medical professionalism in terms meaningful to radiology underlined how ethics lies at the very heart of all we achieve daily as radiology physicians. It has also emphasized education practice as a joint venture where all of us, radiologists, educators, and trainees, need to collaborate and depend on each other to renew our commitment to ethical behavior. The various issues related to a hidden curriculum as powerful levers in education were addressed to stress the importance of a collegial approach to achieve professional excellence.

References

(2004) Charte de l'éthique des facultés de médecine. Pédagog Méd 5:213–17 {English translation available at http://www.sante.univ-nantes.fr/med/ethique/under the index "charte"}

Agliette, Orléan (2000) La théorie économique de la confiance et ses limites. In Laufer R, Orillard M (eds) Cahiers de Socio-Économie. L'Harmattan, Paris

9

Armstrong JD (1999) Morality, ethics, and radiologists' responsibilities Am J Roentgenol 173:279–284

Batalden P, Davidoff F (2007) Teaching quality improvement: The devil is in the details. JAMA 298:1059–1061

Bratman M (1992) Shared cooperative activity. Philos Rev 101(2):327–341

Brazeau-Lamontagne L (2002) L'évaluation de l'éthique médicale des residents. Pédagog Méd 3:152–58 (abstract in English)

Brazeau-Lamontagne L, Barrier JH, Ahern SP (2003) Are academic radiologists evaluating the professional ethics of their residents? Radiology 84:1001–1005

Charter on Medical Professionalism (2002). Project of the ABIM Foundation, ACP-ASIM Foundation, and European Federation of Internal Medicine. Medical professionalism in the new millenium: a physician's charter. Annals of Internal Medicine, 136:243–246 and Lancet, 359:520–523

Collège des médecins du Québec. (2006) Examination on the legal, organizational and ethical aspects of medical practice in Québec (ALDO-Québec). May 2006:102

Cruess RL, Cruess SR (1997) Professionalism must be taught. Br Med J 315:1674–1677

Cruess RL, Cruess SR (2006) Teaching professionalism: General principles. Med Teach 28:205–208

Goold SD, Stern DT (2006) Ethics and professionalism: What does a resident need to learn? Am J Bioeth 6:9–10

Guiberteau MJ (2007) 2006 ACR presidential oration the ring in the radiograph: Profession and principle. J Am Coll Radiol 4:11–17

Gunderman RB (2006) Achieving excellence in medical education. Springer-Verlag, London

Haccoun R (1998) Training in the 21st century: Some lessons from the last one. Can Psychol 39:33–51

Hafferty F, Franks R (1994) The hidden curriculum, ethics teaching and the structure of medical education. Acad med 69:861–871

Hattery R (2002) The physician's charter in the new millennium published by the American Board of Internal Medicine, the American College of Physicians/American Society of Internal Medicine, and the European Federation of Internal Medicine. Ann Intern Med 136:243–246

Ihara CK (1988) Collegiality as a professional virtue. In: Flores A (ed) Professional ideals. Wadsworth, New York

Johnson MS, Marcia N, Gonzales JD, Shelley Bizila MS, CIP (2005) Responsible conduct of radiology research part v: The health insurance portability and accountability act and research. Radiol 237:757–764

Maïmonide MHA. La Priere Medicale. Science et Médecine http://www.lamed.fr/societe/science/459.asp

McKarthy K, Smith C (eds) (2007) The royal college of physicians and surgeons of Canada 2006 annual report. http://rcpsc.medical.org/publications/annual_report_en.pdf

Oljeski SA, Homer MJ, Krackov WS. Incorporating Ethics Education into the Radiology Residency Curriculum: A Model. AJR 2004; 183:569–572

Learning in Practice: New Approaches to Professional Development for Radiologists

10

I.J. Parboosingh, B.P. Wood, L.M. Samson, C.M. Campbell

Radiologists, as other professionals, acquire their expertise from two coexisting learning paradigms. In the first, learning is planned, with observable objectives and performance outcomes to be assessed. This remains the model of traditional formal education, including continuing medical education (CME), a complex and extensive component of lifelong education. The effectiveness of this learning model in today's rapidly expanding and complex environment remains limited (Davis et al. 1995). The second paradigm emphasizes learning from experience and is driven by three motivating forces: practice and performance creates the curriculum; reflection powers the learning process; but one's self controls learning. Unlike formal education, learning and evaluation of learning in practice has not been extensively researched (Kuper et al. 2007). Knowledge-intensive work traditionally relies on learning from practice and has a research literature.

Radiologists' work partners and collaborating physicians are all participants in learning in practice; with additional sources of knowledge such as texts, journals (published or on-line), focused databases, the image and record system, and learning conferences and other group-learning sources. This chapter is focused on the paradigm of practice learning.

10.1
A Department of Radiology Narrative

"Dr. Mary Brown," we shall say, is an assistant professor in a university department of radiology, and is one of 36 faculty radiologists. The department is staffed by 90 support staff, nine nurses, eight coordinators, and three managers. The unit performs 570,000

I.J. Parboosingh (✉)

Obstetrics & Gynecology, and Medical Education, University of Calgary, Calgary, AB, Canada

E-mail: parboo@teusplanet.net

Radiology Education. R.K. Chhem et al. (Eds.)

DOI: 10.1007/978-3-540-68989-8, © Springer-Verlag Berlin Heidelberg 2009

procedures each year, with an expected annual increase of 2%. The department is committed to undergraduate (medical student) and postgraduate (residency) education programs: 24 senior medical students learn in the department annually and 24 residents distributed over their 4 years of training learn from radiologists while fulfilling the Royal College of Physicians and Surgeons of Canada accredited postgraduate curriculum for general and interventional radiology.

10.2
Learning Habits Emphasized During Residency

Dr. Brown accepted a position in the radiology faculty because of her positive experience as a resident. While learning the specialty of radiology was her primary goal, her teachers placed equal emphasis on helping her to become a self-directed learner. This training program encouraged and supports residents' initiative and competence in developing autonomous lifelong learning behavior (Derrick 2003). These learning habits reflect the progressive shifts in postgraduate medical education towards competency in and understanding of lifelong learning skills. Individuals' skills are not always sufficient to sustain continuous learning; therefore, creating and sustaining a learning culture in radiology residency programs is integral to establishing competence in lifelong learning. Dr. Brown was encouraged to develop the framework for learning described by Butler (1996) which has proven useful in her busy practice. In this model, *practice and performance* creates the curriculum, *reflection* powers the learning process, and *self* is the locus of control.

10.3
Programs Supporting Professional Development and Practice Enhancement: A Historical Perspective

A discussion of learning in practice would be incomplete without a brief summary of formal educational initiatives established in North America over the past century. Among them are continuing medical education (CME), continuing professional development (CPD), practice-based learning and improvement (PBLI), and quality improvement (QI).

CME, focused on updating medical knowledge, has attracted a large education industry based on conferences and sponsored largely by pharmaceutical and medical device industries. Practice improvement has been the goal of CME programs, although change in physician behavior and improved patient outcomes is unproven (Davis et al. 1995). CPD, described in the 1980s, reflects a broader base of competencies, sharing of tacit knowledge (Brigley et al. 1997), and incorporating experiential wisdom as well as explicit, research-derived knowledge. The competency of PBLI encourages residents and practicing physicians to demonstrate the principles embraced by CPD. PBLI involves four steps of the learning cycle described by Kolb (1984): identify areas of practice needing improvement, engage in appropriate learning, integrate new knowledge and skills into practice, and check for improvement. QI programs have recently been endorsed by physician organizations. QI programs aim to improve efficiency, create safer patient care, and improve patient health outcomes, while focusing interventions on evidence-based science.

Public demand for both quality care and patient safety emphasizes the endorsement of these programs by professional organizations and attracts participation by physicians. Batalden and Davidoff (2007) emphasize the integration of QI into the daily lives of practitioners in their statement "...everyone who works in health care recognizes that they have two jobs when they come to work every day, i.e., doing the work and improving it". The Royal College of Physicians and Surgeons of Canada's Maintenance of Certification Program (RCPSC 2008) and the American Board of Radiology's Practice Quality Improvement program (Strife et al. 2007) actively support participation in continuing QI in the pursuit of excellence in radiology practice A later section of this chapter discusses the roles and responsibilities of radiologists as individuals and collaborators in QI programs. We will next focus on the components of Butler's framework.

10.4
Practice Models the Lifelong-Learning Curriculum

An increasing and widely dispersed technical and biomedical information base and the increasing technical complexity of imaging methods have resulted in increased patient referrals and subspecialization, so the workplace is diverse and finely focused. Meanwhile the practice of medicine is changing (Coles 2000), with increasingly complex problem solving, clinical judgment, tacit knowledge use, and experiential wisdom in clinical situations that are complex, unique, uncertain, and with conflicting values, a type of work referred to by Johnson et al. (2005) as *tacit work*. Increasing complexity or obscurity of hypotheses with more specific choices of testing in the presence of disease information and the need for efficiency drives today's diagnostic testing procedures.

The practice and knowledge of medicine is more complex as the workload increases, leaving less time for learning. Not surprisingly, physicians are seeking better help with decisions about learning and more efficient and direct methods of learning. Focusing on the knowledge and information most relevant to their practice and immediate professional needs is the result. As radiologists in North America prepare for maintenance of certification they establish a practice profile based on the organ systems, diagnostic categories, patient age, and imaging technologies that are relevant to their consultation patterns. Educational needs that are identified by deficiencies in clinical practice are used to create a learning plan to drive personal learning. Dr. Brown uses multiple information sources to fulfill her learning plan, which she submits annually for maintenance of certification. Features of her practice profile enable Dr. Brown to efficiently focus learning on questions and topics of radiology relevant to her needs. The built-in opportunity to reflect on her own practice experiences and questions and to learn from them shows how Dr. Brown uses practice to create a personal curriculum for learning.

10.5
Reflective Practice Drives the Learning Processes

Coles (2000), studying physicians, and Johnson et al. (2005), reporting on tacit workers in many disciplines, indicate that we learn mainly by reflecting on experiences. Health professionals perceive their practice behaviors as most closely aligned with the three stages of Schön's reflective cycle (Schon 1987).

10.5.1
Knowing-in-Action

Schön describes zones of expertise (ZOE) which differentiate experts from novices. A ZOE is defined by the competencies and capabilities we use routinely to solve problems through a process of *knowing-in-action*. Solving problems by knowing-in-action is routine and mostly automated, requiring little or no critical thinking. Schön describes knowing-in-action as being tacit and thus not possible to record or archive, but it is shared by informal discussions among practitioners in a community of practice. However, many problems are not clear. Routinely using the same solutions can blind us to subtle differences in features of a problem that might lead to a different solution. Knowing-in-action requires vigilance as an element of our expertise.

10.5.2
Reflection-in-Action

When we encounter surprises, unusual or unexplained features, or unexpected factors during routine work, we are led to consider additional factors and diagnoses, seek additional data, and often seek additional information. In our example, Dr. Brown, reviewing the chest radiograph of an elderly patient referred with a clinical diagnosis of pneumonia, recognizes several unusual features that do not fit her mental model that is a categorization of pneumonia features. While seeking additional data, Dr. Brown reviews the patient's medical record and determines that he is a smoker. She consults on the images with a colleague considering the features that fit a diagnosis of lung cancer but not pneumonia, and notifies the care-giving team of additional imaging and other testing that is appropriate to solve the problem. Reflection-in-action often leads to literature searches and confirmation of information hidden in memory. A motivating element of reflection-in-action is that it is a response to an unusual or unexpected feature outside an otherwise characteristic pattern. It is necessary to be alert to recognize and respond to the unexpected or outlier, and to pursue defining sources of information to lead diagnostic decisions.

10.5.3
Reflection-on-Action

In this phase of the reflective cycle, practitioners look back critically over unexpected features and their resolution of the problem. New information may be reviewed and evaluated, a process which can lead to elaboration on our learning. What is newly learned is assimilated as experience, thereby enriching our mental store of categories and their exemplars and ultimately enhancing knowing-in-action. Learning that occurs during clinical care serves to provide us with varied experience and increases expertise. At the same time it reduces the frequency of surprise, a key missed feature, or a mistake in interpretation the next time a similar problem is encountered. Information seeking during the process of reflection-on-action adds to our skills in formulating and searching for information on critical thinking questions, guides accurate location and critical appraisal of scientific evidence, and helps with its appropriate application in similar situations. The final step in this cycle is integration of new knowledge into knowing-in-action. This step often involves interacting with peers and others in a process of collective reflection (Frankford et al. 2000). Radiologists in the USA and Canada may earn credit towards maintenance of certification by submitting documentation of their application of the reflective process in learning during practice.

10.5.4
Research Supports Reflection in Practice

Mann et al. (2007) systematically reviewed and summarized the evidence-based literature on reflective practice. There is evidence that professionals reflect in different ways and to different degrees, and that there may be better learning from those experiences incorporating reflection. Research supports the premise that ability to reflect develops over time, with practice, and in the presence of stimuli such as interaction with colleagues. The work environment and the practices of colleagues and mentors can have an encouraging or inhibiting effect on reflective thinking. Reflection decreases with increasing years in practice, probably because expertise increases. It is speculated that increasing clinical experience with knowing-in-action is most often sufficient to address clinical problems. Evidence is present to support the belief that reflection is inhibited in busy practices or where practitioners tend to work as individuals and do not share practice experiences.

10.6
Embedding Learning in a Practice Environment

10.6.1
Communities of Practice

The adult learner was characterized as self-directed and goal-oriented by Tough (1971) and Knowles (1975). Cole (2000) and Johnson et al. (2002) point out that though "self" remains the locus of control, sharing practice experiences with colleagues and partners provides a major source of learning and knowledge creation for the adult learner engaged in the work of professional practice. The term "communities of practice" (CoPs) refers to groups with shared passion and goals who collectively learn how to perform better through ongoing interaction (Wenger et al. 2002). Through storytelling, for example, they critically reconstruct practice experiences, describe and seek validation of improvisations, and engage in generative dialogue (Pawar 2005) in search of opportunities to enhance practice or performance. Experiences in the knowledge-intensive industries (Wenger et al. 2002; Saint-Onge and Wallace 2003) indicate that CoPs enhance team cohesiveness and outcomes more effectively than do traditional work-related training programs. Gittell et al. (2000) reporting a study in health care showed that quality of communication and relationships among health care providers is associated with improved care for patients undergoing total joint arthroplasty. That health professionals learn well in communities is not new (Parboosingh 2002). What is new is the need for management and accrediting bodies to invest in community as a major vehicle for postgraduate education and continuous practice improvement. National bodies are aggressively promoting the introduction of CoPs in health care organizations, academic departments, and practices. Helping professionals find the time and environment to interact on a regular basis and to focus and improve their communications has presented challenges and slowed progress towards meeting these objectives (Fletcher 2008).

Traditional communication methods used at committee meetings, rounds, and journal clubs tend to advocate best practice, defend positions, and use evidence to achieve closure. The process stifles creative thinking and inquiry. In contrast, newer methods, sometimes called generative dialogue, are aimed at advancing beyond the participants' initial states of knowledge (Pawar 2005). In generative dialogue, participants use stories (narrative) to better understand differing perspectives and interpretations. Doing so builds trust, exploration of concepts, shared understanding and innovative thinking, and raises the collective knowledge of the CoP. However, change and adoption of new patterns of thought requires time, interest, training, and leadership and there are no published reports focused on radiology departments. Pawar (2005) uses case studies to describe efforts to foster CoPs in health institutions. But more traditional methods of knowledge defense, justification, and sharing persist. With the increasing presence of Generation Y in the medical workforce, changes involving collaboration and group learning are certain to increase as this generation is heavily reliant on sharing information, collaboration, and communication in problem-solving situations.

10.6.2
Interprofessional Collaborative Learning

Higher education has consistently viewed community as essential to create collaborative learning (Garrison and Arbaugh 2007). There is increasing information and experience with the role of community in interpersonal and team education, in which trainees of different disciplines learn from each other as they interact in a practice (Suter et al. 2008). In the learning environment we envisage for radiology departments, practicing professionals, students, and residents of all disciplines, referring physicians, and patients are "partners in the organization" and mentor each other using techniques defined by the term *lateral*

mentoring (Polin et al. 2001). In such a culture, residents and students of multiple disciplines are members of CoPs throughout their training where they participate in discussions and learn from the exchange of ideas and practical tips arising during reconstruction and discussion of practice experiences that invariably dominate conversations. As well as learning to respect different perspectives, ideas, and sources of evidence emerging from discussions, students and residents acquire important skills such as clinical judgment, problem solving, and improvisation while solving problems in practice. They additionally learn the value of continuously reexamining data and opinions.

Trainees, educated in classroom environments, are not experienced in the self-management of learning. Indeed, as Candy (1991) states, "spending years in teacher centered educational settings has reduced many professionals to passive learners and deprived them of the confidence to take charge of their learning." We predict it will take time and practice for many trainees and graduates to give priority to planning their own learning.

Nonetheless, introduction of learning groups or learning teams, who have a diversity of experience and opinion, yet are working towards a common goal, will enhance greatly the ability of our trainees to participate in such experiences throughout their professional lives. After working in such environments, learners are confident in expressing their opinions and conclusions, listening to those of others, and modifying their outlook when persuasive points of view are offered. Because the whole is greater than the sum of the parts, they respect the ideas of others and will work together to accomplish common goals.

10.7
Working Towards a Culture of Learning

Individuals alone are not enough to support continuous learning and performance improvement. Building and sustaining a learning culture in today's radiology departments is essential. Berwick (2003) suggests establishing a culture of professionals working in teams to become "citizens in the improvement of their own work." Also promoting culture change, Coiera (2004) states, "The biggest information repository in most organizations sits in the heads of the people who work there, and the largest communication network is the web of conversations that binds them. Together, people, tools, and conversations form the system." According to Westrum (2004), culture determines how information flows in an organization and how information is used determines the culture, which in turn shapes the quality of service and other organizational goals, including professional development and job satisfaction.

Embedding continuous learning in the work environment is essential as the workload and the number of workers from different disciplines increase. While the concept of embedding learning in practice is new in health care, the practice works efficiently in knowledge-intensive industries. The process involves establishing systems that work in the background while practitioners cope with the workload. It will encourage radiologists to focus on providing high-quality, safe patient care knowing that there is a system in place that "manages practice enhancements." Leaders in Westrum's "generative organizations" set reward systems and assign resources to activities that promote interdisciplinary collaborative learning and knowledge generation. This involves appointing a quality improvement officer, allocating

time for meetings and discussion, fostering strategic CoPs, training facilitators for community development and dialogue facilitation, and establishing mentorship and orientation programs for new staff (Saint-Onge and Wallace 2003).

Providing information and communication technologies to enhance collaboration and manage information flow and knowledge creation is an essential component of the infrastructure of departments and clinics working towards embedding learning in practice.

10.8
Practice Assessment and Performance Enhancement

Few physicians understand the complexity of the health care system, yet a comprehending view of the system is critical to understanding changes and advances in knowledge, improved patient health outcomes, quality, and safety. Strife et al. (2007) acknowledge the public demand for high-quality care, while recognizing that a significant proportion of physician practice is not supported by sound scientific evidence. The publication summarizes the QI performance that radiologists must meet for certification. The key characteristics of the American Board of Radiology's Practice Quality Improvement project encourage radiologists to develop proficiency in the systems in which they practice while learning and improving practice (PBLI). The cycle of PBLI actively supported by maintenance of certification programs in Canada and the USA involves four steps: identifying areas for needed improvement through assessment of professional practice gaps, engaging in focused learning, applying the new knowledge and skills to practice, and, finally, checking for improvement in competence, performance, or patient outcomes.

Practice assessment involves measuring practice processes and outcomes through auditing, reflection, and feedback or multisource feedback. Regional and national benchmarks are used to identify gaps between optimal and actual practice and opportunities for improvement. PBLI involves critical analysis of the literature in a search for evidence-based practices and guidelines, and then setting plans for learning that lead to incorporation of changes in practice. Though the PBLI cycle seems simple, Graham et al. (2006) remind us of its subtle complexity and the frequent barriers to implementation of change. Not surprisingly, a review of studies that describe guideline implementation reported by Grimshaw et al. (2004) reveals only a 9% overall improvement in clinical practice.

Innovative methods focus on the goals of continuous QI, which are, according to Erturk et al. (2005), to determine and meet the needs of patients; to approach QI by identifying the underlying cause of poor performance; to apply fact-based management and scientific method; and to empower practitioners to improve quality on a regular basis. Swensen and Johnson (2005) describe the use of a radiology quality map to track the path of a patient through a radiology department in order to identify opportunities for process and outcome improvements.

Another approach to QI recognizes that clinical departments are complex adaptive systems (CAS). A CAS is a collection of individuals (e.g., clinicians, staff, administrators, and patients) whose actions are interconnected such that one person's action changes the

context for other individuals in the system (McDaniel and Driebe 2001). The ability of a CAS to adapt in a manner that allows for change or improvement is enhanced by improving the quality and quantity of communication. A study of organizational features that support innovation in clinical practices found improvement in communication and participation among people at all levels of the practice to be a key feature (Thomas et al. 2005). This approach to QI is consistent with the steps described above to embed learning and continuous improvement in the culture and practice of a department.

10.9
Management of Learning in Practice

Important indicators and documentation of learning in practice are observed by all specialists. Documentation of maintenance of competence and quality of performance demonstrate to society that physicians have met certain quality expectations of accurate, timely, and appropriate care fostered by CPD. Fulfilling guidelines of QI and continuous learning should not be a burden for specialists, heavily committed to efficiency in a busy practice, fulfilling organizational and management responsibilities, and participating in family life. Radiologists must respond to major technology changes, expectations of increased efficiency, and heightened responsiveness to the needs of patients and of referring physicians and peers. At the same time, there are changes in the practice of medicine, the medical record, and ordering and reporting methods. While requiring competence, there are also increasing safety and considerations of appropriateness of a study to answer a clinical question.

Development and use of a *personal development plan* (PDP) confirms that CPD is undertaken seriously and effectively, and is focused on changes within the specialty and the need for regard of radiation issues, patient comfort, and cost of studies. Some categories to be included are competence, management issues, communication, safety, and QI.

10.9.1
Information Sources

In concert with lifelong learning are the principles of efficient and easy access to sources of information and the ability to evaluate, assimilate, and apply knowledge in response to a variety of clinical queries. A folder with this designation is set up to help Dr. Brown organize the avalanche of new information that she must scan to keep up to date. Dr. Brown has subscribed to several pertinent RSS feeds providing new information related to her practice profile and learning plans and uses an RSS reader to direct her reading. She uses RSS feeds from specialty associations, the Royal College (RCPSC) Web sites and select online journals. Dr. Brown uses a book shelf to file full-text articles to which she refers regularly and also an online reference manager.

10.9.2
Learning Plans and Projects

Dr. Brown keeps an electronic learning portfolio of insights extracted from her reading and ideas from meetings and personal learning projects (PLP) which she submits for maintenance of certification (Campbell et al. 1996).

10.9.3
Networks

Dr. Brown belongs to a number of working groups (communities of practice) that meet regularly, using listservers and online discussion boards to discuss select aspects of practice and professional life. Dr. Brown finds her online communities, many of which are task-oriented and include professionals from disciplines other than radiology, to be an efficient way of exchanging new information and ideas for practice enhancement.

10.9.4
Recognition of Expertise

In this folder of her PDP, Dr. Brown keeps an updated curriculum vitae and requirements for maintenance of certification and validation of license to practice. Dr. Brown records and electronically submits on an ongoing basis PLPs and the results of practice audits, in addition to participation in rounds and conferences to the Royal College (RCPSC) to fulfill her requirements for maintenance of certification.

10.10
Conclusions

As the twenty-first century enfolds, we are witnessing a shift in emphasis in CPD from provider-dominated to learner-centered practice-based learning and, at the same time, a shift in the vision of the radiologist from that of an autonomous independent learner to one who is "connected" with colleagues, works in a learning environment, and whose CPD activities are focused on performance enhancement. In spite of these subtle shifts in CPD, learning activities still require the ability to self-monitor, to use educational resources appropriately, to be selective in the adoption of new practices, and to be knowledgeable of the changes peers are introducing into their practices. In addition, there are increasing pressures for leadership that not only fosters a learning culture even in the busiest radiology clinic, but that also provides resources that assist radiologists to embed continuous practice enhancement in their daily activities.

References

Batalden P, Davidoff F (2007) Teaching quality improvement: The devil is in the details. JAMA 298:1059–1061

Berwick DM (2003) Improvement, trust, and the healthcare workforce. Qualit Saf Heal Care 12:448

Brigley S, Young Y, Littlejohns P, McEwen J (1997) Continuing education for medical professionals: A reflective model. Postgrad Med J 73:23–26

Butler J (1996) Professional development: Practice as text, reflections as process, and self as locus. Aust J Ed 40:265–283

Campbell C, Parboosingh J, Gondocz T, Babitskya G, Lindsay E, De Guzman R, Klein L (1996) Study of physicians' use of a software program to create a portfolio of their self-directed learning. Academ Med 71:s49–s51

Candy PC (1991) Self-direction for lifelong learning, Jossey-Bass Higher and Adult Education Series. Jossey-Bass, San Francisco

Coiera E (2004) Four rules for the reinvention of health care. BMJ 328:1197–1199

Coles C (2000) Developing our intuitive knowing: An alternative approach to the assessment of doctors. In: Bashook PG, Miller SH, Parboosingh J, Horowitz SG (eds) Credentialing physician specialists: A world perspective: Proceedings of the conference held in Chicago. The Royal College of Physicians and Surgeons of Canada, Ottawa and the American Board of Medical Specialties, Evanston

Davis DA, Thomson MA, Oxman AD, Haynes RB (1995) Changing physician performance. A systematic review of the effect of continuing medical education strategies. JAMA 274:700–705

Derrick GM (2003) Creating environments conducive for lifelong learning. New Dir Adult Cont Educ 100:5–15

Erturk SM, Ondategui-Parra S, Ros PR (2005) Quality management in radiology: Historical aspects and basic definitions. J Am Coll Radiol 2:985–991

Fletcher SW (2008) Chairman's summary of the conference. In: Hager M (ed) Continuing education in the health professions: Improving healthcare through lifelong learning, 2007 Nov 28 – Dec 1, Bermuda. Josiah Macy Jr. Foundation, New York

Frankford DM, Patterson MA, Konrad RT (2000) Transforming practice organizations to foster lifelong learning and commitment to medical professionalism. Acad Med 175:708–717

Garrison R, Arbaugh JB (2007) Researching the community of inquiry framework: Review, issues, and future directions. Int High Educ 10:157–172

Gittell JH, Fairfield KM, Bierbaum B, Head W, Jackson R, Kelly M et al. (2000) Impact of relational coordination on quality of care, postoperative pain and functioning, and length of stay; a nine-hospital study of surgical patients. Medical care 38(8):807–819.

Graham ID, Logan J, Harrison MB, Straus SE, Tetroe J, Caswell W and Robinson N (2006) Lost in knowledge translation: Time for a map. J Contin Educ Health Prof 26:13–24

Grimshaw J, Eccles M, Tetroe J (2004) Implementing clinical guidelines: Current evidence and future implications. J Contin Educ Health Prof 24(Sp1):S31–S37

Johnson BC, Manyika JM and Yee LA (2005) The next revolution in interaction. The McKinsey quarterly: The Online Journal of McKinsey & Co, Volume 4: http://www.mckinseyquarterly.com/article_page.aspx?ar=1690&L2=18&L3=30&srid=27&gp=0 Accessed 24 April 2008

Knowles MS (1975) Self-directed learning: A guide for learners and teachers. Associated Press, New York

Kolb D (1984). Experiential learning. Prentice-Hall, Englewood Cliffs

Kuper A, Reeves S, Albert M, Hodges BD (2007) Assessment: Do we need to broaden our methodological horizons? Med Educ 41:1121–1123

Mann K, Gordon J, MacLeod A (2007) Reflection and reflective practice in health professions education: a systematic review. Adv Health Sci Educ. doi:10.1007/s10459-007-9090-2

McDaniel R, Driebe D (2001) Complexity science and health care management. In: Blair JD, Fottler MD and Savage GT (eds) Advances in health care management vol 2. JAI Press, Stamford

Parboosingh J (2002) Physician communities of practice: where learning and practice are unseparable. J. Continuing Education in Health Professions. 24(4):230–236.

Pawar M (2005) Committees and boards in healthcare organizations: Barriers to organizational learning? Reflect 6:12–22

Polin L et al (2001) Lateral mentoring. Pepperdine University Online Master of Arts in Educational Technology, unpublished PDF

RCPSC (2008) RCPSC Maintenance of Certification Program Guide 2008. The Royal College of Physicians and Surgeons of Canada, Ottawa http://rcpsc.medical.org/opd/moc-program/index.php. Accessed 24 April 2008

Saint-Onge H, Wallace D (2003) Leveraging communities of practice for strategic advantage. Butterworth Heinemann, an imprint of Elsevier

Schon DA (1987) Educating the reflective practitioner. Jossey Bass, San Francisco, CA

Strife JL, Kun LE, Becker GJ, Dunnick NR, Bosma J, Hattery RR (2007) The American Board of Radiology Perspective on maintenance of certification: Part IV—Practice quality improvement in diagnostic radiology. RadioGraph 27:769–774

Suter E, Arndt J, Arthur N, Parboosingh J, Taylor E, Deutschlander S. Role understanding and effective communication as core competencies for collaborative practice. J. Interprofessional Care 2008. In press.

Swensen SJ, Johnson CD (2005) Radiologic quality and safety: Mapping value into radiology. J Am Coll Radiol 2:992–1000

Thomas P, McDonnell J, McCulloch J, While A, Bosanquet N, Ferlie E (2005) Increasing capacity for innovation in bureaucratic primary care organizations: A whole system participatory action research project. Ann Fam Med 3:312–317

Tough A (1971) The adult learning projects: A fresh approach to theory and practice in adult learning. Ontario Institute for Studies in Education, Toronto, Canada

Wenger E, McDermott R, Snyder W (2002) Cultivating communities of practice: A guide to managing knowledge. Harvard Business School Press, Boston

Westrum R (2004) A typology of organizational cultures. Qual Saf Health Care 13:22–27

Acquiring Competencies in Radiology: The CanMEDS Model

11

R.K. Chhem, L.M. Samson, J.R. Frank, J. Dubois

11.1
Introduction and History of CanMEDS

Over the past decade and a half, the CanMEDS initiative has become the Royal College of Physicians and Surgeons of Canada's flagship standards document in Canada. Described fundamentally as an initiative focused on improving patient care, the framework evolved through ongoing collaboration with hundreds of Royal College Fellows, family physician educators, educationalists, and other contributors (Frank 2005). In 2001, a diagram of CanMEDS was created to capture both the elements and the interconnectivity among the elements (see Fig. 1).

The CanMEDS initiative first began in the early 1990s through a desire to reform medical education and ensure that Canadian physicians were prepared to thrive in a changing health care environment (Frank 2005). As early as the late 1980s, Royal College Fellows began to write to the Royal College to raise their concerns about the changes in health care and the resulting need to train physicians to adapt to these changes. The types of changes that were particularly prominent at the time included, for example, "patient consumerism, government regulations, financial imperatives, access to medical information on the Internet, litigation, technology and the explosion of medical knowledge" (Frank 2005).

Thus, in direct response to the evolving health care environment and the mounting concerns of its Fellows, "the College's Health and Public Policy Committee created a Societal Needs Working Group (SNWG) to 'identify the core competencies generic to all specialists to meet the needs of society'" (Frank 2005).

The initial concept of identifying the tasks or behaviors required of physicians, and then organizing these into distinct roles, emerged from the work of the Educating Future Physicians

R.K. Chhem (✉)
Department of Medical Imaging, Schulich School of Medicine
and Dentistry, University of Western Ontario, London, ON, Canada N6A 5C1
E-mail: rethy.chhem@lhsc.on.ca

Radiology Education. R.K. Chhem et al. (Eds.)
DOI: 10.1007/978-3-540-68989-8, © Springer-Verlag Berlin Heidelberg 2009

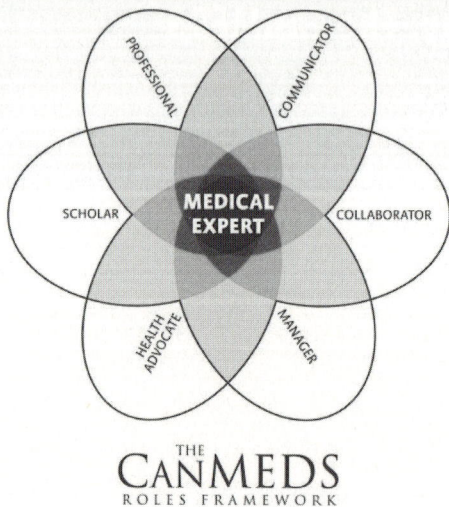

Fig. 1 A diagram was created in 2001 to illustrate the elements and the interconnections of the Can-MEDS roles embodied by competent physicians: medical expert (the central role), communicator, collaborator, health advocate, manager, scholar, and professional. This diagram, also known as the CanMEDS "cloverleaf," "daisy," "flower," and "illustration," was officially trademarked in 2005 and was revised to more accurately reflect the fluidity and overlap amongst the CanMEDS roles

for Ontario (EFPO) project, whose goal has been to make education in Ontario more responsive to evolving health needs of the province. As EFPO's focus was on Ontarians and all physicians providing health care for that population, it was necessary to reexamine the issues to make them more germane to the tasks required of specialist physicians serving patients across Canada. The process began with extensive reviews of the relevant published and unpublished literature, including consumer surveys and focus groups. From this information, general competencies of specialists were extracted and these were clustered into seven major roles (Frank et al. 1996).

In order to understand the concept of CanMEDS, it is important to first clarify how the terminology being used is defined.

11.2
What Is Educational Competency?

The paradigm shift from structure- and process-based to competency-based education and outcomes evaluation was considered as a second "Flexnerian revolution" by Carraccio hearkening back to the first "revolution" triggered by the Flexner report on medical education in 1910 (Carraccio et al. 2002). Carraccio et al. (2002) describe "competency" as a "complex set of behaviors built on the components of knowledge, skills, attitudes, and competence as personal ability."

Albanese (2008) further proposed five criteria which can be used to define a competency:

1. It focuses on the performance of the end product or goal state of instruction.
2. It reflects expectations that are external to the immediate instructional program.
3. It is expressible in terms of measurable behavior.
4. It uses a standard for judging competence that is not dependent upon the performance of other learners.
5. It informs learners, as well as other stakeholders, about what is expected of them.

The definition of competency is much more complex than a simple learning objective and demands a certain level of integration. For example, a physician who is competent in his patient communication skills will need to integrate several additional elements that inform this competency, such as empathy, synthesis of the information to be communicated, avoidance of medical jargon, and active, effective listening, to name a few. Also, in order to ensure that the communication is effective, the physician needs to mobilize his/her internal resources (knowledge, skills, and attitude) as well as his/her external resources (appropriate environment, office and administrative assistance). Indeed, the physician needs to adapt this competency into a specific clinical situation: communicating with a trauma patient in the emergency room calls for a different set of skills than communicating with intensive care unit patient's relatives. This notion of "situation" or "family of situations" determines the choice of the appropriate resources and capacities used in effective communication.

11.3
What Is Outcome-Based Education?

From the early 1990s, the concept of learning outcomes has been recognized and considered in physician education by the General Medical Council in the UK, the Association of American Medical Colleges in the USA, the Royal College of Physicians and Surgeons of Canada, and significantly by the Accreditation Council for Graduate Medical Education (Harden 2002a, b). In a structure- and process-based model, the driving forces of curriculum and process are the content and the teacher. In a competency-based model, the driving forces are the outcome and the learner (Carraccio et al. 2002).

"Outcome-based education is defined as (Harden 2002a):

> The development of clearly defined and published learning outcomes that must be achieved before the end of the course
> The design of a curriculum, learning strategies and learning opportunities to ensure the achievement of the learning outcome
> An assessment process matched to the learning outcomes and the assessment of individual students to ensure that they achieve the outcomes
> The provision of remediation and enrichment for students as appropriate"

The emphasis on learning outcomes is helpful to both students and teachers. The approach helps students plan for their learning effectively as it makes "it clear what students can

11

hope to gain from following a particular course" (Harden 2002a). Similarly learning outcomes also ensure that the teacher begins with the "end" in mind, thereby allowing appropriate planning decisions to flow from how they will best assist the teacher and student to achieve the desired outcomes. This includes decisions around that end to plan the content of the teaching, design the teaching material more effectively, set a blueprint for examination using the outcomes, and finally ensure that appropriate assessment strategies are selected (Jenkins and Unwin 2001). Harden makes very clear the difference between instructional objectives and learning outcomes that are related to "the detail of specification, the level of specification where the emphasis is placed, the classification adopted and interrelationships, the intent or observable result, and the ownership of the outcomes" (Harden 2002b).

11.4
What is CanMEDS?

CanMEDS is the acronym for Canadian Medical Education Directions for Specialists. This framework seeks to answer a fundamental question raised by the Royal College of Physicians and Surgeons of Canada in the early 1990s: "How can we best prepare physicians to be effective in this environment and truly meet the needs of their patients?" (Frank 2005). Why is there a need to establish CanMEDS? The main reason is the rapid changes of medical practice due to the evolution of biomedical and social changes in addition to the aging of the Canadian population (Frank 2005). The framework structure of CanMEDS is composed of seven thematic groups of competencies. Among them, the "medical expert" is the central integrative role. The competencies are divided in two main groups: the first are key competencies; the second are defined as enabling competencies.

11.5
CanMEDS and Radiology Competencies

The seven core CanMEDS competencies have been established for interventional radiologists (Baerlocher and Asch 2006). Because interventional radiologists are involved heavily with patient care by conducting complex procedures at all stage of disease management (from diagnostic to therapeutic, including follow-up with patient hospitalization), their profile is similar to that of any other attending clinicians. Therefore, the CanMEDS guidelines for this radiological practice include a comprehensive pattern of the seven core competencies and may serve as a baseline template for any other radiological specialties.

The typology of competencies is displayed on the CanMEDS Web site (Frank 2005). For the purpose of this review chapter, we will describe only the key competencies, along with some examples to illustrate either a key competency or enabling competencies.

11.5.1
Medical Expert

In order to fulfill his/her role as medical expert, the physician should be able to:

1. Function effectively as a consultant, integrating all of the CanMEDS roles to provide optimal, ethical, and patient-centered medical care
2. Establish and maintain clinical knowledge, skills, and attitudes appropriate to his/her practice
3. Perform a complete and appropriate assessment of a patient
4. Use preventive and therapeutic interventions effectively
5. Demonstrate proficient and appropriate use of procedural skills, both diagnostic and therapeutic
6. Seek appropriate consultation from other health professionals, recognizing the limits of her expertise (Frank 2005)

11.5.2
Communicator Role

In order to fulfill his/her role as communicator, the physician should be able to:

1. Develop rapport, trust, and ethical therapeutic relationships with patients and families
2. Accurately elicit and synthesize relevant information and perspectives of patients and families, colleagues, and other professionals
3. Accurately convey relevant information and explanations to patients and families, colleagues, and other professionals
4. Develop a common understanding on issues, problems, and plans with patients and families, colleagues, and other professionals to develop a shared plan of care
5. Convey effective oral and written information about a medical encounter (Frank 2005)

Similar to all other medical specialists and family medicine physicians, radiologists need to master communication skills since encounters with patient and family are numerous. Interventional radiologists, whether they perform vascular, nonvascular, neuroangiographic procedures practice like attending physicians with admission privileges and patient management responsibilities. This is even more critical in pediatric radiology, where communication with parents and family is a key parameter for success in their radiological "care." For interventional procedures, Baerlocher and Asch (2006) suggest that the physician as a communicator should be able to establish and maintain a therapeutic relationship with patients involving trust, empathy, understanding, and confidentiality, to elicit relevant information from patients, their families, friends, community, and other members of the health care team, and to effectively discuss care with patients, their personal supporters, and other members of the health care team.

Given the multicultural pattern of Canadian demography, radiologists need also to develop some cultural competencies in order to be able to communicate effectively with patients and colleagues from diverse backgrounds. Specific needs and expectations must be explicitly outlined in the residency program. Teaching strategies for developing communication skills must be integrated into the curriculum and assessed accordingly.

Confidentiality is of paramount importance and should be emphasized within the communication competency of a radiologist. The picture archiving and communication system workstation has become a nexus for case discussion between radiologists, residents, medical students, and attending physicians. In some cases, these workstations are located in close proximity to the patient waiting room. Care must be taken to ensure the patient's personal information is handled in a way that respects his/her privacy. Similarly, a specific set of communication skills are required to enable a radiologist to speak to a patient and procure informed consent to conduct a procedure. Critical information about the procedure, its advantages, and limitations, as well as potential complications must be disclosed and discussed with the patient, in clear, jargon-free language. For example, a radiologist must be able to explain the procedure for conducting an arthrography or bone biopsy to his/her patient in sufficiently clear language that would allow the patient to give informed consent for the procedure.

11.5.3
Collaborator Role

In order to fulfill his/her role as collaborator, the physician should be able to:

1. Participate effectively and appropriately in an interprofessional health care team
2. Effectively work with other health professionals to prevent, negotiate, and resolve interprofessional conflict (Frank 2005)

Examples of collaboration in radiology include contributions to interdisciplinary health care activities such as research, teaching, committee work, and consultation (i.e., during a bone tumor board). As a consultant in this example, the goal is to establish a management and therapeutic strategy for a patient with a bone tumor. The radiologist must be able to present a logical sequence of imaging files from the patient. He/she must also be able to establish efficient collaboration with other health care professionals, including imaging technicians, other radiologists, and clinicians.

11.5.4
Manager Role

In order to fulfill his role as manager, the physician should be able to:

1. Participate in activities that contribute to the effectiveness of the health care organizations and systems
2. Manage his/her practice and career effectively
3. Allocate finite health care resources appropriately
4. Serve in administration and leadership roles, as appropriate (Frank 2005)

The resident in radiology would be able to adjust to the workload and establish an efficient time management between reading conventional radial dossiers at workstations, while supervising computed tomography or magnetic resonance imaging and/or ultrasound at the same time. He/she should be able to conduct bone biopsy and arthrography. Also the radiologist should be able to review cases, do dictation, and sign reports. Finally, he/she would be able to also establish a schedule for academic activities either alone or with residents or medical students.

11.5.5
Health Advocate Role

In order to fulfill his/her role as health advocate, the physician should be able to (Frank 2005):

1. Respond to individual patient health needs and issues as part of patient care
2. Respond to the health needs of the communities that he/she serves
3. Identify the determinants of health of the populations that he/she serves
4. Promote the health of individual patients, communities, and populations

In radiology, the radiologist or senior resident should be able to explain to the patient, lay person, or physicians the principles of radiation protection and suggest reasonable options for the least-invasive X-rays or procedures for a specific clinical situation. The radiologist should be able to discuss technological advances and trends to understand the future of medical imaging and its impact on medical practice. Radiologists should be able to design a computed tomography protocol minimizing radiation and yet provide the relevant data for diagnosis to inform and educate other health care professionals about guidelines and standards for radiological practice.

11.5.6
Scholar Role

In order to fulfill his/her role as scholar, the physician should be able to (Frank 2005):

1. Maintain and enhance professional activities through ongoing learning
2. Critically evaluate information and its sources, and apply this appropriately to practice decisions
3. Facilitate the learning of patients, families, students, residents, other health professionals, the public, and others, as appropriate
4. Contribute to the creation, dissemination, application, and translation of new medical knowledge and practices

The radiologists should be able to contribute to collaborative clinical research with orthopedic surgeons, sport and exercise physicians, and rheumatologists, for example, or in clinical trials using imaging as a biomarker. Radiologists must have a working knowledge of epidemiology. They may contribute to teaching and learning during rounds, journal clubs, and teaching medical students. They must be able to discuss ethics in research, offer a critical appraisal of literature in the field, and practice evidence-based radiology.

11

11.5.7
Professional Role

In order to fulfill his/her role as professional, the physician should be able to (Frank 2005):

1. Demonstrate a commitment to his/her patients, profession, and society through ethical practice
2. Demonstrate a commitment to his/her patients, profession, and society through participation in profession-led regulation
3. Demonstrate a commitment to physician health and sustainable practice

In radiology, this means that the radiologist must maintain a transparent, ethical relationship with the medical imaging industry. It also means that radiologists must accept the responsibility for maintaining a healthy work–life balance for themselves and their professional colleagues.

11.6
Evaluation

Once the learning objectives and outcomes have been established according to the curriculum's requirement, it is fundamental to identify the most relevant and optimal tools for a valid and accurate assessment. The Royal College of Physicians and Surgeons of Canada has published a comprehensive introductory guide to assessment methods for CanMEDS competencies (Table 11.1). A detailed description of this evaluation and assessment process is beyond the scope of this chapter, however some key points will be stressed. In the context of assessment, reliability means "a way to deliver consistent results in the same situation time after time." Validity means "assessing intended knowledge, attitudes, skills or behaviours, that are accepted as legitimate by teachers and learners" (Bandiera et al. 2006). This assessment process should be placed in "a concrete, observable learner behaviours or well-defined components of a learner's knowledge base" (See p. 4 in Bandiera et al. 2006). The assessment items must be as explicit and descriptive as possible. Finally, some experts advocate the role and use of portfolio learning for personal and professional development (Snadden and Thomas 1998; Gordon 2003; Cole 2005).

11.7
Challenges for Implementation of the Competency Framework of CanMEDS

The successful implementation of the CanMEDS framework in the training of specialists requires a strategy that would involve four main domains:

Table 11.1 Key tools for assessing the CanMEDS competencies (Bandiera et al. 2006)

Medical expert	Communicator	Collaborator	Health advocate	Manager	Scholar	Professional
1. Written tests (MCQ, SAQ)	+++	+	++	++	+	++	+
2. Essays	++	+	+	+++	+	+	+
3. Oral exam	+++	+	+	+	*	*	+
4. Direct observation and ITER	+++	+++	+++	+++	+++	+++	+++
5. OSCE/SP	+++	+++	+++	++	*	*	+
6. Multi-source feedback	++	+++	+++	+++	+++	++	+++
7. Portfolio	++	++	+	+++	++	+++	+++
8. Simulations	+++	+	+++	*	++	*	++

1. Standard for curriculum teaching and assessment. The residency education objectives, program accreditation, residents' sessions, certification examinations, and maintenance of competence must be established to incorporate CanMEDS competencies. Their College Examination Board is using CanMEDS domains to create assessment blueprints to guide examination item development. Here CanMEDS must become the essential ingredient in residency education and continuing professional development.
2. Faculty development for CanMEDS. It is essential to ensure a genuine inclusion of the CanMEDS approach in teaching, learning, and assessment in residency teaching. CanMEDS workshops have been established to support the need for education for university, hospital departments, and a group of faculty members.
3. Research and development resources. The Royal College has created research and development grants to support scholarship related to CanMEDS implementation.
4. Outreach and communication. Finally, it is essential to establish an effective communication team to reach stakeholders (and to identify CanMEDS champions) in order to promote the implementation of CanMEDS on a national scale.

In addition to these four domains, one must keep in mind that in the context of globalization, establishing partnerships and collaboration across the globe is encouraged by openly sharing CanMEDS intellectual property worldwide. Further, interaction must be established with related health professionals that include nurses, chiropractors, physicians' assistants, pharmacists, and veterinarians. Many of those professions have adopted CanMEDS in their jurisdiction. The paradigm shift from process-based medical education to a competency-based and outcome evaluation requires an immense cultural change that would need a genuine commitment of all strata of the radiology training program (postgraduate studies vice-dean, program directors, faculty members, and the residents themselves). Profound cultural change means alteration of behavior, which is actually the ultimate goal of any educational intervention. Importantly, it appears that what began as a desire to develop a framework to support improved patient care has inspired a dialogue stimulating people to think deeply about their practice and values. Promoting reflection in this way aligns more

11

closely with Glassik's standards for scholarship (Glassik 2000) and is more likely to generate new knowledge and theory, stimulating further growth in the profession that promises to
ultimately improve patient care.

References

Albanese MA, Mejicano G, Mullan P, Kokotailo P, Gruppen L (2008) Defining characteristics of
    educational competencies. Med Educ 42:248–255
Baerlocher MO, Asch MR (2006) The interventional radiologist as "Clinician": What does it
    mean? CanMEDS for the interventional radiologist. CARJ 57:25–29
Bandiera G, Sherbino J, Frank JR (2006) The CanMEDS assessment tools handbook. An intro-
    ductory guide to assessment methods for the CanMEDS competencies. The Royal College of
    Physicians and Surgeons of Canada, Ottawa
Carraccio C, Wolfsthal SD, Englander R, Ferentz K, Martin C (2002) Shifting paradigms: From
    Flexner to competencies. Acad Med 77:361–367
Cole G (2005) The definition of "portfolio". Med Educ 39:1141
Frank JR (2005) The CanMEDS 2005 physician competency framework. Better standards, better
    physicians, better care. The Royal College of Physicians and Surgeons of Canada, Ottawa
Frank JR, Vanoss D (2007) The CanMEDS initiative: In preventing and outcomes-based frame-
    work of physician competencies. Med Teach 29:642–647
Frank JR, Jabbour M et al (1996) Skills for the new millennium: Report of the societal needs
    working group: CenMEDS 2000 project. The Royal College of Physicians and Surgeons of
    Canada, Ottawa
Glassik CE (2000) Boyer's expanded definitions of scholarship, the standards for assessing schol-
    arship, and the elusiveness of the scholarship of teaching. Acad Med 75:877–880
Gordon J (2003) Assessing students' personal and professional development using portfolios and
    interviews. Med Educ 37:335–340
Harden RM (2002a) Developments in outcome-based education. Med Teach 24:117–120
Harden RM (2002b) Learning outcomes and instructional objectives: Is there a difference? Med
    Teach 24:151–155
Jenkins A, Unwin D (2001) How to write learning outcomes. http://www.ncgia.ucsb.edu/educa-
    tion/curricula/giscc/units/format/outcomes.html. Accessed 15 December 2002
Snadden D, Thomas ML (1998) The use of portfolio learning in medical education. Med Teach
    20:190–199v

Technologies for Teaching: Exploring the Use of PACS, Databases, and Teaching Files

12

R.N. Rankin

12.1
Introduction

A radiologist sits at his workstation reviewing imaging procedures obtained from medical imaging machines in a variety of places, including his own institution, and others on the same geographical network. He comes to one procedure which shows an unusual combination of findings which bring to mind a number of questions which it would be prudent to answer before he commits his report to the patient's electronic chart, thereby giving the patient an irrevocable label of disease. Some of his questions can be answered by obtaining information from this patient's medical chart, which he does by direct access from the workstation at which he is sitting. Other questions may be answered by referring to information sources dealing with the particular diseases he is considering for the diagnosis and differential. Some of this information is textual, some pictorial as befits his role as an imaging specialist. The information sources may reside on his local network, or indeed anywhere else in the Internet-connected world. Using teaching files accumulated at his own and other institutions for image comparison, and textual information from databases reached via Internet search engines, he is able to refine his report to accurately indicate to the referring physician the preferred diagnosis in this case with a high degree of certainty.

The clinical report finished, he then selects the best representative images from the procedure and sends these off, together with some diagnostic information, but securely and suitably anonymized to conform with current laws regarding individuals' health and personal information, to the departmental archival database used for teaching purposes – the electronic equivalent of the old "film teaching file" or "film museum." At a later time, when there is respite from the urgency of clinical work, he can access this file, edit

R.N. Rankin
Department of Medical Imaging, Schulich School of Medicine
and Dentistry, University of Western Ontario, London, ON, Canada
E-mail: rankin@uwo.ca

Radiology Education. R.K. Chhem et al. (Eds.)
DOI: 10.1007/978-3-540-68989-8, © Springer-Verlag Berlin Heidelberg 2009

12

the images or text, and add important information from other specialties such as pathology, and reference material in Portable Document Format and other forms. In this way, and over time, he has managed to put together an impressive collection of interesting cases which he is now able to use in various forms for teaching purposes.

The departmental teaching file database is but one of several that reside on a local server, and from which this radiologist can pick cases for teaching purposes. These files can be made available to students at any time for ongoing learning purposes. Any of these images can be transferred directly from the database into standard programs used for teaching purposes (PowerPoint, Keynote). They can also be bookmarked into collections used for specific teaching episodes, and can further be used in this teaching file program or other programs used for assembling electronic learning sessions which students can be directed to use. When the students each complete a session, the radiologist/teacher is e-mailed with the results of that session, giving a direct assessment of the student's skills. The results of a group of students' review of these cases can further be used to direct a group learning session built around the case collection.

As the radiologist signs off on this case he also signs onto the MAINPORT Web site of the Royal College of Physicians and Surgeons of Canada (RCPSC). There he enters into his own personal database a record of this clinical encounter and the learning he attained through it. This becomes a part of his official record of professional development as an item of structured point of care learning, essential to his maintenance of licensure and recognition as an expert in his field. His use of the teaching files and structured learning sessions can also be recorded in the same way to confirm his roles of communicator and scholar.

This scenario reflects the potential of the current state of the art of the practice of radiology and nuclear medicine in most leading teaching centers in the Western world. The advent of digital imaging and the use of picture archiving and communication systems (PACS) for display and storage of all procedures in imaging departments, completely displacing the use of film, has led to major changes in the way in which both clinical practice and academic practice are performed. The potential for linkage of clinical information to academic resources is a benefit of this change, and opens up a number of possibilities in the further development of education in the imaging sciences. These changes advance the learning process for both students and the teacher. The important features of these changes are:

1. The availability of information to both the teacher and the student
2. The currency of information availability
3. The ability to use the information in a variety of ways to suit differing learning opportunities
4. The ability to provide feedback during learning sessions to enhance this process
5. The ability to provide feedback to the teacher for student assessment
6. Provision of a record of learning for the teacher/medical practitioner to support his roles as medical expert, professional, communicator, and scholar.

Each of these changes will be examined in greater detail and the importance of each change to the learning process detailed.

12.2
Information Availability and Its Currency

The "premise of resource-based learning is that as students become able to select their own learning materials from information resources, they become active, independent learners" (Breivik 1998). The students in medical imaging range from undergraduate medical students to postgraduate residents with a similar range in the imaging sciences associated with radiology and nuclear medicine. It should be assumed that they already have skills in using modern information resources, but need to learn about the quantity and quality of information sources available for their chosen profession. In this context, the radiologist is also a lifelong learner for whom the wide availability of information resources is a significant advance.

The range of local and other resources now available, because of the development of the digital imaging world and electronic networks, has increased significantly over the last two decades. Because most practice is now performed at a networked workstation, these resources are potentially available at any time during the performance of clinical work, or during review sessions with trainees at the workstation. This is a major change from the traditional "view-box" practice of radiology, leading to a much greater ease of learning in an ongoing practice situation for both the teacher and the student. This immediacy of availability of information is at the core of the changes to the learning environment, increasing relevancy for learning purposes. Even in a more structured learning session such as with a group of students these changes are still relevant. This is because it is likely that the equipment used to display teaching material is a standard networked workstation adapted for group teaching purposes with suitable electronic displays, and located in a classroom adapted for this purpose.

For the teacher the major change is in learning how to assess the importance of various information resources, and then how to best use these in the variety of learning situations in which they may be encountered. There is a wide choice of database software which can be used to build the "teaching files" on which much radiological learning takes place (Scarsbrook et al. 2005). The ideal teaching file software, according to Scarsbrook et al., would have the major features of versatility, accessibility, ease of use, compatibility, and flexibility. A Google search on "radiology teaching file software" gives about 42,900 hits, giving some idea as to the breadth of software available. Which particular type of software to use will depend very much on local decisions related to PACS, networks, and information technology support. Other internally located databases and external resources accessed over the Internet can be used in similar ways to the local teaching file archive. Some of these may already have a recognized stamp of authenticity (i.e., the American College of Radiology teaching file collection), but others may need individual assessment by the teacher using their own abilities as an expert in their field to do this.

There is no recognized guide to either the authenticity or the value of any of the many available teaching file resources. Each individual radiologist/teacher will have to apply his knowledge as an expert, scholar, and communicator to the use of any information resource in each learning opportunity. Probably of most use in this assessment will be knowledge of the source (i.e., an accredited university department), personal recommendation (i.e., knowledge of the author(s)), proven use in relevant clinical or teaching situations, and use of his skills as an expert in the field.

12.3
Information Use to Suit the Learning Opportunity

Take the example of a clinical case used for teaching in both undergraduate and postgraduate situations. The example we will use is based on a patient's chest X-ray showing abnormalities related to cardiac disease. For the patient this leads to additional clinical and radiographic workup.

For the undergraduate learning situation the information presented by the use of the initial chest X-ray should lead to learning about basic abnormalities which may be found in cardiac disease on chest X-ray, and an initial investigative pathway to further the diagnosis and treatment of the condition suspected.

For the postgraduate student the use of the chest X-ray in a learning situation should present the opportunity to describe in detail all the abnormal findings on the examination and workup a favored diagnosis and relevant differential diagnoses. The student should also be able to accurately define further investigations, particularly those related to his specialty, and to then assess the results of those investigations to confirm the actual diagnosis.

In either case this scenario could happen in a clinical situation at the workstation, or in a more structured individual or group learning session, or in a situation of knowledge assessment. In any of these situations, use of information resources available at the site of learning may enhance the learning opportunity. In the digital imaging world, with its multiplicity of available information sources, these can be accessed and used as part of the learning process. A key component of this scenario is the availability of a fully integrated network, so all resources are available at the primary workstation. It is also important for the teacher in these situations to be able to assess the information accessed to ensure it is relevant to the level of knowledge of the student, and is used in an appropriate manner. It is this assessment which presents challenges to the teacher which were not present previously. As with the general availability and immediacy of information access, the teacher has to develop methods of assessment of the information sources, such that the information used in the learning sessions has sufficient and relevant value for the student.

12.4
Feedback for Students and Teachers

The process of learning in both undergraduate and postgraduate medicine has a basis in both traditional classroom instruction and an apprenticeship where learning by example and feedback are paramount. In either situation, it is important for the learners, particularly as they are now adult learners, to know how well they are assimilating their new knowledge. It is also important for the teacher to know how well the student is developing, and whether this development is according to the objectives of the teaching program.

Feedback to the student takes place in both informal and formal ways in the variety of teaching situations encountered in the medical learning environment. The availability of information and its use has certainly changed the opportunities available for informal feedback.

The use of formal feedback generated by electronic sessions should not, however, supplant the more informal and face-to-face feedback mechanisms already in place. But more of interest here is formal feedback and how the use of electronic teaching formats changes the ways in which this can be utilized to enhance the learning process.

The use of electronic teaching files to structure learning sessions for individuals and groups of students, according to the capabilities of the software used, gives the basis for using feedback in a variety of ways. A learning session can now be constructed in which information can be presented to the student to elicit a response, upon which the software can be set to respond in a variety of ways, the intent of which is to reinforce the knowledge presented and used. If the student's response is incorrect, further information can then be presented to correct the knowledge deficit. A summary of responses and their value can also be presented to the student on completion of the learning program. Until the advent of the complete digital imaging environment this sort of learning resource was much more difficult to construct. Now with clinical and academic resources networked it becomes reasonable to expect that teachers in the imaging sciences will produce electronic teaching programs designed for a variety of student capabilities, given the right tools and time to use them. This is a significant enhancement of the academic radiologist's role of scholar and communicator.

With a number of elements of a teaching program now in electronic format, the possibility arises for standardized assessment and automated transmission of those assessments to the teacher. Performing and collecting student assessments has always been a problem in medical education. With more structured electronic learning opportunities becoming available, it is now possible to have equivalent structured assessments built into the learning sessions, and with modern software capabilities to have these assessments saved to a database or sent to the teacher for use as part of a more comprehensive student evaluation. As teachers in imaging become more familiar with these techniques, the value of student assessments should be increased, as long as those assessments are additive to the more traditional methods.

12.5
The Record of Expertise

In 2000 the RCPSC introduced the continuing professional development (CPD) framework for all specialist physicians in Canada (Parboosingh 2005). This framework recognizes the competencies of the physician in a number of roles which had previously been enunciated as the CanMEDS roles by a group of physicians, in the Educating Future Physicians for Ontario project. In order to maintain their standing with the RCPSC, and in some jurisdictions their licensure, all specialist physicians in Canada have to subscribe to the CPD framework by recording educationally valuable activities in order to accumulate a record of sufficient items to prove their ongoing expertise in these roles. Some of these items are allotted a greater value than others – such as practice audits and structured point of care learning – while other activities which do not have the same direct relevance to practice and active learning opportunity, such as attendance at a conference, receive only a minimal value score.

Almost all medical jurisdictions now have requirements for continuing medical education; however, most simply require the recording of attendance at educational events, some of which will be accredited by a medical professional organization. The strength of the RCPSC framework is that the educational events are evaluated according to recognized educational values, giving weight to those events which have features which are known to lead to greater and more relevant learning in practice.

The advent of PACS and a networked environment, as we have seen, has significantly changed the way in which an imaging specialist works. Not only has it led to a better teaching environment for the teacher and the student, but it has also led to improvement of the environment for the imager to continue his own learning within his practice situation. The widespread use of networked electronic databases for clinical and academic purposes enables the performance of audits, practice, and case reviews. The availability and immediacy of knowledge resources enables the better use of the specialist's knowledge and learning in place which occurs with use of these resources in a practice setting. The further use of the many electronic tools and resources available for teaching purposes enables the practitioner to then claim and confirm his roles as medical expert, professional, communicator, and scholar.

12.6
Summary

Sweeping changes have taken place in the medical imaging workplace, dependent on the development of digital imaging and the software and networks on which this resides. These changes have led to significant changes to education in the specialty, with real enhancements to the roles of the teacher and the relevancy of available information to the learner. These changes are ongoing, and with good educational guidance will transform teaching in imaging. Finally, a cautionary note should be sounded. The teaching environment in imaging is multifacetted, and the enhancements offered by the digital imaging environment should not be allowed to overwhelm those already-proven teaching methods already used. A good teaching program still requires that a curriculum is set out, and followed by regular assessments of learner, teacher, and teaching environment. In this way the tools available will be used to best advantage.

References

Breivik PS (1998) Student learning in the information age: American Council on Education series on higher education. Oryx Press, UK

Parboosingh J (2005) CPD and Maintenance of Certification in the Royal College of Physicians and Surgeons of Canada. Obstet Gynaecol 5:43–49

Scarsbrook AF, Foley PT, Perriss RW, Graham RNJ (2005) Radiological digital teaching file development: An overview. Clin Radiol 60:831–837

Portable Imaging Systems for Interactive Teaching of Radiography, Computed Tomography and Ultrasound Imaging Principles

13

J.J. Battista, T.L. Poepping

13.1
Introduction

In this age of rapid medical and technological advancements, institutions are recognizing the need for interdisciplinary training. In a recent article (Hendee 2007), the need for more extensive physics education during a clinical residency in diagnostic imaging has been emphasized. Corrective measures have been recommended by the American Association of Physicists in Medicine and the Radiological Society of North America to address the growing gap between knowledge base and digital-imaging technology.

Currently, classroom lectures typically are used to teach medical physics residents specializing in diagnostic imaging (i.e. diagnostic radiology or nuclear medicine), where the fundamental aspects of medical imaging systems, such as computed tomography (CT) and ultrasound, are often illustrated through a collection of graphical slides. These topics are usually taught by a team of imaging scientists or engineers, who focus on basic physics and complex mathematics, and then by medical imaging specialists, who focus on clinically interesting images of pathological findings. What appears to be missing is a bridge between the two educator disciplines, and thus the resident or student currently is expected to somehow make the connections between theory and practice.

An interesting parallel is seen at the university undergraduate level. Science students are exposed to physical principles, for example, but rarely are exposed to the end-user practical applications. Conversely, medical residents are more familiar with the clinical applications, and need to link these back to the underlying basic sciences. Undergraduates are accustomed

J.J. Battista (✉)
Department of Medical Biophysics, The University of Western Ontario, Ontario,
Canada
E-mail: j2b@uwo.ca

Radiology Education. R.K. Chhem et al. (Eds.)
DOI: 10.1007/978-3-540-68989-8, © Springer-Verlag Berlin Heidelberg 2009

13

to classroom lectures with simple concurrent laboratory demonstrations that demonstrate the basic physics, whereas imaging residents more typically are accustomed to applied, case-based learning *without* companion laboratory demonstrations. We believe that there is a discontinuity in these forms of teaching. This gap has inspired us to develop some introductory laboratory demonstrations that can be used to facilitate the knowledge transfer, but acting in different directions for the two types of students: for undergraduate students, we aim to motivate them for further learning in physics by demonstrating more clearly the relevance and impact of physics in life-science applications; and for residents, we hope to provide a real-time display of the relevant experimental physics in an exemplifying and systematic way.

This approach is reflective of recent calls for reform in scientific education that have pointed towards more active learning strategies to engage students better, such as through group problem solving, inquiry-based laboratory experiments and interactive computer modules (Handelsman et al. 2004). While problem-based learning has been strongly embraced by medical and professional schools, it has been slow to be adopted at the undergraduate level. However, some ongoing examples are interactive computer modules for teaching electronics and engineering (Ertugrul 1998), first-year physics courses focusing on life-science problems and applications for medical and biological science students (Zinke-Allmang 2009) or focusing on the hottest topic of today – the environment (Lin 2008).

One of the obstacles to incorporating classroom demonstrations of medical physics is the lack of devices for practical demonstrations at an intermediate level between very basic physics (e.g. waves and springs) and state-of-the-art imaging systems (e.g. CT scanner). Hence, for the training of residents, the hands-on demonstrations are often delayed until access to a clinical system can be arranged during non-clinical hours of operation. However, these later sessions tend to focus more on clinical diagnostic procedures at an image-display workstation rather than demonstrating the image-formation process. Also, these full-scale systems are "black boxes" that cannot readily be manipulated solely for educational purposes. When they are used for teaching, there is pressure to guarantee a machine state of readiness should a clinical emergency arise. The internal workings of the imaging systems are rarely exhibited or altered without running the risk of inducing an equipment malfunction or exposure to ionizing radiation (e.g. X-ray CT). It is our goal to narrow the gap in knowledge transfer by introducing laboratory devices that are compact and safe enough to be used in classroom or laboratory learning.

Initially, we have focused on demonstrating the principles and imaging performance (resolution, contrast, attenuation, scattering) of radiography, CT and ultrasonic imaging. The CT system uses light rays instead of X-rays and therefore encourages repeated experimentation without introducing a radiation hazard. The ultrasound system uses a portable, hand-held unit and numerous test objects that can be imaged interactively. The two systems are economical, and relatively "open" so that the student can safely perform experiments and manipulate the data with software available on-line or off-line. Residents can perform simple optical and ultrasonic imaging experiments with minimal preparation and supervision. They are invited to participate interactively in troubleshooting sessions and produce images in real time under a wide range of imaging conditions with easily controllable parameters. This experience is expected to enrich the learning experience and improve the grasp of underlying physical principles that are taught previously or concurrently through lecturing. The two devices that we describe can be viewed as small-scale "toy" systems with enough similarity to full-scale clinical imaging systems to offer unique instructional advantage.

13.2
Small-Scale Imaging Systems

13.2.1
Optical CT Imaging System

Small-scale CT systems based on using light instead of X-rays have been developed for non-educational applications (Doran and Krstaji 2006; Sharpe et al. 2002). The CT scanner we describe here was originally developed in our laboratory for gel dosimetry purposes (Babic et al. 2008) and is now a commercialized device (Modus Medical Devices, London, Canada). In most respects, identical principles apply to the data acquisition and to the image reconstruction from multiple radiographic views of a specimen obtained by either light or X-rays. The table-top optical CT system is shown in Fig. 1a, with its internal components shown schematically in Fig. 1b. The illuminator (right) consists of an array

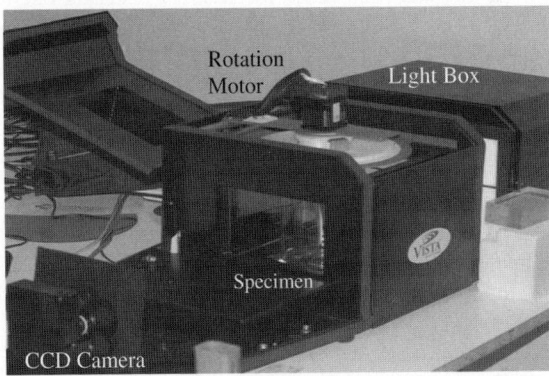

a

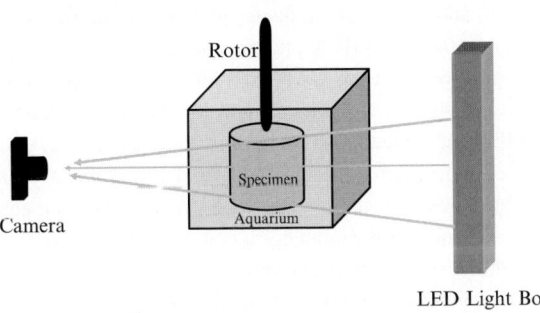

b

Fig. 1 An example of an optical computed tomography (CT) scanner (Modus Medical Devices, London, ON, Canada). The light box (LED panel) fully illuminates the specimen and transmitted light rays are detected by the camera (CCD). In radiography mode, the specimen remains stationary. For CT reconstruction, the specimen is rotated in steps and the camera "snaps" a picture for each viewing or projection angle. Such portable systems can be purchased at a cost of less than Canadian $20,000. **a** A photograph of the actual system; **b** the internal components

of light-emitting diodes that emit photons with selectable wavelengths of 633 or 590 nm towards a diffusing front plate. The specimen to be imaged is immersed in an aquarium that holds a liquid with refractive index properties that minimize light refraction and reflection. These effects would bend the light paths and produce image artefacts if the specimen were to be imaged openly in air.

This imaging system can be operated in radiography mode or CT reconstruction mode. In radiography mode, a translucent object placed at the centre of the scanner is illuminated by the light panel (right), and its shadow is captured by the video camera (left). A single view taken by the camera strongly resembles a radiograph. It should be noted that this 3D optical system is based on cone-beam geometry as used in traditional radiography and specialized CT scanners (Yang et al. 2007). If desired, a more traditional fan-beam CT geometry can be achieved by placing a rectangular slit aperture at the front face of the light box. In CT reconstruction mode, a large number of radiographic images are acquired consecutively while the specimen is rotated by the motor at the top centre of the scanner chassis. Rays that travel through the specimen in a conelike geometry are captured by a digital camera, and the captured frames are recorded by a standard personal computer. This computer also controls the rotation of the specimen in small angular increments with brief pauses between the image frame captures and transfers. Three-dimensional CT reconstruction can be accomplished using a standard backprojection algorithm (Kak and Slaney 2001).

There is one obvious salient difference between this optical system design and that of an X-ray-based system. The geometry is reciprocally inverted in that the light rays originate in a broad uniform beam at the light box (right), traverse the specimen (centre) and finally pass through a small aperture within the camera lens assembly (left). In X-ray CT, X-rays originate instead from a small point source in the X-ray tube, traverse the specimen and finally diverge to reach the detector. In brief, optical and X-ray photons travel in opposite directions, but they are similarly attenuated along the traversed ray paths. The imaging principle and reconstruction concept is identical.

The radiographic or tomographic images can be viewed, manipulated and analysed quantitatively in 2D or 3D space, with software that is very similar to that available on clinical image-display workstations. Raw and processed image data can also be exported to other programs (e.g. Excel, ImageJ, MATLAB) for subsequent analysis. This feature is important for composing student assignments and for formal evaluation of the depth of understanding and efficiency of learning. We have developed test objects and an associated set of basic physics experiments that demonstrate underlying physical principles of CT (see Sect. 13.3.1). These include demonstrations of spatial resolution, contrast resolution and linearity of reconstructed attenuation coefficients that are closely related to CT numbers (Hounsfield units) used on clinical systems. For example, students can set the "level and window" on the attenuation values for optimal display of an optical density range, much like on a diagnostic workstation.

Table 13.1 lists the resolution capabilities of the optical CT scanner. It can be operated in low- and high-resolution modes. In these modes, the sampled element (voxel) size can be adjusted in the range from 2 mm down to 0.25 mm. Consequently, the reconstructed 3D image data sets occupy 1 MB at low resolution and up to 525 MB in high-resolution mode. The number of radiographic projections required to produce these CT images ranges from

Table 13.1 Spatial-resolution settings for the optical scanner

Esolution	Image voxel size (mm per side)	Approximate size of reconstructed 3D image data set (MB)	Approximate time to reconstruct on a PC (min)
Low	2	1.0	3
Medium	1	8.0	7
High	0.5	65	15
Very High	0.25	525	45

Data provided courtesy of Modus Medical Devices (London, Canada)

86 up to 512, with CT image reconstruction times that range from 3 to 245 min at high resolution. The ability to change these parameters offers the student learning opportunities in understanding the compromise between spatial resolution and computer resource consumption.

13.2.2
Ultrasound Imaging System

Figure 2 shows the system that we have assembled for demonstrations of ultrasound imaging principles. It incorporates a small, commercially available ultrasound unit coupled to a transducer probe (Sonosite 180PLUS, with an L38/10–5 MHz linear-array transducer), which serves as both the ultrasound source (transmitter) and the detector (receiver). The system shown uses a central frequency of 5 MHz, corresponding to a wavelength of approximately 0.3 mm in water and soft tissue, and allows a maximum image depth of approximately 7 cm.

The control unit allows variation of basic parameter settings (e.g. gain, depth, focus) that affect image quality, and it can easily be interfaced to a laptop or personal computer using an "image grabber" for in-class digital projection and for subsequent data exportation and off-line analysis (e.g. using Excel or MATLAB). Students can manipulate the system parameters, visually observe the direct impact on imaging performance, and through off-line analysis can also quantitatively determine the impact on image-quality metrics.

We have developed a set of basic experiments that demonstrate the underlying physical principles of ultrasound imaging (e.g. attenuation, scatter, reflection). Various test objects with accurately known acoustic properties and dimensions demonstrate specific concepts and the effects on different aspects of image features and quality (e.g. accuracy, artefacts). Typical ultrasound tissue-mimicking material (TMM) consists of strong, water-based gels with components to adjust the acoustic properties (e.g. speed of sound, acoustic attenuation and backscattering) in order to mimic that of different types of tissue (Poepping et al. 2004; Rickey et al. 1995). Samples of solutions (e.g. glycerol) or solids (e.g. plastics) also provide a wide range of acoustic properties for emphasis of various physical effects and induced image artefacts.

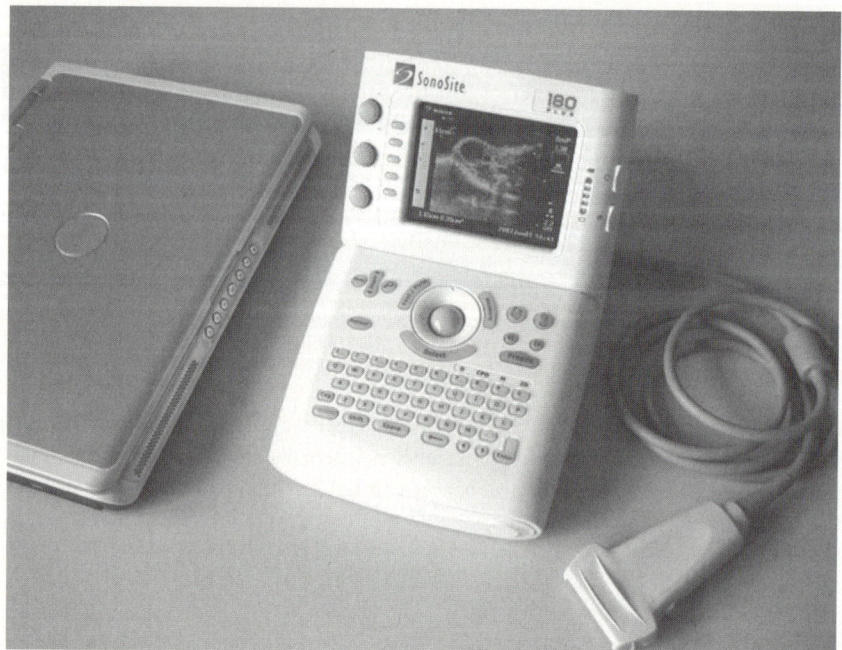

Fig. 2 An example of a portable ultrasound system (Sonosite 180PLUS) beside a standard laptop for size comparison. Portable ultrasound systems cost in the range of Canadian $10,000 to Canadian $20,000, including the linear-array transducer.

13.3
Educational Sessions

13.3.1
CT Imaging Experiments

13.3.1.1
Image Reconstruction

Figure 3 shows a photograph and CT reconstruction of a test phantom consisting of a fluid-filled plastic container in the shape of a miniature bear. The 3D surface is presented either as a maximum-intensity projection (MIP) (Fig. 3b) or as a surface rendering (Fig. 3c). Clinically, the MIP technique is often used in CT angiography (Hyde et al. 2007). These results provide an instant appreciation of the 3D nature of CT reconstruction. This can be further explored through multiplanar views of the interior of the specimen. Figure 4a shows, for example, a transverse section through the eyes of the miniature bear. Figure 4b shows a sagittal cross-section and reveals small air bubble adhesions within the head.

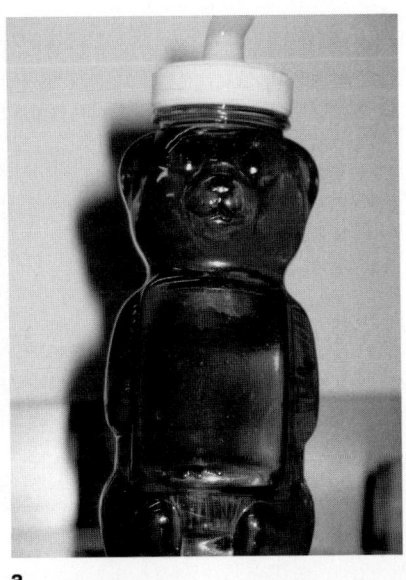

Fig. 3 Miniature bear specimen used to demonstrate 3D CT imaging. (**a**) Photograph of plastic "bear" container filled with blue liquid; (**b**) 3D viewing using maximum intensity projection algorithm; (**c**) 3D viewing using a surface-rendering algorithm.

13

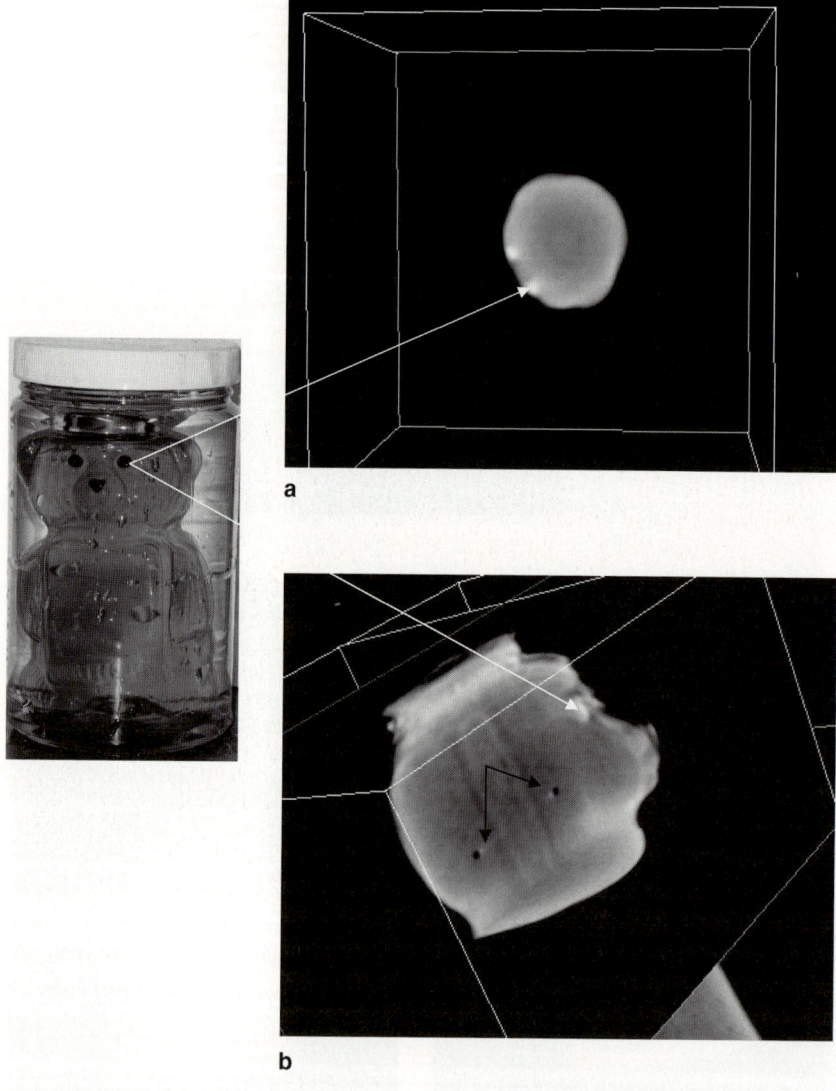

Fig. 4 CT images of the miniature bear phantom. The instructor or students can select any of these cross-sections in three dimensions interactively on the computer screen. (**a**) Transverse section revealing the eyes. (**b**) Sagittal section showing the eyes (white arrows) but also small air-bubble adhesions (black arrows) in the head

13.3.1.2
Spatial Resolution

Figure 5 shows the tests of the spatial resolution of the radiography and CT system using a transparency sheet (Fig. 5a) with a series of line pairs in vertical and horizontal directions. Figure 5b shows a transparency of the USAF Resolution Test Chart (Earl 2002) centred

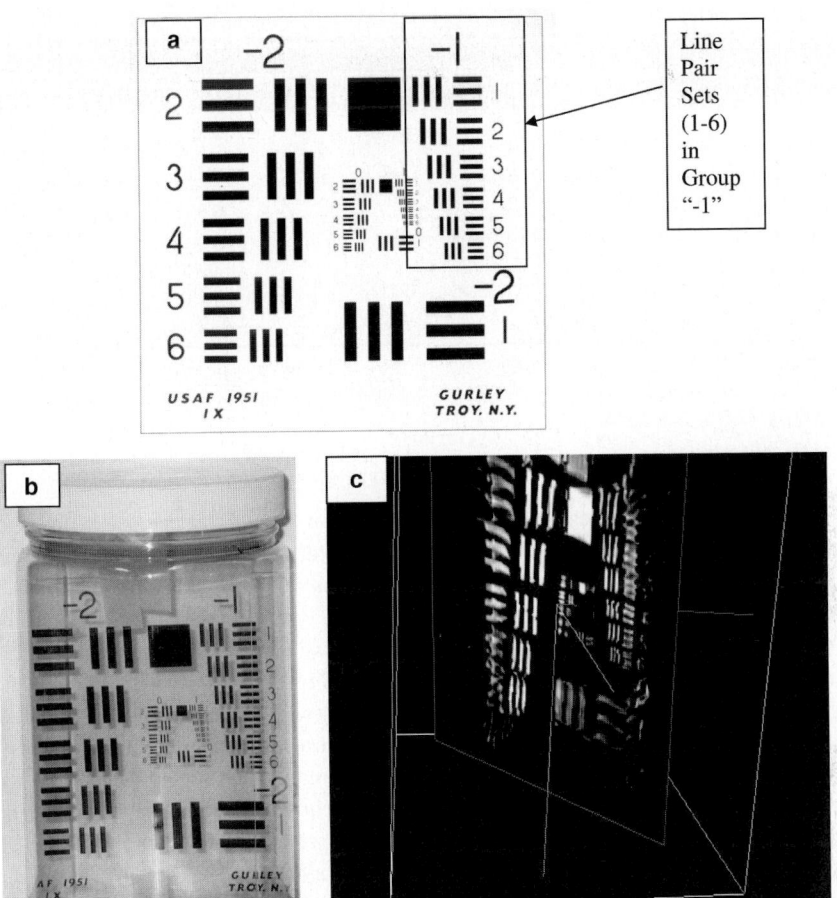

Fig. 5 USAF Resolution Test (see Table 13.2). (**a**) Photograph of the test chart which is divided into line-pair "sets" from 1 to 6 and "groups" of −2, −1, 0 and +1 with different magnification levels. (**b**) Transparency of the photograph shown in Fig. 6a, placed in empty jar for CT test. (**c**) CT image in an oblique central plane showing a resolving power of 1 mm.

within a cylindrical jar for insertion into the optical scanner (Fig. 5c). Table 13.2 lists the line widths and their matched spacings, ranging from 0.22 to 3.20 mm.

With the optical system, it is possible to visualize set 5 of group "−1", both vertically and horizontally, corresponding to approximately 1 mm isotropic resolution. However, a significant number of optical artefacts are also seen in the peripheral zones because this sheet was imaged "in air", without immersion in a refractive-index-matching liquid. Students can be challenged to explain these artefacts.

Table 13.2 Spacings and matching line widths in the USAF Resolution Test Chart (Earl 2002)

Set	Group			
	−2 (mm)	−1 (mm)	0 (mm)	1 (mm)
1	3.20	1.60	0.80	0.40
2	2.85	1.43	0.71	0.36
3	2.54	1.27	0.63	0.32
4	2.26	1.13	0.57	0.28
5	2.02	1.01	0.50	0.25
6	1.80	0.90	0.45	0.22

13.3.1.3
Contrast Resolution

Figure 6 demonstrates a test of CT contrast resolution. The object that was scanned is shown in Fig. 6a and consists of five finger-shaped tubes each loaded with a different optical attenuation liquid (i.e. different concentrations of blue ink). Figure 6b shows a transverse section through the different tubes. Tube 1 offers the most contrast (5 mL of ink per litre of water, $\mu = 2.40\,\mathrm{cm}^{-1}$) while tube 6 offers 32 times (2^{-5}) less contrast and is much more difficult to visualize without adjusting the display "level and window" settings. Figure 6c demonstrates the linearity of the optical CT scanner. It shows a plot of the linear attenuation coefficient (μ) as determined by CT reconstruction versus the concentration of blue ink dyes. It demonstrates that a CT image is "more than just a pretty picture". It is a quantitative map of local attenuation coefficients (i.e. per voxel) throughout the 3D image space, resulting from the light (or X-rays) acting as a probing energy. The analogy to CT numbers (in Hounsfield units) is related to these linearity curves:

$$N_{CT} = 1000(\mu - \mu_0)/\mu_0, \tag{13.1}$$

where the μ values are calculated for each voxel via the CT reconstruction algorithm, and μ_0 is chosen to be in the midrange of the expected attenuation of the materials scanned. This is similar to X-ray CT numbers that are calibrated to have a baseline value of zero for water – a good central reference material for human tissues, approximately midway between the values for air and compact bone. In optical CT scanning, μ_0 can be similarly referenced to a stable liquid of intermediate attenuation and calibrated independently by a spectrophotometer.

13.3.2
Ultrasound Imaging Experiments

The portable ultrasound system (Fig. 2) is used, along with basic test objects, to demonstrate the underlying physical principles of ultrasound and the effects of different parameter settings. The instructional motivation is to uncover the "black box" of clinical systems and reveal a deeper understanding of how different material acoustic properties and system

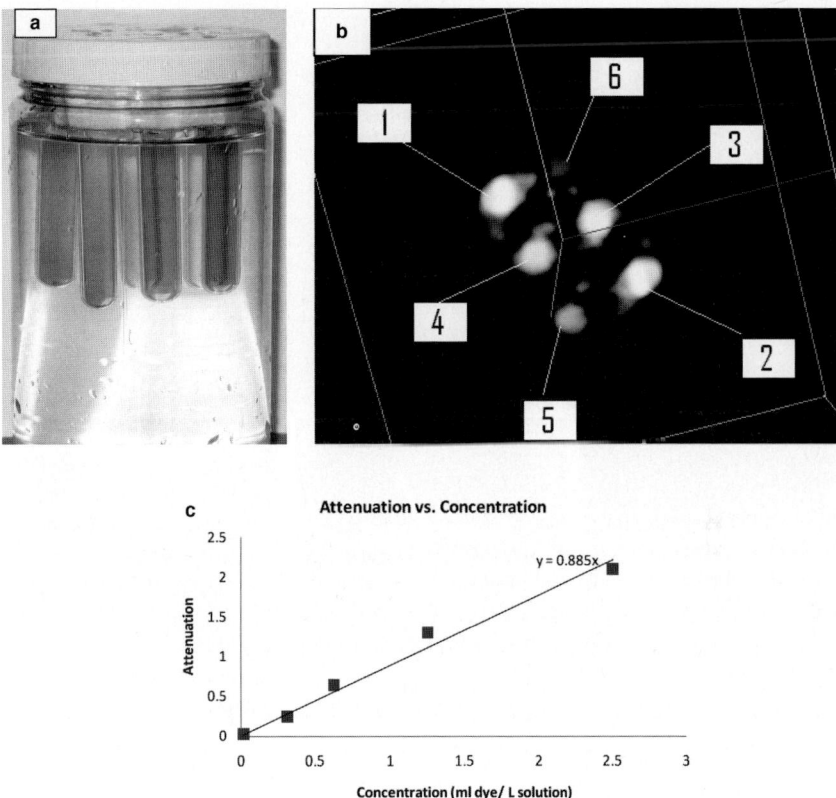

Fig. 6 CT contrast resolution "finger" phantom. (**a**) Photograph of the "finger" phantom showing six inner tubes filled with coloured liquids. (**b**) Axial CT image showing the various contrast targets. (**c**) CT linear attenuation coefficient (per centimetre) versus concentration of blue ink

parameter settings can affect an image. Students are able to image test "phantoms" made of materials with known acoustic properties and known dimensions.

13.3.2.1
Acoustic Velocity (Speed of Sound)

Diagnostic ultrasound imaging systems assume or incorporate an average speed of sound based on a well-accepted average value for soft tissues (i.e. $1,540 \, \mathrm{m \, s^{-1}}$). Images are formed, by displaying signal intensity as a function of depth, on the basis of echo return time (distance = $1,540 \, \mathrm{m \, s^{-1}} \times$ time) *assuming* the average speed in soft-tissue. This assumed value can lead to incorrect depth calculation results for tissues in which the acoustic waves traverse at a different speed of sound. Figure 7 demonstrates the spatial displacement due to differences in the speed of sound in different solutions within an object of known dimension. This example shows a comparison of dimensions as measured

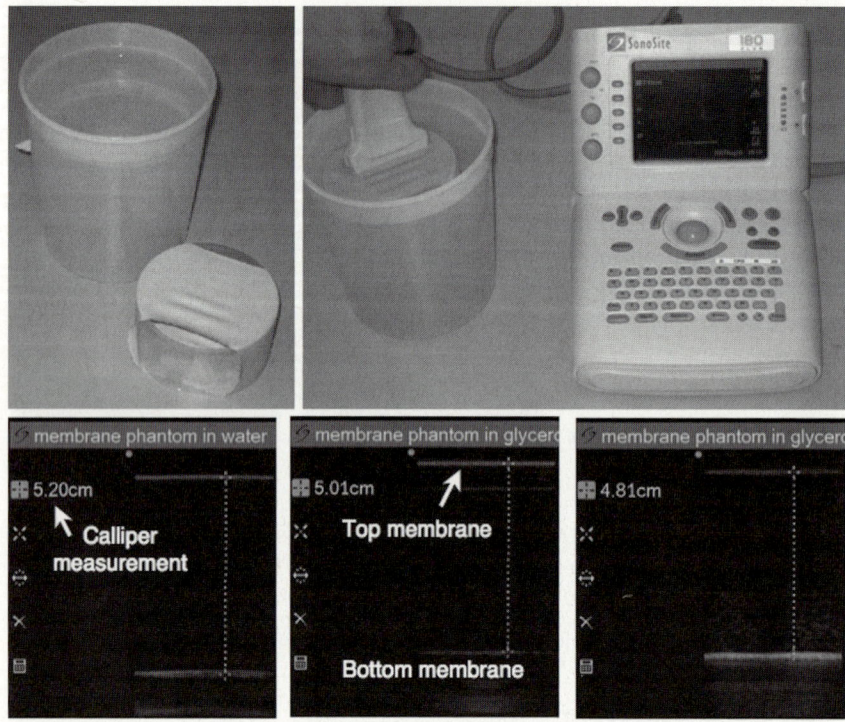

Fig. 7 A membrane phantom for demonstrating the effect of a material with speed of sound different from that of the soft-tissue average value of 1,540 m s^{-1}. The phantom consists of a hollow cylinder, covered by rubber layers to form top and bottom membranes separated by a known fixed distance (5.0 cm), which can be submerged in fluids of different speed of sound (1,480 m s^{-1} for water, 1,540 m s^{-1} for 8.84% glycerol solution, 1,600 m s^{-1} for 18.13% glycerol solution). On-screen callipers allow measurement of the apparent distance of separation.

by the ultrasound machine (i.e. apparent distances seen on the displayed image) with the actual known distance (5.0 cm).

13.3.2.2
Reverberations

Intense secondary reflections from layers of tissue or materials with significant differences in the acoustic impedance can "echo", or bounce back and forth multiple times, before being received at the transducer. These multiple echoes are misinterpreted, owing to the prolonged return time, as arising from deeper in the material. They appear as reverberations, or "ghost" layer boundaries, on the image. This is demonstrated convincingly in Fig. 8 by imaging a plastic disk in water.

Fig. 8 Reverberations produced by multiply reflected ultrasound echoes are demonstrated using a thin disk of plastic immersed in water. In this image, the paths of the ultrasound echoes (angled only for clarity) and the resulting reverberation artefacts are illustrated using colour-matched arrows

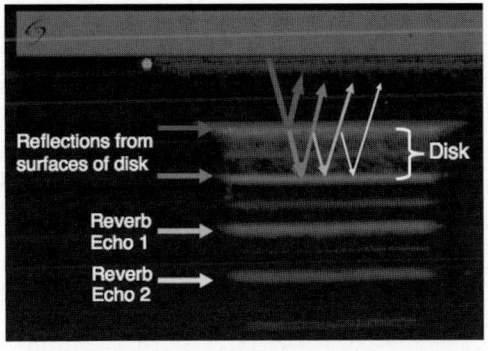

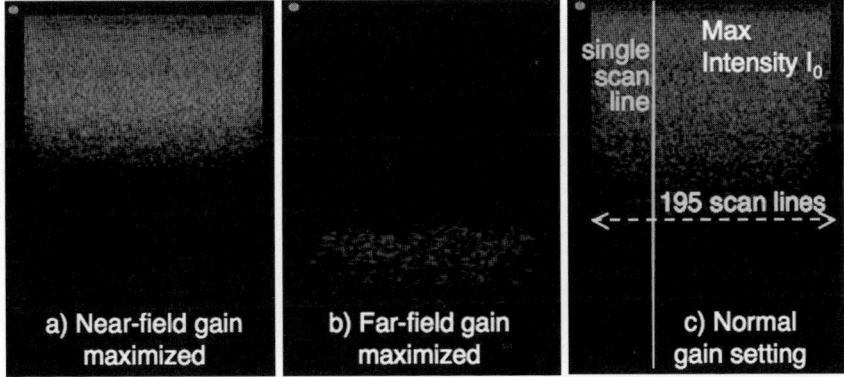

Fig. 9 Images demonstrating the attenuation of the ultrasound intensity with depth and the effect of using the different gain (i.e. intensity amplification) controls to compensate for the intensity decrease. Images were taken of a solid block of agar-based tissue-mimicking material (TMM) with known uniform attenuation, using different gain settings to maximize (**a**) near-field intensity, (**b**) far-field intensity and (**c**) overall intensity. The vertical line marks a single scan line, such as shown in the intensity versus depth plot in Fig. 10.

13.3.2.3
Attenuation

Attenuation is the loss in ultrasound intensity due to scattering and absorption interactions, resulting in an exponential decrease in ultrasound signal intensity with depth or distance in an absorber. The system gain control is used to compensate for low detected signal – due to low reflection or high attenuation – by amplifying the returned echo signal. Figure 9 shows the effect of different gain adjustments on an image of a uniform tissue-substitute (TMM) block, with homogeneous distribution of particles producing a known attenuation

13

coefficient (approximately 3.5 dB cm^{-1} at 5 MHz) (Poepping et al. 2004, Rickey et al. 1995). Figure 10 demonstrates data extracted from the image using off-line processing to plot the signal intensity as a function of depth. Intensity is shown along a single scan line in the image, as indicated in Fig. 10c. Multiple lines can be averaged, thus smoothing out the inherent fluctuations due to noise and speckle. The plot also clearly demonstrates the linear decrease in signal intensity, rather than an exponential decrease. This is due to the internal signal processing and depth-dependent gain that typically is applied to the image displayed by an ultrasound system.

13.3.2.4
Acoustic Impedance, Reflection and Scatter

Reflections occur owing to differences in acoustic impedances of the insonated materials. Figure 11 demonstrates the specular reflection that occurs at smooth boundaries between materials and the diffuse reflection (backscatter) from distributed scattering sites of different concentrations of dispersion densities. The phantom uses layers of two materials with different acoustic impedance. Both materials have small particles homogenously dispersed through-out, with a particle concentration of 0.5% in the outer layers and varied particle concen-

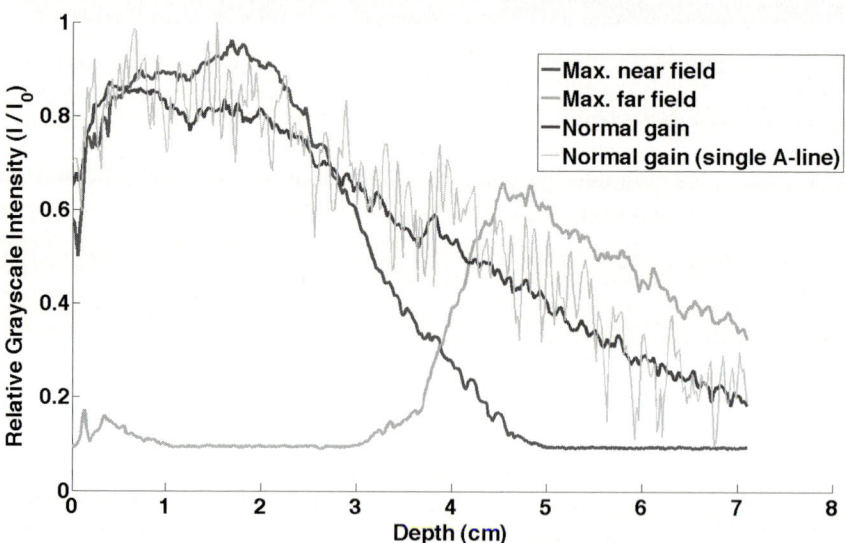

Fig. 10 Plots of the ultrasound signal intensity as a function of depth can be generated from off-line analysis of the images. Intensity from a single vertical A-line within Fig. 9c is shown, along with an averaged intensity line from all 195 vertical scan lines across each of the three images in Fig. 9.

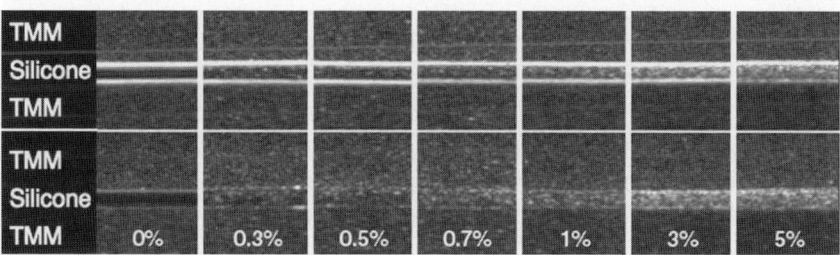

Fig. 11 Different forms of reflection are demonstrated using a phantom with a thin silicone layer, seeded with small particles ranging in concentration from 0% (*left image pair*) to 5% (*right*), embedded in standard TMM with 0.5% particle concentration. Strong specular reflection is observed (*top panel of images*) when the transducer is nearly perpendicular to the boundary. For non-perpendicular incidence (as used for *bottom panel of images*), the middle silicone layer can be distinguished by the difference in diffuse backscatter when the particle concentration is different from that of the surrounding material. (Reprinted with permission from Ultrasound in Medicine and Biology/Elsevier)

trations in the middle layer, progressing from 0% (left) to 5% (right), as labelled. Figure 11a shows the intense echo signal from the material boundaries due to specular reflection, which is only detected when the reflection is directed back towards the transducer, namely when the transducer axis is perpendicular to the boundary. Figure 11b demonstrates the effect of imaging with an oblique insonation angle; here the different material layers can still be distinguished owing to different levels of diffuse backscattering because of the different scattering particle concentrations. This increase in scatter also leads to increased attenuation as is evident from the reduced intensity in the bottom layer of the phantom images as one progresses from left to right in the image sequence.

13.3.2.5
In Vitro and In Vivo Imaging

Finally, to appreciate how all of the different interactions contribute to general ultrasound imaging, students can have access to the system to image an assortment of more realistic or complex unknown objects. Students can image easily accessible sites on themselves, such as the carotid artery in the neck (Fig. 12) or the muscles in the forearm. The volume, area and distance software measurement tools can be used and tested. The accuracy of such measurements can be demonstrated by using "mystery" objects, such as a hard-boiled egg embedded in TMM (Fig. 13), where the dimensions and volume were accurately determined beforehand.

13.4
Summary and Conclusion

In the course of teaching physics to undergraduate science students, particularly those in the life sciences, and to clinical residents in the imaging specialties, we have perceived a need for developing hands-on practical demonstrations of fundamental

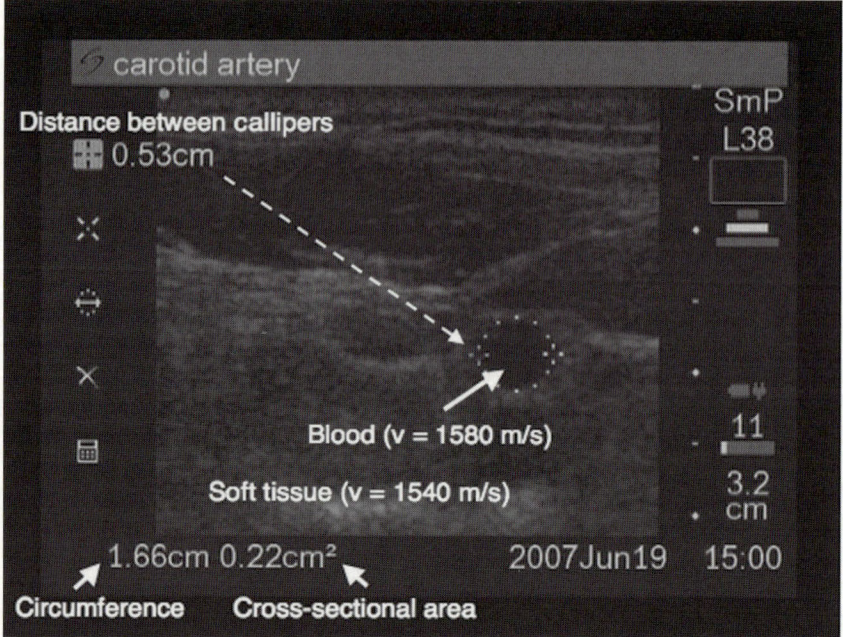

Fig. 12 Students can image themselves in order to relate the different image features studied using phantoms back to a more realistic scenario, such as an image of the carotid artery. Artery diameters and cross-sectional areas can be measured, and compared across different individuals, using the on-screen callipers

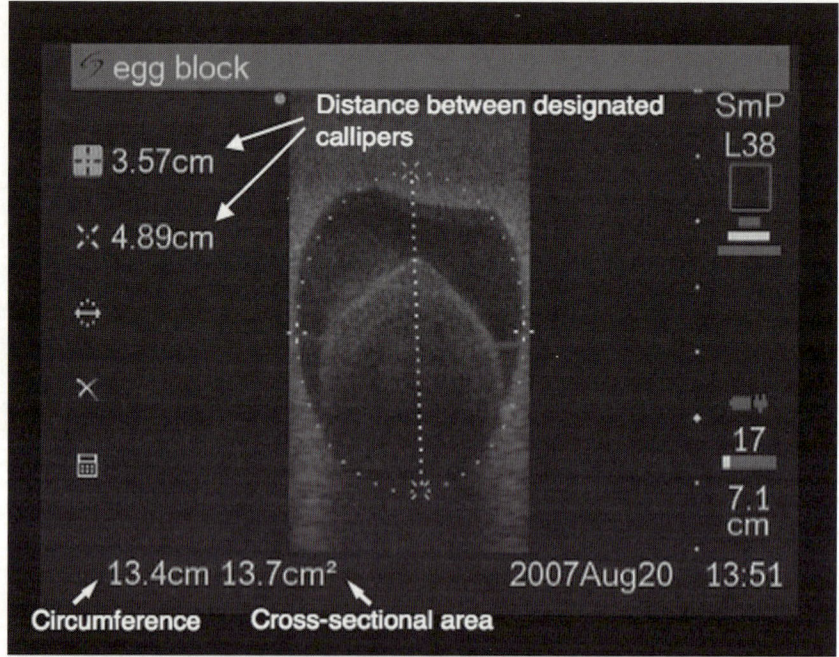

Fig. 13 Mystery test objects, such as a hard-boiled egg of a predetermined size and volume, embedded in visually opaque TMM, can be used to test area and volume measurements using the on-screen callipers. Notice the shadow created by the highly attenuating yolk of the egg

medical imaging concepts. The "learning gap" is due, in part, to the interdisciplinary teaching done by two types of educators – scientists and medical application specialists. Split lectures and limited, or delayed, access to clinical imaging equipment introduce temporal and interdisciplinary gaps between learning of the fundamental physical theory and witnessing practical medical applications. We believe that concurrent lectures with interactive laboratory demonstrations will enhance learning and allow students to recognize and apply this knowledge more broadly across multiple imaging methods. Here, we have introduced two portable devices that can be used in teaching the fundamental physics of CT and ultrasound imaging interactively to residents in a classroom or laboratory setting. These are low-cost table-top (less than Canadian $20,000) imaging systems whose components are visible, tangible and hazard-free. Students can explore the hardware and software components and be prepared with a better understanding of the physics before accessing the full-scale clinical diagnostic systems. The system controls can be manipulated (i e. "knobology") by the instructor or student to assess the experimental impact of changes made in imaging parameters and tissue conditions. A set of simple experiments have been devised to use commonly available tissuelike materials, and require minimal training and preparation to demonstrate the underlying concepts of imaging science. We intend to introduce these imaging devices and experiments in our undergraduate science curriculum and diagnostic-imaging residency programmes at the University of Western Ontario. Our goal is to narrow the gap between the learning of fundamental physics and exciting applications to imaging technologies used in modern diagnostic medicine.

13.5
Conflict of Interest Statement

J.J Battista, as former employee of Cancer Care Ontario, is party to a licensing agreement with Modus Medical Devices (London, ON, Canada), the company that manufactures the optical CT scanner described in this chapter.

Acknowledgements

This project was made possible with funding from the students of the University of Western Ontario (Undergraduate Science Students' Council) and the Fellowship for Teaching Innovation (supported by Foundation Western). We also acknowledge the hard work of two undergraduate students, Reginald Taylor and Joel Cox, who developed many of the laboratory experiments during the summer of 2007. We appreciate many fruitful discussions with our colleagues Kevin Jordan, Ian MacDonald and Blaine Chronik. We also wish to acknowledge the technical assistance of John Miller and Jennifer Dietrich of Modus Medical Devices, and Hristo Nikolov at the Robarts Research Institute.

13

References

Babic S, Battista J, Jordan K (2008) Three-dimensional dose verification for intensity-modulated radiation therapy in the radiological physics centre head-and-neck phantom using optical computed tomography scans of ferrous xylenol-orange gel dosimeters. Int J Radiat Oncol Biol Phys 70:1281–1291

Doran SJ, Krstaji N (2006) The history and principles of optical computed tomography for scanning 3-D radiation dosimeters. Fourth international conference on radiotherapy gel dosimetry, Institute of Physics. J Phys Conf Ser 56:45–57

Earl GF (2002) Technical note: USAF 1951 and microscopy resolution test charts (30 Nov. 2002) http://www.efg2.com/Lab/ImageProcessing/TestTargets/#USAF1951, Accessed March 3, 2007

Ertugrul N (1998) New era in engineering experiments: An integrated interactive teaching/ learning approach and real time visualisations. Int J Eng Educ 14:344–355

Handelsman J, Ebert-May D, Beichner R et al (2004) Scientific teaching. Science 304:521–522

Hendee WR (2007) Improving physics education in radiology. J Am Coll Radiol 4:555–559

Hyde DE, Habets DF, Fox AJ, Gulka I, Kalapos P, Lee DH, Pelz DM, Holdsworth DW (2007) Comparison of maximum intensity projection and digitally reconstructed radiographic projection for carotid artery stenosis measurement. Med Phys 34:2968–2974

Kak AC, Slaney M (2001) Principles of computerized tomographic imaging, published by Society of Industrial and Applied Mathematics (SIAM) and available on-line at http://www.slaney.org/pct/pct-toc.html Accessed March 3, 2007

Lin B (2008) Nothing too theoretical about this physics class. UBC Reports 54(3). http://www.publicaffairs.ubc.ca/ubcreports/2008/08mar06/physics.html Accessed April 3, 2008

Poepping TL, Nikolov HN, Thorne ML, Holdsworth DW (2004) A thin-walled carotid vessel phantom for Doppler ultrasound flow studies. Ultrasound Med Biol 30:1067–1078

Rickey DW, Picot PA, Christopher DA, Fenster A (1995) A wall-less vessel phantom for Doppler ultrasound studies. Ultrasound Med Biol 21:1163–1176

Sharpe J, Ahlgren U, Perry P, Hill B, Ross A, Hecksher-Sørensen J, Baldock R, Davidson D (2002) Optical projection tomography as a tool for 3D microscopy and gene expression studies. Science 296:541–545

Yang WT, Carkaci S, Chen L, Lai C, Sahin A, Whitman G, Shaw C (2007) Dedicated cone-beam breast CT: Feasibility study with surgical mastectomy specimens. Am J Roentgenol 189:1312–1315

Zinke-Allmang M (2009) Physics for the Life Sciences. Nelson Education Ltd, Toronto, ON, Canada.

Medical Education Research: Challenges and Opportunities in the Scholarship of Discovery

J. Collins

Narrative

In 1990, the Accreditation Council for Graduate Medical Education (ACGME) changed the requirements for diagnostic radiology residency to require residents to have 6 months of radiology training prior to taking independent call. In 2007, the requirements were again revised, requiring residents to have 12 months of radiology training prior to taking independent call (Rumack 2007). The change was justified as follows: during 6 months of training, residents cannot be exposed to standard 4-week rotations in all subspecialty areas of radiology, and residents are more accurate in formulating preliminary interpretations if they have 12 months rather than 6 months of exposure to the specialty. Resident results in the American College of Radiology in-service examination, which show a steady increase in scores with each year of training, were used to justify the latter. Furthermore, other medical specialties required constant supervision for first-year residents by more senior residents or in-house supervision of residents by faculty members.

The ACGME requires all residency review committees to review program requirements for training programs every 5 years and revise them as necessary. Proposed changes by the Radiology Residency Review Committee, including the 12-month rule, were presented at national meetings and on the Radiology Residency Review Committee Web site. Numerous comments were received from the American College of Radiology, the American Board of Radiology, the American Medical Association, the Association of Program Directors in Radiology, and individual radiology chairpersons, radiologists, program directors, and residents (Amis 2008). Many of the comments expressed concern regarding the new requirement for 12 months of training in diagnostic radiology before a resident is allowed to participate in independent call.

J. Collins
Department of Radiology, University of Wisconsin School of Medicine and Public Health, Madison, WI, USA
E-mail: jcollins@uwhealth.org

Radiology Education. R.K. Chhem et al. (Eds.)
DOI: 10.1007/978-3-540-68989-8, © Springer-Verlag Berlin Heidelberg 2009

14

Surveys of radiology program directors and radiology chief residents showed that the majority of respondents from both groups were opposed to the change (Gunderman and Delaney 2007; Berger et al. 2007). Those opposed to the change cited the following reasons: (1) beginning to take call is always challenging at first, regardless of when it occurs; (2) the proposal is not evidence-based; (3) the change would impose an increased burden on other residents and faculty members; (4) the current system functions well; (5) increasing upper-level on-call duties would undermine recruitment; (6) programs should improve preparation for on-call duties rather than change their timing; (7) such a change would necessitate violation of the ACGME's duty hours regulations; (8) other medical specialties do not impose such a waiting period; and (9) the change would interfere with board examination preparation by fourth-year residents. Respondents agreed that patient safety was a priority in making decisions regarding trainee education. However, the survey results indicated that one of the most frequent objections of program directors to the rule change was the lack of evidence that increasing the length of training before residents take independent call would actually improve patient care. Multiple studies were cited, showing that few discrepancies were found between preliminary residents' after-hours interpretations and later final interpretations made by attending radiologists (Carney et al. 2003; Wechsler et al. 1996; Wysoki et al. 1998). Limitations of these studies included lack of a gold standard and small numbers of residents. Additionally, these were not large multi-institutional studies and therefore generalizability of conclusions across training programs could not be assumed. This is an important consideration given that the number of residents in radiology training programs varied from as few as eight to over 50. The surveys showed that, in general, programs with fewer residents tended to have residents take call on a more frequent basis, and because of this, it was likely that no single solution would be appropriate for all programs.

In the majority of programs surveyed, residents took call after 4–6 months of radiology training, indicating that the new requirement would affect a large number of programs. The surveys also showed that the majority of respondents disagreed that the American College of Radiology in-service examination reliably indicated the degree of resident on-call competency. Respondents commented that no study had compared the on-call accuracy of residents at 6 and 12 months of training, or showed that residents perform below the level of the community standard of care while on call. An alternative proposal suggested by respondents was that residents not be allowed to participate in call responsibilities until they had formal instruction related to on-call responsibilities and performed satisfactorily in examinations related to that instruction. In fact, many respondents reported that they already provided some form of preparation course, most commonly on-call specific lecture series or conferences.

The above narrative illustrates a scenario where a change was made in residency training requirements that led to a divide in opinion among constituents and large-scale opposition to the change. This is not unexpected when a change affects a large number of individuals and programs in a substantial way, and there are claims of insufficient objective evidence to justify the change. Many of the issues discussed in the remainder of this chapter represent challenges in medical education that are illustrated by this narrative.

14.1
Introduction

Medical education research includes any investigation related to the education of medical professionals, including research related to undergraduate (medical school), graduate (residency), and continuing medical education. Medical education research can focus on any number of topics, including curriculum development, teaching methods, student evaluation, teacher evaluation, course evaluation, faculty development, admission and preparation of candidates for medical training, factors influencing career choice, research methods, and use of technology in education.

Research has internal validity if its outcome is a function of the approach being tested rather than of other causes. It has external validity if its results will apply in the real world. A common problem in medical education research that affects internal validity is the fact that human beings change over time as a function of the normal course of development and the acquisition of experience. Undergraduate medical education is a 4-year process and residency training can take several years. Trainees are exposed to many educational experiences during their training. Research that involves taking measurements at two different times, before and after an intervention, must take into account the changes that naturally occur over time that are not due to the intervention. A common threat to external validity is the difference in student and patient populations amongst different institutions and regions of the country. The results of an investigation performed with one resident group at one institution may not be generalizable to other resident groups at other institutions.

In the world of medical education research, complete experimental control is often difficult or impossible because of limitations in the ability of the researcher to assign subjects and manipulate conditions. This is only one reason why the medical education literature is full of editorials, narrative descriptions, surveys, and preexperimental studies.

Randomized trials represent an ideal study design, but in the field of education, contamination is a frequent concern (i.e., students randomly assigned to different groups talk to each other or share study materials). In addition, it is often not ethically acceptable to provide treatment to only some of the learners. Understanding these challenges and how to work around them is critical to the success of medical education research. Although more quantitative educational research is needed, qualitative methods are indicated in certain circumstances (e.g., focus groups leading to the development of survey questions or generating hypotheses for subsequent testing). Too much medical education research falls short because of small sample sizes. This is a particular problem when the focus of the research is targeted to a specialty area and does not combine institutional resources through collaboration with other investigators. This chapter addresses these and other challenges in medical education research, the characteristics of successful medical education research centers, trends, and opportunities in medical education research, and the future of radiology education research.

14.2
Challenges in Medical Education Research

Wartman (2004) described four major challenges facing the field of health professions education research: conceptual difficulties, pressures on the curriculum, financial concerns, and the need to link education to outcomes. Conceptual difficulties refers to methodological challenges in conducting medical education research. One of these challenges is the time between learning and important outcomes, which may be so long that the effects of the curriculum are obscured or that the link is indirect. Wartman has called this challenge the "educators' uncertainty principle" (Wartman 1994): "Since education itself can play only a part in the overall outcome it is expected to affect, we cannot know the precise effect of education on the outcomes of education."

Pressures on the curriculum include frequent changes in regulatory requirements that affect accreditation of undergraduate, graduate, and continuing medical education by the Liaison Committee on Medical Education, the ACGME and the Accreditation Council for Continuing Medical Education, respectively. Medical education can be viewed as a continuum from medical school to residency to posttraining continuing professional development. The curriculum must change with the health care system and societal expectations. Regulatory-driven curriculum changes can introduce challenges to ongoing research under controlled conditions. Changes in the curriculum will affect the educational experiences among groups of trainees, which can render a study invalid.

The greatest challenge in medical education research is linking the content and method of medical education to the quality of physician care and patient health outcomes. Currently, medical students are evaluated by their performance in examinations and programs are evaluated by the success rate of student and resident graduation and certification. The introduction of the competency requirements by the ACGME and maintenance of certification programs by the American Board of Medical Specialties are examples of how regulatory bodies have begun to require that physicians demonstrate a higher level of accountability to the public. However, few studies have demonstrated that differences in quality of patient care can in fact be attributed to individual physicians' education, certification, and performance (Tamblyn et al. 1998; Prystowsky et al. 2002).

Another important challenge to the field of medical education research is lack of a critical mass of skilled education researchers. Many clinical departments operate with a budget deficit that is being addressed by increasing the clinical productivity of their clinician-educators, which serves to erode the already limited protected time for educational research. This slows the academic advancement of clinician-educators, resulting in a paucity of senior mentors (Thomas et al. 2004).

Educational research rests heavily on social science research methodology. Proficiency with this methodology requires training and experience (van der Vleuten et al. 2004). Researchers often try to apply methods that are successful in biomedical research to medical education, which either does not work or forces the researchers to adapt the research question to the method instead of the other way around (Schuwirth and van der Vieuten 2006). Although evidence-based medicine is important to the understanding of the application of medical interventions, educational research methods should be geared to the idiosyncrasies of the educational domain. Unlike much of medical research, educational research neither can nor should always use controlled experimentation as the method of preference. Most clinical faculty members do not have the expertise to design appropriate educational research studies and will need to acquire these skills or collaborate with medical education specialists who do have the expertise.

Because educational research is often qualitative, rarely involving randomized controlled trials, and outcomes are often difficult to evaluate and not detectable until years after the event, physician teachers are often suspicious of medical education research (Petersen 1999). If medical education research is to inform more teachers it must become accessible, comprehensible, convincing, and demonstrably related to the real issues faced by medical teachers at the bedside, clinic, or imaging monitors. Medical educationalists must present ideas in clear, jargon-free format to show that research methods are designed for the task and competently carried out, and convince their colleagues that the evidence base is as important in educating new physicians as it is in assessing a new chemotherapy or imaging modality.

14.3
Funding of Medical Education Research

In a recent article (Carline 2004), Carline addressed the underfunding of medical education research. In 1998, the US education budget was $300 billion and less than 0.01% was spent on research (USHCS 1998). In 1994, the amount of federal spending on health professions education research was less than 0.001% of the total amount of direct federal spending on graduate medical education (Goldstein 1994).

Over 15 years ago, Wartman and O'Sullivan (1989) recommended the creation of a national center for health professions education research. In his more recent publication, Wartman (2004) again declared, "health professions education as an enterprise has lacked the solid research and development needed to create the infrastructure and support systems necessary to support the full scientific advance of the field" and "the need for such a national center is urgent and compelling." The status and future of medical education research were discussed at a conference jointly sponsored by the Bureau of Health Professions and the Association of American Medical Colleges in 1993 (BHPr-AAMC 1994). Recommendations from this conference included a proposal for the development of a study section in the National Institutes of Health (NIH) devoted to medical education research and the establishment of centers for medical education research in several medical schools.

A recent study determined how published medical education research studies were funded and the approximate costs of conducting these studies (Reed et al. 2005). The authors selected studies from two journals encompassing all medical specialties (*JAMA, New England Journal of Medicine*), four medical education journals (*Academic Medicine, Medical Education, Teaching and Learning in Medicine, Medical Teacher*), and seven journals representing the core specialty areas of internal medicine, general surgery, pediatrics, family medicine, obstetrics and gynecology, and emergency medicine. A total of 665

14

medical education articles were published in the 13 peer-reviewed journals from September 1, 2002 to December 31, 2003, of which 290 met all study inclusion criteria. Authors of 243 studies responded to a survey of items related to the percentage of the authors' total work commitment devoted to the study, resources used and their costs, attainment of funding, and the first author's estimated cost of conducting the study. The cost of each study was calculated by multiplying the percentage effort of each author for the duration of the study by the national median salary for each author, according to specialty and academic rank, and then adding the costs of the resources used. The median calculated cost of conducting the 243 studies was $24,471. The median authors' estimate of study cost was $10,000. Funding was obtained for 29.6% of the studies, with the median amount of funding being $15,000. The median calculated cost of funded studies was $37,315, resulting in a deficit of $22,315 per funded study. Factors independently associated with attaining funding were training in grant writing and the number of medical education studies published by the first author.

Reed et al. (Reed et al. 2007) developed a reliable and valid instrument to measure the methodological quality of educational research studies and applied the instrument to a sample of 210 medical education research studies, to identify relationships between funding and study quality. The instrument, called medical education research study quality instrument (MERSQI), included ten items, reflecting six domains of study quality: study design, sampling, type of data (subjective or objective), validity, data analysis, and outcomes. MERSQI scores were correlated with global quality ratings from two independent experts who were nationally recognized authorities in medical education research and current or former editors of leading medical education journals. The association between MERSQI scores and the 3-year citation rate (number of times the study was cited in the first 3 years after publication) was measured. Additionally, the association between MERSQI scores and the impact factor of the publishing journal in the year the study was published was measured. Of the 210 studies evaluated, 149 (71%) did not have any funding, 30 (14%) had between $1 and $19,999 in funding, and 31 (15%) had $20,000 or more in funding. In bivariate analysis, attainment of $20,000 or more in funding was significantly associated with an increase in total MERSQI score. Higher MERSQI scores were found in studies conducted by first authors with higher numbers of overall previous peer-reviewed publications and higher numbers of previous peer-reviewed medical education publications. Few studies in the sample measured patient or health care outcomes, highlighting the need to advance outcomes research in medical education. The authors of the study theorized that funding allowed researchers to conduct more-rigorous studies, but felt it was conceivable that the process of applying for funding, rather than the funding itself, was responsible for the observed associations.

In his review of research reports from two leading education journals, *Academic Medicine* and *Teaching and Learning in Medicine*, Carline found that of 70 articles published, 45 did not include an acknowledgment of funding (Carline 2004). Of the 25 articles that did acknowledge funding, five indicated support from departmental or faculty development funds. A total of 30 individual agencies were acknowledged in the listing of external funding for the remaining 20 articles, including the NIH, Health Resources and Services Administration, the Fund for the Improvement of Postsecondary Education, the Centers for Disease Control and Prevention, the Canadian Institutes of Health, the Association of

American Medical Colleges, the National Board of Medical Examiners, the Society of General Internal Medicine, the American Academy of Family Physicians, the Royal College of Physicians and Surgeons of Canada, the Robert Wood Johnson Foundation, and the W.K. Kellogg Foundation.

It is clear that the majority of medical education research is carried out without support of external funding. Faculty development programs and career awards from federal or private foundation grants support educational research, although not always with direct financial support to cover faculty time. Equipment and supplies needed for medical education research, such as handheld computers, laptop computers, standardized patients, or video equipment, have often already been purchased by the institution. The research to determine how to implement and measure the effectiveness of such technology requires faculty time and expertise as well as information technology support personnel and other support staff. However, many intramural and external education research grants limit or disallow budgeting for faculty time. Medical school faculty members who engage in educational research typically have substantial clinical and in some cases administrative responsibilities that consume the majority of their time. Although there are nonphysician medical education researchers with master's or doctoral degrees, they generally collaborate with physicians. Dedicated time for educational research may be difficult to justify in an environment of decreasing revenue. When educational research is a priority of departments and institutions, they subsidize faculty salaries to allow time for such research.

Million-dollar grants for medical educational research, such as the Undergraduate Medical Education for the twenty-first Century project, are limited to funding of major medical school reforms. Training grants from the Bureau of Health Professions or the NIH that support evaluation and research usually represent a small portion of the total funding. Most of these large grants do not fund medical education research per se, but provide opportunities to develop and evaluate educational programs as well as to learn and develop skills in research methods (Carline 2004). These granting institutions do not typically have medical education as a primary focus. To get around this, faculty creatively fold in educational issues in the context of disease-based research. Unless there are dramatic changes in government policy, such as the creation of a federally funded educational research grants program, medical education will continue to be seen as a local, institutional responsibility, and medical education research will remain a predominantly locally funded activity. Because of the general dearth of external funding available for educational research, most research projects have been underfunded, have involved secretarial and faculty time indirectly donated by the divisions, and have been accomplished on shoestring budgets (Thomas et al. 2004).

Many societies offer funding for medical education research. These are generally smaller grants ranging from $5,000 to $15,000 (e.g., the American College of Emergency Physicians, the Emergency Medicine Foundation, the Society for Academic Emergency Medicine, the Association of Professors of Gynecology and Obstetrics). The Foundation for Anesthesia Education and Research awards educational research grants of up to $50,000 a year for up to 2 years for research in anesthesia education (FAER 2006). Recipients of these grants must be guaranteed 40% nonclinical time to carry out the research. However, even if the entire $50,000 was allotted for faculty salary, it would not come close to providing 40% of an anesthesiologist's salary. The Association for Surgical Education awards grants of up to $100,000 for up to 3 years in education development and research in surgical education (CESERT 2008). These grants are only available to members of the Association of Surgical Education (given priority) or other national surgical organizations.

Grants of up to $150,000 for 2 years are available through the Edward J. Stemmler, MD Medical Education Research Fund (Stemmler Fund, 2007). Proposals must be based on research or development of innovative assessment approaches that will enhance the evaluation of those preparing to continue to practice medicine. Multi-institutional collaboration is encouraged.

There are a variety of grants databases available on the Web with free access, such as GrantsNet, funded by the American Academy of Science. However, these databases are generally geared towards basic science and not educational research. If the terms "radiology education" are entered into GrantsNet, pages of grant programs (GrantsNet 2008) that seem to have little to do with research in radiology education appear. Looking for funding via this route is an inefficient way of acquiring support for medical education research. One of the problems with such databases is that they do not include search terms appropriate for medical education research.

14.4
Characteristics of Successful Medical Education Research Centers

A series of case studies of medical education research groups (Arnold 2004) outlines the similarities and differences of eight highly productive groups: Dartmouth Medical School (Nierenberg and Carney 2004), Johns Hopkins University School of Medicine (Thomas et al. 2004), University of Kentucky College of Medicine (Elam 2004), University of Maastricht Faculty of Medicine (van der Vleuten et al. 2004), University of Michigan Medical School (Gruppen 2004), University of California, San Francisco, School of Medicine (Irby et al. 2004), University of Toronto Faculty of Medicine (Hodges 2004), and the University of Washington School of Medicine (Wolf et al. 2004). The groups vary in age (5–30 years), size, and composition (three full-time equivalents spread over ten researchers, three full-time equivalent staff, and 18 PhD candidates in one instance, to eight core faculty, five staff, 12 fellows and professors, and 100 affiliates in another instance). However, the groups share several characteristics. Their educational research goal is closely aligned with their institutional missions. Leaders who themselves are accomplished educators and/or researchers in medical education champion these groups. All describe constrained or limited funding, but enough to support a critical mass of highly skilled education researchers and important infrastructure to support the research mission. The groups emphasize the importance of collaboration as essential to medical education research for several reasons. Most medical education problems require the synthesis of content expertise provided by faculty members in basic science or clinical departments, with the educational, behavioral, and social science expertise provided by faculty members in a medical education research unit (Gruppen 2004). Collaboration enables investigators to accomplish more together than they could separately, and to expand the impact of the research beyond small numbers. Faculty development was part of the infrastructure of all groups (through local institutional programs, and in some cases through encouragement of faculty to participate in the Association of American Medical Colleges' Fellowship in Medical Education Research, the Harvard Macy Scholars Program, and the American Academy of Physician and Patient).

The success of these groups was measured by their publications and funding. At Dartmouth Medical School, the total number of manuscripts submitted per year rose from four in 2000–2001 to between 15 and 20 in 2002–2003 (Nierenberg and Carney 2004). At Johns Hopkins University School of Medicine, 57 peer-reviewed educational research publications since 1995 were identified (Thomas et al. 2004). The University of Maastricht Faculty of Medicine reported an average of 32 publications per year over the prior 5 years (van der Vleuten et al. 2004). Faculty in the Department of Medical Education at the University of Michigan published 83 peer-reviewed articles from 2000 to 2004 and were awarded a total of $839,574 in grant funding (Gruppen 2004). Since its establishment of an Office of Medical Education, the University of San Francisco has seen a fourfold increase in peer-reviewed publications in educational research (Irby et al. 2004). In the first 6 years of operation, the Wilson Centre at the University of Toronto saw grant funding increase from Canadian $800,000 in 1997 to Canadian $5,400,000 in 2003 and over 100 publications in major education journals annually (Hodges 2004). Direct external grant and contract support for which department faculty are the principal investigators grew from over $135,000 per year in 1997 to over $680,000 per year in 2002, and topped $1.2 million per year in 2003 at the University of Washington (Wolf et al. 2004).

14.5
Trends in Medical Education Research

On the basis of a MEDLINE review, the total number of medical education research articles published in English increased steadily from about 1,329 in 1980 to 2,907 in 2003 (Wartman 2004). The top-three medical education research journals (*Academic Medicine, Medical Education, Family Medicine*), which have a combined circulation of just under 14,000, accounted for just over 20% of all medical education articles published in English from 1994 to 2003 (Wartman 2004). Of the top-nine medical education research journals (Wartman 2004), none are radiology journals. The number of articles published in these nine journals from 1994 to 2003 ranged from 234 (*The Lancet*) to 2,699 (*Academic Medicine*), with a total of 24,028. From his review of medical education research, Wartman concluded "the field of health professions education research is growing, articles on internship and residency predominate, and the major journals dedicated to the field have modest circulations" (Wartman 2004).

In another review of the medical education research literature, Regehr (2004) focused on four journals that are central to the medical education research enterprise: *Academic Medicine, Advances in Health Sciences Education, Medical Education*, and *Teaching and Learning in Medicine*. All are dedicated to health professional education questions and focus on all aspects of the medical education enterprise rather than specializing on a level (e.g., graduate medical education) or specialty (e.g., radiology). From his review of the research articles in these journals since 2000, he identified four content themes: (1)

applied curriculum and teaching issues (2) skills and attitudes relevant to the structure of the profession (3) students' characteristics, and (4) evaluation of individuals. One of the largest and fastest growing areas in curriculum design and evaluation was the integration of simulation into the curriculum as a mechanism for teaching without direct contact with patients (e.g., standardized patients, bench models, and virtual reality simulators) (Regehr 2004). Another active topic was the use of technology as a vehicle for curriculum delivery (e.g., videoconferencing, Web-mediated collaborative learning environments, or CD-ROM or Web-based databases of educational information). The core competencies elaborated by the ACGME and the Royal College of Physicians and Surgeons of Canada have recently been the focus of increasing study. In particular, a substantial number of researchers have sought to understand "professionalism" as regards how it is taught at various levels of medical education, and how to dependably measure students' competence in this area. Studies of student characteristics have focused on individual differences in learning styles and motivation, and the effects of age, gender, and race or ethnicity on differences in medical school experiences. The results of such studies can be used to inform admissions committees (i.e., in selecting students who will be successful and admitting an increased number of underrepresented populations) and lead to a better understanding of career choice and practice patterns. Greater attention is being paid to evaluation of individuals in concert with new requirements to develop and utilize dependable measures to assess clinical competence. Two tools under current investigation are portfolio assessments and objective structured clinical examinations (Regehr 2004).

More recently, Todres et al. (2007) reviewed research published in 2004 and 2005 in two general medical journals, the *BMJ* and *The Lancet*, and two leading medical education journals, *Medical Education* and *Medical Teacher*. None of the 390 research papers published in *The Lancet* was in the field of medical education. Only 11 of the 399 papers published in the *BMJ* related to medical education. Very few papers reported studies using experimental designs, with case-control studies and randomized controlled trials each accounting for less than 3% of the sample. No meta-analyses were found. 116 (30%) of the 387 papers stated that the study had external funding, 47 had internal funding, and 224 gave no information on funding. Less than half of the studies were collaborative ventures between two or more institutions. The authors of the study likened the research landscape in medical education to that of primary care and health services research 20 years ago, when there was a paucity of trained researchers, who used primitive research methods, and struggled for funding. They went on to lament that undergraduate and postgraduate curriculum reforms over the past 20 years have resulted in major changes in the way that students and postgraduates are taught, "often on the basis of nothing more than pragmatism, fashion, and whim."

A structured longitudinal review of the undergraduate medical education literature from nearly four decades characterized historical and current study methods and evaluated whether participation of medical education departments or centers was associated with more rigorous methods (Baernstein et al. 2007). The annual number of publications increased over time from one (1969–1970) to 147 (2006–2007). Recruitment of participants from more than one institution was present in only 6% of publications. A little more than half of the publications (54%) used a comparison group. Validated outcomes were reported in only 16% of publications. The interval between the intervention and the last assessment was less than 1 month in the majority of publications, and rarely was the statistical power of the study or the cost of the intervention reported. None measured benefit to patients as an outcome and rarely was outcome measured in terms of behavior change in the workplace. Less than half reported receiving funding. Educators considering a curricular change need to know the cost as well as the potential benefits of the program they are considering. Although calculating the cost of an educational program requires considerable effort, some costs, such as equipment or standardized patient salaries, can be estimated. However, only 3% of recent publications reported the cost of any part of the relevant programs.

Despite a well-developed body of clinical literature in radiology and an extensive literature in the field of education, there are relatively few articles regarding radiology education in professional journals. The number of radiology education articles published increased from 9.2 articles per year from 1966 to 1986 to 12.6 articles per year from 1987 to 1997 (Calhoun et al. 1988; Collins et al. 2001). The percentage of experimental studies increased from 8.7 to 12.3%. However, in both periods, the majority of articles were expository and in the latter period only 31.2% of experimental articles were truly experimental, substantiating a lack of hypothesis-driven research. The most common topic in both periods was program description and the fastest-growing topic of study was technology. The top-three journals publishing radiology education articles in the period 1987–1997 were *Investigative Radiology* (5.73 articles per year), *American Journal of Roentgenology* (3.18 articles per year), and *Radiology* (1.17 articles per year). Although *Academic Radiology* only published 0.45 articles per year, it did not begin publication until 1994. A more recent assessment would likely show a large percentage of radiology education papers being published in *Academic Radiology*, as it has been a major forum for publication of radiology education papers since its inception. Another relatively new venue for publication of radiology education papers is the *Journal of the American College of Radiology*. The increased number of articles addressing radiology education is encouraging. However, there still remains a dearth of empirical research in radiology education.

14.6
Opportunities in Medical Education Research

It is rare for medical education research to show a relationship with health outcomes. Many obstacles prevent this from being easily accomplished. The time between delivery of an educational program and measurement of patients' or health outcomes can be very long, especially when the focus is on medical students (Shea et al. 2004). Intervening events, such as residency training and varying kinds of independent learning, act as variables that influence outcomes. Other factors unrelated to the educational intervention that influence patient outcomes include patient mix, patients' values and preferences, severity of disease, and health care delivery systems. Documenting the relationship between education and patient outcomes represents one of the biggest challenges and greatest opportunities in medical education research. Continuing medical education programs have focused on patient outcome measures (e.g., blood pressure control, smoking cessation). However, the link between patients' outcomes and residents' or medical students' education is less direct and more difficult to measure.

A major opportunity for medical education research is examination of the outcomes resulting from the implementation of educational interventions directed towards the new competency requirements of the ACGME (1999). The description of the six competencies and requirements for individual and program assessment are part of an ACGME initiative aptly referred to as the "Outcome Project." Many questions related to outcomes assessment will need to be answered. For example, do changes in the resident curriculum affect a physician's preparedness to deliver patient care? Do they influence the quality of patient care? Do they affect the costs (both manpower and dollar costs) associated with patient care?

The growing demand for accountability in health care emphasizes the need to promote research that examines the linkages between medical education and quality health care (Chen et al. 2004). The Commonwealth Fund report (CFTFAHC 2002), *Training Tomorrow's Doctors: The Medical Education Mission of Academic Health Centers*, found that "the available data are insufficient to judge the performance of academic health centers in discharging their educational responsibilities beyond establishing a minimum level of competency." The Task Force recommended that the federal government support research to produce valid and reliable measures of the costs and quality of medical education, and specifically requested $25 million in public funding to develop and implement improved measures of performance in medical education.

14.7
The Future of Radiology Education Research

Opportunities in radiology education research are opening up both within and outside the radiology specialty. The Radiological Society of North America, in collaboration with the Association of University Radiologists, the Association of Program Directors in Radiology, and the Society of Chairmen of Academic Radiology Departments, offers an annual Radiology Educational Research Development Grant (RSNA 2008). This grant program fills a void where no previous program existed by providing funding for radiology education research to all levels of investigators to investigate any area related to radiology education. These 1-year grants of up to $10,000 can be used to pay for the costs of research materials, research assistant support, and investigator salary support (up to half of the grant award). Applicants must be a member of one of the sponsoring organizations. Other Radiological Society of North America grants related to radiology education include Fellowship Training (providing $50,000 salary support for 1 year), Educational Scholar (2-year grant up to $75,000 per year to pursue advanced training in the discipline of radiology education), and Education Seed (1-year grant up to $30,000 to pursue radiology education research).

The Society of Pediatric Radiology offers seed grants of up to $10,000 for 1 year to support research and education in pediatric radiology (Society for Pediatric Radiology 2005). No salary support is provided. However, they also offer the N. Thorne Griscom Award for Education in Pediatric Radiology, to support projects involved in pediatric radiology education. This award of $40,000, offered only in even-numbered years, is to be used to support investigator salary and benefits.

The paucity of funding available for radiology education research is one of the challenges facing efforts to advance the science of radiology education. As with the medical field in general, much of the educational research in radiology continues to be done with volunteer time and materials. This is not an adequate model to build or sustain a viable radiology education research enterprise. In addition to the funding limitations, there is not a critical mass of radiology educators who have the skills and resources (including funded time) to nurture and train new radiology educators. The lack of a formal organized funding program results in most radiology education research being noncohesive, institution-specific, and involving small samples. Multi-institutional studies involving large sample sizes and adequate study periods require substantial and sustained infrastructural support.

Nonradiology organizations offer medical education programs that are available to radiologists. The American Association of Medical Colleges Medical Education Research Certificate program is a new initiative designed to provide a basic foundation in research principles relevant to educational research in medical education (AAMC 2008). The program is open to all who are interested in improving their educational research skills and is targeted to those with a background in medical education but relatively less experience in conducting educational research. The International Association of Medical Science Educators offers a Webcast audio seminar series on educational research and scholarship (IAMSE 2008). Archives of the spring 2002 to fall 2007 sessions are available on their Website.

The AAMC has offered a fellowship in medical education research for many years (Collins and Salas 1997). Many medical schools offer intramural educational research grants that have proven benefits (Albanese et al. 1998). These and other faculty development and grant programs that are available to radiologists are not enough to elevate radiology education research to the level afforded to basic and clinical science research. An organized approach championed by skilled radiology educators is needed. One of the ways this might be accomplished is through the development of radiology fellowship programs in medical education within select radiology departments where there exists the infrastructure necessary to support such a program. Many academic radiology departments are associated with a major university where such fellows would have access to colleges of education, psychology, and related fields. With a year dedicated to studying and practicing radiology education research, under the auspices of experienced investigators, a fellow could take advantage of the many training and funding opportunities offered by radiology and nonradiology societies. These fellowships could be funded by departments through the clinical income the fellow generates by spending a percentage of his/her time practicing clinical radiology. Eventually, such fellowship programs would result in a critical mass of radiology education investigators that could substantially impact on the support allocated for such research within the field of radiology.

In 2002, Elias Zerhouni, Director of the NIH, convened a series of meetings to chart a roadmap for medical research in the twenty-first century (NIH 2008). Participants were asked a series of four questions:

> What are today's scientific challenges?
> What are the roadblocks to progress?
> What do we need to do to overcome roadblocks?
> What can't be accomplished by any single Institute – but is the responsibility of NIH as a whole?

14

It is through this type of collaborative thinking and informed decision-making that a national research agenda is developed. These same questions could be asked of radiology education researchers if brought together as one group to determine a common mission and "roadmap" for radiology education research. Through this process, the most critical areas of radiology education research could be prioritized and a strategy for implementation designed. The questions might be reworded as follows: What are the challenges in radiology education (e.g., documenting the link between education and patient outcomes)? What are the roadblocks to success (e.g., underfunding, lack of sufficient investigators, nonunified research agenda)? What do we need to overcome these roadblocks (e.g., establish a national center for health professions education research, develop fellowships in radiology education research, establish a formal society of radiology education researchers)? What cannot be accomplished by any single institution or investigator (e.g., the need for multi-institutional, multidepartmental, multispecialty collaboration)? Elias Zerhouni asked working groups to address the following questions in relation to the proposed initiatives:

> ➤ Can the NIH afford *not* to do it?
> ➤ Will the initiative be compelling to our stakeholders, especially the public?

Again, a parallel argument can be made for radiology education research that as a specialty we cannot afford *not* to develop a viable educational research mission because our stakeholders (i.e., patients) demand answers to the questions that such research must address.

14.8
Summary

Current radiology education research is predominantly a volunteer effort on the part of faculty who have considerable clinical and administrative responsibilities. There is no common voice for radiology education researchers and no national research agenda. As a result, the investigations tend to focus on short-term outcomes with small sample sizes and yield results that are usually not generalizable to the general radiology community. Studies often lack appropriate control groups and use subjective and unvalidated instruments to assess outcomes. The questions that must be answered regarding the effectiveness of radiology education and its effect on the quality of patient care are no less important than any of the questions addressed by basic and clinical science research. Medical education research can be made more meaningful by planning prospective studies with mechanisms for following participants over many years, making better use of rigorous retrospective studies, and clarifying linkages between educational processes and patient health outcomes. Building a critical mass of radiology education researchers through education fellowship programs specific to radiology and mobilizing the existing radiology education researchers into one group with a shared vision are opportunities that will enable radiologists to take better advantage of existing funding and training opportunities and advance the science of radiology education.

References

AAMC Medical Education Research Certificate (2008) http://www.aamc.org/members/gea/merc. htm. Accessed 30 January 2008

ACGME Outcome Project (1999) http://www.acgme.org/outcome/comp/compMin.asp. Accessed 30 January 2008

Albanese MA, Horowitz S, Moss R, Farrell P (1998) An institutionally funded program for educational research and development grants: it makes dollars and cents. Acad Med 3:756–761

Amis ES Jr (2008) New program requirements for diagnostic radiology: update and discussion of the more complex requirements. Am J Roentgenol 190:2–3

Arnold L (2004) Preface: case studies of medical education research groups. Acad Med 79:966–968

Baernstein A, Liss HK, Carney PA, Elmore JG (2007) Trends in study methods used in undergraduate medical education research, 1969–2007. J Am Med Assoc 298:1038–1045

Berger WG, Gibson SW, Krupinski EA, Morals JD (2007) Proposed ACGME change in length of radiology residency training before independent call. Results of a survey of program directors and chief residents. J Am Coll Radiol 4:595–601

Calhoun JG, Vydareny KH, Ten Haken JD, Blane CE (1988) Journal publications in radiology education: a review of the literature, 1966–1986. Invest Radiol 23:62–67

Carline JD (2004) Funding medical education research: opportunities and issues. Acad Med 79:918–924

Carney E, Kempf J, DeCarvalho V, Yudd A, Nosher J (2003) Preliminary interpretations of after-hours CT and sonography by radiology residents versus final interpretations by body imaging radiologists at a level 1 trauma center. Am J Roentgenol 181:367–373

Center for Excellence in Surgical Education, Research and Training (2008) http://www.surgical-education.com/mc/page.do?sitePageId = 28551&orgId = ase. Accessed 30 January 2008

Chen FM, Bauchner H, Burstin H (2004) A call for outcomes research in medical education. Acad Med 79:955–960

Collins J, Salas AA (1997) Fellowship in medical education research: an opportunity for academic radiologists. Acad Radiol 4:700–702

Collins J, Kazerooni EA, Vydareny KH, Blane CE, Albanese MA, Prucha CE (2001) Journal publications in radiologic education: a review of the literature, 1987–1997. Acad Radiol 8:31–41

Commonwealth Fund Task Force on Academic Health Centers (2002) Training tomorrow's doctors: the medical education mission of academic health centers. The Commonwealth Fund, New York

Edward J. Stemmler (2007) MD Medical Education Research Fund of the National Board of Medical Examiners 2007–2008 Call for Proposals, http://www.nbme.org/PDF/2007–2008 StemmlerFundCFP.pdf. Accessed 30 January 2008

Elam CL (2004) Medical education research at the University of Kentucky College of Medicine. Acad Med 79:985–989

Foundation for Anesthesia Education and Research (2006) http://faer.org/programs/grants/options. html. Accessed 30 January 2008

Goldstein BP (1994) Where do we go from here? Afterword to the Proceedings of the BHPr-AAMC Conference, "Research in Medical Education: Policies for the Future." Acad Med 69:625–626

GrantsNet Funding Directory. (2008) http://www.grantsnet.org/search/fund_dir.cfm?global_indv_key=100167032&global_indv_type=pgm_public&global_pgm_levl=All&global_session_id=719455. Accessed 30 January 2008

14

Gunderman RB, Delaney LR (2007) Should 12 months of training be required before diagnostic radiology residents take independent call? A survey of the Association of Program Directors in Radiology. J Am Coll Radiol 4:590–594

Gruppen LD (2004) The Department of Medical Education at the University of Michigan Medical School: a case study in medical education research productivity. Acad Med 79:997–1002

Hodges B (2004) Advancing health care education and practice through research: the University of Toronto, Donald R. Wilson Centre for Research Education. Acad Med 79:1003–1006

International Association of Medical Science Educators (2008) http://www.iamse.org/development/index.htm. Accessed 30 January 2008

Irby DM, Hodgson CS, Muller JH (2004) Promoting research in medical education at the University of California, San Francisco, School of Medicine. Acad Med 79:981–984

NIH Roadmap (2008) http://nihroadmap.nih.gov/overview.asp. Accessed 30 January 2008

Nierenberg DW, Carney PA (2004) Nurturing educational research at Dartmouth Medical School: the synergy among innovative ideas, support faculty, and administrative structures. Acad Med 79:969–974

Petersen S (1999) Time for evidence based medical education. Br Med J 318:1223–1224

Proceedings of the BHPr-AAMC Conference (1994) "Research in Medical Education: Policies for the Future". Acad Med 69:601–626

Prystowsky JB, Bordage G, Feinglass JM (2002) Patient outcomes for segmental colon resection according to surgeon's training, certification, and experience. Surgery 132:663–670

RSNA R&E Foundation Educational Grant Programs (2008) http://www.rsna.org/Foundation/EducationGrants.cfm. Accessed 30 January 2008

Reed DA, Kern DE, Levine RB, Wright SM (2005) Costs and funding for published medical education research. J Am Med Assoc 294(9):1052–1057

Reed DA, Cook DA, Beckman TJ, Levine RB, Kern DE, Wright SM (2007) Association between funding and quality of published medical education research. J Am Med Assoc 298:1002–1009

Regehr G (2004) Trends in medical education research. Acad Med 79:939–947

Rumack C (2007) Special section – first year residents taking call: changing radiology resident call. J Am Coll Radiol 4:602–603

Schuwirth LWT, van der Vieuten CPM (2006) Challenges for educationalists. Br Med J 333:544–546

Shea JA, Arnold L, Mann KV (2004) A RIME perspective on the quality and relevance of current and future medical education research. Acad Med 79:931–938

Society for Pediatric Radiology R&E Scholarships and Award Opportunities. (2005) http://www.pedrad.org/displaycommon.cfm?an=1&subarticlenbr=38. Accessed 30 January 2008

Tamblyn R, Abrahamowicz M, Brailovsky C, et al (1998) Association between licensing examination scores and resource use and quality of care in primary care practice. J Am Med Assoc 280:89–996

Thomas PA, Wright SM, Kern DE (2004) Educational research at Johns Hopkins University School of Medicine: a grassroots development. Acad Med 79:975–980

Todres M, Stephenson A, Jones R (2007) Medical education research remains the poor relation. Br Med J 335:333–335

United States House Committee on Science (1998) Unlocking our future: toward a new national science policy. http://www.house.gov/science/science_policy_report.htm. Accessed 30 January 2008

van der Vleuten CPM, Dolmans DHJM, de Grave WS, van Luijk SJ, Muijtjens AMM, Scherpbier AJJA, Schuwirth LWT, Wolfhagen IHAP (2004) Education research at the Faculty of Medicine, University of Maastricht: fostering the interrelationship between professional and education practice. Acad Med 79:990–996

Wartman SA (1994) Research in medical education: the challenge for the next decade. Acad Med 69:608–614

Wartman SA (2004) Revisiting the idea of a national center for health professions education research. Acad Med 79(10):910–917

Wartman SA, O'Sullivan PS (1989) The case for a national center for health professions education research. Acad Med 64:295–299

Wechsler RJ, Spettel CM, Kurtz AB, et al (1996) Effects of training and experience in interpretation of emergency body CT scans. Radiology 199:717–720

Wolf FM, Schaad DC, Carline JD, Dohner CW (2004) Medical education research at the University of Washington School of Medicine: lessons from the past and potential for the future. Acad Med 79:1007–1011

Wysoki MG, Nassar CJ, Koenigsberg PA, Novelline RA, Faro SH, Faerber EN (1998) Head trauma: CT scan interpretation by radiology residents versus staff radiologists. Radiology 208:125–128

Developing a Radiology Curriculum for a New Medical School in Singapore

15

Kiang-Hiong Tay, Robert Kamei, Bien-Soo Tan

15.1
Preamble

Radiology over the past several years has become an increasingly integral component of patient management, not only in helping clinicians coming to a diagnosis through a wide range of imaging modalities, but also in treatment of diseases. Interventional radiology has, in many instances, replaced conventional medical or even surgical therapy as the new standard of care.

Despite this increasingly critical role in clinical medicine, there continues to be relatively little emphasis on radiology education in the curriculum of most medical schools. As a result, many interns and residents are not well trained in interpreting simple radiographs and scans or even in requesting the appropriate imaging modality to resolve a particular clinical problem.

Despite imaging being such a critical component of day-to-day clinical practice, the lack of clinical radiology training is clearly undesirable and should therefore play a bigger role in medical student education.

In 2005, a unique opportunity to develop an innovative teaching program integrating radiology training with core medical education arose when the Singapore Government announced the setting up of a second medical school in Singapore. This new medical school was a partnership between Duke University School of Medicine and the National University of Singapore (NUS), and was to be sited within the campus of Singapore General Hospital (SGH). It was created with the understanding that the majority of the teaching

Kiang-Hiong Tay (✉)
Associate Professor and Radiology Thread Leader, Duke-National University of Singapore
Graduate Medical School Singapore, 2 Jalan Bukit Merah, Singapore 169547, Singapore
E-mail: tay.kiang.hiong@sgh.com.sg

Radiology Education. R.K. Chhem et al. (Eds.)
DOI: 10.1007/978-3-540-68989-8, © Springer-Verlag Berlin Heidelberg 2009

15

faculty would come from SGH and several specialty centers within the campus. The education leadership at the new medical school, the Duke-NUS Graduate Medical School Singapore, recognized the valuable role of radiology in teaching medicine and decided to integrate radiology education into its curriculum.

This article describes the background of the setting up of the new medical school and the challenges we face in developing the new school's radiology curriculum.

15.2
Background for Setting Up a New Medical School

In 2000, the Singapore Government launched a Biomedical Sciences Initiative that had a twofold plan: firstly, to make Singapore the biomedical hub of Asia and, secondly, to attract both research and health sector manufacturing capabilities to Singapore. Incentives have been offered to attract companies to Singapore, and the government is funding research institutes devoted to genomics, bioinformatics, bioengineering, nanotechnology, molecular and cell biology, and cancer therapies.

In 2001, a Medical Education Review Panel evaluated the plan and subsequently recommended that Singapore establish a graduate medical school to produce the highly trained physician-scientists needed to support the Biomedical Sciences Initiative.

The new graduate medical school was intended to complement NUS's existing undergraduate medical school. Students enter medical school after completing their Singapore–Cambridge General Certificate of Education advanced level examinations (or equivalent) and then pursue a 5-year curriculum towards a medical degree.

In April 2005, Duke University and NUS signed a formal agreement under which the two institutions would partner to establish a new medical school in Singapore which would be named the Duke-NUS Graduate Medical School Singapore. Graduates from Duke-NUS receive a joint Doctor of Medicine (MD) degree from both Duke University and NUS.

Duke-NUS Graduate Medical School Singapore is located in central Singapore on the grounds of SGH, the flagship public hospital in Singapore. Known as the Outram campus, the National Cancer Centre, National Dental Centre, National Heart Centre, and Singapore National Eye Centre are in the vicinity and are closely affiliated with Duke-NUS. Duke-NUS faculty are also affiliated with other health centers located elsewhere in Singapore, including the KK Women's and Children's Hospital, Changi General Hospital, and the National Neuroscience Institute (Duke-NUS GMS Web site).

15.3
Duke-NUS Graduate Medical School Curriculum

The Duke-NUS Graduate Medical School follows the American model of postbaccalaureate medical education in which students begin their medical studies after earning undergraduate or postgraduate degrees in any discipline other than medicine.

Duke-NUS Graduate Medical School offers a rigorous 4-year graduate entry medical education program with a distinctive focus on medical research, education, and patient care.

The curriculum, based on that of Duke University School of Medicine's, is vastly different from other MD training programs within the USA and elsewhere. Duke-NUS students cover basic science in 1 year, which gives them the opportunity to care for patients a full year earlier than their peers from other medical schools. The third year is almost fully devoted to independent scholarship and research, with the opportunity to work with renowned scientists. The rationale and evolution of this unique curricular model at Duke University is chronicled in detail in a recent article by Grochowski et al. (2007).

The first year of the Duke-NUS curriculum is a rigorous immersion in the basic sciences, the building blocks of medicine. The content is integrated into four interdisciplinary courses, each of which covers a range of subjects while placing them into a larger context. The four courses include molecules and cells (integration of biochemistry, genetics, and cell biology), normal body (integration of gross anatomy, microanatomy, physiology), brain and behavior (integration of neurobiology and human behavior), and body and disease (integration of microbiology, immunology, pathology, and pharmacology).

Each course is conducted by expert clinicians from respective medical fields in Singapore, which gives the opportunity for the students to gain first hand, up-to-date information. In addition, faculty members from Duke University visit Duke-NUS to conduct some of the courses and share their knowledge and research experiences.

Clinical skills and understanding investigative methods are also core curricular components in the first year. Students attend each week a course named "Practice Course," in which they learn and practice their communications skills. These include history taking, interviewing patients, and conducting physical examinations in a simulated clinical environment involving standardized patients. Standardized patients are individuals who are carefully trained to portray patient roles. These simulated physician–patient encounters are closely monitored under the guidance of Duke-NUS faculty members and are recorded/video-taped for the purpose of learning and assessment. During the initial months, students learn how to take patient histories, conduct a physical examination, and establish good physician–patient relationships, among other clinical skills.

The practice course dovetails with the first-year basic science curriculum, giving students a holistic view of their studies and helping them translate knowledge learned in the classroom into real-life situations.

Students also attend monthly sessions reviewing journal articles as a means of becoming critical readers and understanding the basic investigative methods and tools needed to conduct research.

Duke-NUS students begin their clinical rotations full time during the second year. Basic science components they learned during the first year and clinical skills from the practice course are essential background information necessary when seeing patients.

The second year, which begins with an orientation, focuses on a series of core clerkship rotations designed to develop students' clinical problem-solving skills and their ability to appropriately use resources to diagnose and treat patients. The duration of each rotation is 8 weeks. Core rotations include medicine, surgery, obstetrics and gynecology, pediatrics,

15

neurology, and psychiatry. Upon completion of clerkships, students are given the opportunity to take electives during a period of 4 weeks to explore subspecialties that were not covered during clerkships.

In addition, there are five 1-week clinical cores during the second year. Students discuss integrative topics such as patient safety, geriatrics/palliative care, and evidence-based medicine in this course. Also, approximately three times per month, students also return for Practice Course 2. This course is devoted to the themes of professionalism, ethics, end-of-life issues and advanced clinical skills and communications.

Duke-NUS's unique third year provides students with an unparalleled opportunity to study an area of particular interest in depth. Designed to prepare students for leadership roles in medical care and research, the third year allows students to gain scholarly experience in using their critical thinking skills and creativity to develop a research project and further explore their interests in shaping up their long-term career goals in medicine. At the end of their third year, Duke-NUS students are expected to submit a thesis.

Third-year students are also expected to complete their family medicine clerkship during this year unless they are precluded from doing so by their scholarly experience requirements. If they do not complete the family medicine clerkship in the third year, the students must complete it either at the end of their third year or in their fourth year.

The fourth year at Duke-NUS enhances students' preparation for their internships and residencies through clinical rotations. Students complete 42 elective clinical science credits, including one subinternship, one critical care elective, and a capstone course. Students must also complete a continuity clinic experience, if they did not complete it in the third year.

The course of study in the final year is tailored according to each student's career goals. The advisory dean and faculty mentors assigned to each student will help personalize a fourth-year program from a wide range of clinical electives. The year ends with the 4-week-long capstone course, which covers topics such as clinical skills for internship, communication skills, health care systems, advanced basic science topics, financial planning, personal wellness, and medical/legal issues. (Duke NUS GMS Website)

15.4
Radiology in Duke-NUS Graduate Medical School: Getting Started

With the start of the new medical school, the leadership of the SGH radiology department saw an opportunity to have radiology play a greater role in the medical student education and training.

The first challenge was to advocate to the leadership at Duke-NUS the need for more radiology education in the curriculum. As mentioned earlier, the curriculum is modeled closely on that of Duke University School of Medicine and in that curriculum, the main radiology teaching is in elective postings to the radiology department at the end of years 2 and 4. Radiology was therefore not part of the initial focus when the school set out to recruit the teaching faculty.

Since many of the first-year basic science modules were taught by practicing clinicians, they were very interested in using radiological images to teach topics such as anatomy,

neuroscience, and pathology. A few radiologists were approached in these classes to provide the radiological images, but their efforts were not coordinated.

However, it was realized that radiology teaching could be integrated into the entire 4-year curriculum in novel ways, and not only in the clinical rotations. A faculty position of Radiology Thread Leader was created at the school to develop, implement, and coordinate a radiology program throughout Duke-NUS Graduate Medical School's 4-year curriculum.

15.5
Defining the Role of Radiology in the Graduate Medical School Curriculum

Broadly speaking, we believed that radiology could contribute to Duke-NUS's teaching program in two ways: (1) by using radiology to teach other subjects and (2) by teaching of Radiology.

15.5.1
Using Radiology to Teach

Advances in imaging and information technology have produced new ways to depict the structure and function of the human body. Three-dimensional, virtual endoscopy, and dynamic displays are now the norm. Some medical schools have incorporated the use of radiological images to complement cadaveric dissection to teach anatomy, with some new schools going as far as discarding cadaveric dissection altogether (Miles 2005).

For the first-year Duke-NUS curriculum, the basic sciences are taught in integrated courses with frequent cross references to clinical practice. Computed tomography (CT) and magnetic resonance imaging (MRI) images, in particular three-dimensional reconstructed images, of the various body regions, were used by many faculty members to teach anatomy. Although our radiology department was not directly involved in the teaching of these modules, we hope to integrate the teaching of radiological anatomy by radiologists in these modules in the future.

15.5.2
Teaching of Radiology

The Duke-NUS leadership acknowledged that radiology plays an important role in modern medicine and recognized that basic radiological competency is a valuable skill set for all Duke-NUS students to acquire.

After discussion with the deans and teaching faculty, it was decided that radiology teaching should be integrated with the various clinical clerkships throughout year 2 of the Graduate Medical School curriculum, in addition to the radiology electives at the end of years 2 and 4.

The objectives of the radiology program were defined as follows. At the end of the program, the Graduate Medical School student should have:

- Basic knowledge of the various imaging modalities, including X-rays, fluoroscopy, ultrasound, CT, MRI, and nuclear medicine as well as their indications and limitations
- Basic knowledge of radiation safety and principles of radiation protection
- Basic knowledge of the various contrast media, their indications, contraindications, and complications
- Basic competency in interpreting chest, abdominal, and skeletal radiographs
- The ability to select the most appropriate and cost-effective radiological investigation for clinical situations and understand the imaging strategies of common clinical problems
- Basic knowledge of interventional radiology as well as its role and applications in modern medicine.

15.6
Developing the Radiology Program for Duke-NUS

Having articulated and defined radiology's role and objectives, the next step was to develop a radiology curriculum and schedule that would fit into the Duke-NUS curriculum.

Because there was no radiology curriculum from Duke University to use as a starting point, a literature search on radiology education in medical schools was done and revealed some rather startling findings.

We discovered that most medical schools in the world do not have a formal radiology curriculum. In two separate surveys published in 1994 and 2000, less than a third of medical schools in the USA have mandatory core radiology clerkships and the vast majority (72%) of the medical schools offer radiology teaching only in the form of an elective posting. This is despite the fact that 87% of clinicians in a separate survey felt that radiology education should be mandatory in medical school (Collins et al. 2002).

The methods of teaching radiology are also highly variable in different schools, ranging from didactic lectures to small-group tutorials to problem-based learning. In some schools, radiology teaching is integrated into the clinical clerkships. More recently, there is a trend towards using electronic media and computer-aided and Web-based e-learning tools to teach radiology. Many institutions have designed interactive electronic or Web based materials for radiology teaching and assessment, and in some institutions, their radiology program is designed on the Internet for independent, self-directed learning. It seems like no two schools are alike in terms of teaching method and content. We were unable to find any publications on the effectiveness of the various teaching methods.

The Web sites of the Royal College of Radiologists (RCR) as well as of the Association of University Radiologists and the Alliance of Medical Student Educators in Radiology (AMSER) suggested a curricular framework and core topics for a radiology teaching program in a medical school. It is, however, unclear how many medical schools in the USA and UK, where these guidelines originate, adopt the recommendations of these professional bodies.

The unique curriculum design of Duke-NUS Graduate Medical School makes it extremely challenging to introduce any new programs into the curriculum. The curriculum is very full and compact as the basic sciences and clinical clerkships have been shortened to create time for a research year. It was decided that radiology be given time in the orientation to the clinical year to introduce the basics of radiology, and several days to cover safety issues in radiology as well as to teach the basics of interpretation of chest, abdominal, and skeletal X-rays. This is followed by weekly or biweekly tutorial sessions in radiology throughout all the clerkships to cover radiology topics specific to the clerkships. For example, radiology in trauma, radiology in acute abdomen, and mammography will be covered during the surgery clerkship, while neuroimaging will be covered in the neurology clerkship. The topics and teaching methods will follow closely the recommendations of the RCR and the AMSER.

The radiology electives at the end of years 2 and 4 will be used for more in-depth coverage of the various subspecialties of radiology.

15.7
TeamGMS and Self-Directed Learning

Another unique feature of the Duke-NUS Graduate Medical School curriculum is the use of a modification of the "team-based-learning" educational technique, which is dubbed "TeamGMS (Haidet 2002)." Students work in teams to solve problems posed by faculty in a highly interactive teaching session. These problems require the students to use the information they have been asked to learn independently before class. TeamGMS allows the faculty to focus their teaching time in class on expanding, illustrating, and demonstrating the application of the knowledge the students have just acquired rather than simply delivering content via lectures. Students must become actively engaged with the material and are challenged by the faculty to develop the critical-thinking and communication skills that are important for future academic careers (Michaelsen 2005). Feedback thus far has shown the technique to be well received by both the Duke-NUS students and faculty. To our knowledge, TeamGMS technique has not been applied for the teaching of radiology. We are quite excited by the technique and are currently exploring using it to teach some modules of the radiology program.

Duke-NUS students are expected to attend all radiological rounds held in conjunction with the various clinical departments. The rounds will provide the students with real-life experience of how radiology is used in the diagnosis and even treatment of the patients' conditions. Duke-NUS students will be encouraged accompany their patients to the radiology department to observe how a radiological examination is performed on their patients and to discuss the radiological findings with the attending radiologists. The students will also be allowed to scrub up and assist in interventional radiology procedures.

Self-directed learning will be encouraged to complement and reinforce the radiology program at Duke-NUS. The digital nature of radiological images makes it well suited for self-learning. There is a wealth of electronic film libraries and electronic teaching material available online and many of the Web sites providing this material offer free access. Duke-NUS students will additionally be directed to existing radiology education resources available on the Internet.

15

We are also keen to develop our own electronic film library as well as electronic/Web-based teaching, self-learning, and assessment tools, not just for use by our medical students but also to serve the needs of radiology residents/fellows as well as other health care professionals on Outram campus who desire to learn more about radiology. We are currently evaluating a few platforms and are looking at partnering relationship to help us develop a product relevant to our local settings and needs.

15.8
Radiology and the Research Year

Since the Duke-NUS students devote the entire third year to research, this provides another opportunity for a small group of students to undertake a more extensive individual project in radiology. Biomedical imaging research is one of the key areas in the Government's Biomedical Sciences Initiative. Advances and innovations in radiological/imaging hardware and software as well as interventional radiological instrumentation and therapies are progressing at a rapid pace. SGH and other institutions on the Outram campus operate many state-of-the-art imaging instruments. For example, there are seven MRI scanners on the Outram campus, the latest being the Siemens Magnetom Verio 3T MRI scanner (fourth installation in the world), seven CT scanners, including two 64-slice instruments and one dual-source CT instrument, a positron emission tomography (PET)–CT instrument with an onsite cyclotron as well as micro CT and micro PET instruments for animal imaging. Several Duke-NUS medical students have advanced degrees in engineering and signal processing. There are many outstanding researchers and clinician scientists who will be able to serve as research mentors to Duke-NUS students for their third-year project. Involvement in this program will certainly expand radiology scholarship in Singapore.

15.9
Graduate Medical School Radiology Faculty

Recruiting the radiology teaching faculty for the school has been another challenge. Duke-NUS has a strict budget which limits the number of radiology faculty members that can be appointed. As the amount of work involved in building a completely new radiology program for Duke-NUS was going to be significant and there was initially no clear indication of the type and amount of support for the faculty, many radiologists were hesitant to come forward to teach, given their already heavy service workload. Nevertheless, a small group of radiologists who were accomplished in their respective subspecialty fields with a keen interest in teaching eventually stepped forward to take up the challenge.

Although all of the faculty members had been previously involved in teaching radiology residents as well as medical students, most did not have formal training in education. To help design and implement the radiology program at the school, the Radiology Thread Leader attended the First International Conference on Scholarship in Radiology Education

in August 2007 in London, Ontario, Canada. The conference proved to be very useful, not just in learning about education strategies, scholarship, and education research, it was also a great opportunity to network with educators from universities around the world. Subsequently, a faculty development workshop specifically tailored to education in the radiology setting was held in Singapore and was well received.

15.10
Moving Forward

It is rather disconcerting to discover from our literature search that in many medical schools around the world (including those in Singapore), medical student radiology education has clearly not kept pace with the tremendous clinical advancements of radiology in modern medicine. Radiology curriculum and pedagogy are highly variable throughout various medical schools, even among those from the same countries. Faculty training, development, and support (time and remuneration) are also variable, but we appear to lag behind our clinical counterparts in these aspects. Electronic and Web-based teaching/learning have flourished in the last couple of years, but the effectiveness of these learning technologies has not been studied. In fact, evidenced-based radiology education and radiology education research are glaringly lacking.

Our involvement in teaching radiology in the new school has forced us to take a closer look at radiology education in Singapore. Although it is comforting to know that many of our colleagues around the world face the same issues, recognizing these educational gaps in training has been an important first step for us to set in motion a series of initiatives to improve the scholarship of radiology education in Singapore. Developing the radiology program for Duke-NUS marks the beginning of this journey.

References

Association of University Radiologists – Alliance of Medical Student Educators in Radiology (AMSER) website – National Medical Student Curriculum in Radiology Available at: (http://www.aur.org/amser/AMSER_curriculum.html)

Collins J, Dottl SL, Albanese MA (2002) Teaching radiology to medical students: an integrated approach. Acad Radiol 9:1046–1053

Duke–NUS Graduate Medical School Web site. Available at: (http://www.gms.edu.sg) Accessed 24 April 2008

Grochowski CC, Halperin EC, Buckley EG (2007) A curricular model for the training of physician scientists: the evolution of the Duke University School of Medicine curriculum. Acad Med 82:375–382

Haidet P, O'Malley KJ, Richards B (2002) An Initial Experience with "Team Learning" in Medical Education. Academic Medicine. 77(1):40–44

Michaelsen L and Richards B (2005) Drawing Conclusions from the Team-Learning Literature in Health-Science Education: A Commentary, Teaching and Learning In Medicine, 17:1,85–88

15

Miles KA (2005) Diagnostic imaging in undergraduate medical education: an expanding role. Clin Radiol 60:742–745

Royal College of Radiologists website – Radiology for Medical Students. Available at: (http://www.rcr.ac.uk/index.asp?PageID=703)

Leadership in Radiology Education

16

R.B. Gunderman

Nothing fails like success, because we do not learn from it. We learn only from failure.
— Kenneth Boulding

The fates of radiology departments and other radiology organizations have always hinged on the quality of their leadership, but leadership is becoming an ever more important capability for radiologists. The rapid pace of changes in medical science and technology, the various medical disciplines, the organization and financing of healthcare, and the political system are making it more vital than ever that we educate learners to assume leadership roles.

Yet it is not sufficient that we merely prepare learners to lead, if by preparing learners to lead we mean teaching leaders how to tell other people what to do and then get them to do it. It is equally vital that we prepare leaders to learn. In his essay "Learning from failure," Major Doug Crandall of the Department of Behavioral Sciences and Leadership at the US Military Academy at West Point outlines the vital role of learning in leadership (Crandall 2007).

When it comes to education, some learning opportunities are more important than others. Crandall regards leaders' failures less as curses than blessings, because they represent essential learning opportunities. He divides leadership failures into three types:

1. Level one: failures in what we do
2. Level two: failures of who we are
3. Level three: failures of who we want to be

Crandall argues that to prepare future leaders to meet the leadership challenges they will face, we must prepare them to be more self-reflective and self-critical. He describes one of the most important habits future leaders can develop as "taking a hard look at themselves and thus bearing the fruit of improvement that comes from this personal pruning."

R.B. Gunderman
Education Division, Department of Radiology, Indiana University School of Medicine,
702 Barnhill Dr, RI 1053, Indianapolis, IN 46202-5200, USA
E-mail: rbgunder@iupui.edu

Radiology Education. R.K. Chhem et al. (Eds.)
DOI: 10.1007/978-3-540-68989-8, © Springer-Verlag Berlin Heidelberg 2009

16

16.1
Level One: Failures in What We Do

As Crandall sees it, the mission of leadership educators is not to teach learners how to lead but to help them learn how to teach themselves to lead. The key is not to follow certain rules or techniques of leadership, but to help learners relate new knowledge to their past, present, and future experiences in a lifelong journey of leadership development.

The best students of leadership are not the ones who have memorized the most words of advice from leadership textbooks, but those who have made the most of their failures. The most promising leaders of the future are the people who learn the most every day from the text of their own experience. There is no better guidebook, rule book, or policy and procedure manual than our own daily experiences, and our mission in developing leaders is to help them become dedicated and insightful readers of this text.

Consider level-one failures. In many leadership situations, we get feedback on how well we have done, and we categorize these results as successes or failures. Examples include ubiquitous radiological activities such as protocoling, performing, and interpreting imaging examinations, as well as less stereotypical activities such as making formal presentations, composing manuscripts, and devising call schedules.

When we get the diagnosis right, or at least include it in our differential diagnosis, we have succeeded. If we have failed to consider the right diagnosis, received a rejection notice for a manuscript, or left a clinical service uncovered, the feedback on failure tends to be relatively unambiguous. If we approach such feedback appropriately, we can make changes in the way we do things to decrease the probability that we will experience such setbacks in the future.

16.2
Level Two: Failures in Who We Are

Crandall argues that level-one learning is insufficient. We need to look beyond failures of what we do to level two, failures of who we are. Level-two failures are much easier to ignore than level-one failures. For one thing, they strike much closer to home, less at our actions than our identity. This identity is composed of our biological makeup, our rearing as children, our education, our experiences, and our own past self-reflection.

When we make a level-one failure, we need to look beyond what we did to the reasons that led us to do it. Did an error result from our impatience or carelessness? Are we insufficiently curious, attentive, or compassionate? Are we afraid of change, or so weakly committed to the status quo that we leap at any opportunity to do things differently?

Failures of who we are usually less obvious, but we will also go out of our way to hide them from others and ourselves. We would rather blame external forces than face up to our own internal weaknesses. Radiologists who always blame someone else when things go wrong will find it impossible to learn some of the most important lessons their experience has to offer. As a result, they will tend to perform poorly compared with more self-reflective leaders.

It is tempting to blame adverse outcomes on external factors, but in so doing, we deprive ourselves of the opportunity to look inward and thereby improve ourselves. What we need to do, and to help the next generation of leaders learn to do, is to hold up a mirror to ourselves, and ask how our own character and work habits may have contributed to the disappointment.

This is why the military so widely employs such techniques as after-action review, the purpose of which is to encourage the participants in a completed project or mission to reflect retrospectively and introspectively on what they have been through, looking for lessons by which to improve future performance. (Gunderman and Chan 2007) The principal purpose of holding up such a mirror is not to assign blame, but rather to help us understand ourselves better.

In perhaps the greatest novel ever written, Cervantes's Don Quixote recommends drama as an important adjunct to moral education. The play "places before us at every step a mirror in which we may see vividly portrayed the actions of human life; nothing indeed more truly portrays us as we are and as we would be than the play and the players" (Cervantes 2003). Human beings are gifted with the ability to learn not only from firsthand experience, but vicariously as well.

Therefore leadership educators can foster learning from failure by encouraging learners to read. Valuable in this regard are biographies and autobiographies, especially those composed by authors who are willing to discuss their subject's failures as well as successes. Novels are another great source of vicarious insight into failure, because they give us the opportunity to know the inner psychological lives of characters. We see up close and personal the deleterious effects of a lack of self-reflection, as well as the benefits that accrue to those who are able to scrutinize themselves.

Because we are much less likely to get candid feedback on who we are than on what we do, we need to seek out such appraisals. We need to cultivate a reputation for honesty and humility, so others know we can handle criticism as well as praise. If subordinates think we will react angrily or even vengefully to criticism, we will receive too little important feedback, and we may hear nothing of problems until they reach the disaster stage.

Excessive defensiveness is a prescription for leadership disaster. Yet it is not enough to admit our imperfection, no matter how laudable this may be. We also need to show others that we are sincerely committed to improvement, and that we will put their input to use in becoming better leaders. Lack of fear reduces subordinates' disincentive to offer a critical appraisal, but the hope that it will be used to good effect is an even more powerful positive incentive.

16.3
Level Three: Failures of Who We Want To Be

Level-three failures, failures of who we want to be, are the most important of all learning opportunities. Crandall argues that such failures violate one of two vital leadership commitments: our core leadership values or our core purposes. An example of an infringement of core leadership values is a leader who sincerely espouses a participative model of strategic planning but fails to share with colleagues key knowledge and perspectives on the challenges and opportunities before the organization. Decisions can be only as good as the knowledge on which they are based, and a leader who seeks to engage colleagues in decision making needs to be a good sharer of knowledge.

16

An example of a violation of core purpose is a leader who forgets the primary commitment to the long-term welfare of patients and the community and begins to make decisions based strictly on the short-term financial interests of the group. In the short term, such an approach may improve financial performance, but in the long term, it tends to erode personal commitment and professional fulfillment.

We need to encourage learners to ask themselves a vital question: Why do we want to lead? Is it to fatten our own wallets? Is it to draw more attention to ourselves? Is it because we enjoy bending others to our will? Or do we seek to lead because we genuinely care about how patients, colleagues, and our organizations are faring and want to do whatever we can to help them fare even better?

The best leaders are not the ones who regard others as levers by which to raise themselves. The best leaders are the ones whose primary orientation is service, a commitment to helping others perform at their best. In this sense, the best leaders operate less by a model of command and control than by a model of education, helping others to discover and in practice realize their full potential.

If we fail to help future leaders learn to look in the mirror and see not only who they are but also who they want to be, then we are selling them short. If they learn to weigh both what they do and who they are against their ideal vision of themselves, they will be prepared to learn the most essential leadership lessons and become the best leaders they can be.

Crandall quotes a former instructor from his department. Our most important message is not what we say or even what we do. Our most important message "is our lives." Our leadership style reflects far more than the books we have read and the leadership courses we have attended. Our leadership style reflects our ultimate aspirations as physicians and human beings.

This spirit of leadership is reflected in the words and actions of some of the greatest leaders of the twentieth century, such as Mohandas Gandhi and Martin Luther King Jr. Consider, for example, King's 1963 "I have a dream" speech (King 1992). Instead of railing against the faults of others, he invoked a vision of a universal brotherhood against which all human beings, including King himself, could assay themselves. King not only indicted us for our faults, he inspired us to dream of a better life and so become better than we are.

Are we trying to make everyone else conform to our vision, or are we educating others to discover and work to be their best, both individually and collectively? To say that our life is our message means, as Gandhi said, that we need to be the change we want to see in the world. It also means being mindful of the fact that everyone has made mistakes. Real credibility lies not in the illusion of infallibility, but in the capacity for honest self-reflection, the willingness not only to admit our mistakes but also the determination to learn from them.

References

Cervantes M (2003) Don Quixote, trans. Starkie W, Signet Classic, New York

Crandall D (2007) Learning from failure. In: Crandall D (ed) Leadership lessons from West Point. Jossey-Bass, San Francisco, CA

Gunderman RB, Chan S (2007) Where is the action in organizational learning? Radiology 242:650–653

King ML Jr (1992) I have a dream. In Washington JM (ed) I have a dream: writings and speeches that changed the world. Harper Collins, New York

The Business of Radiology Education Scholarship

17

L.A. Matheson

17.1
Introduction

A radiology department at a large Canadian university recently established a Centre for Education focused on supporting the education of physicians and students with a clear vision of changing the traditional approach to medical scholarship and education. The academic chair in this radiology department challenged the notion of education as a separate entity or activity from the practice of medicine. In many ways, he was a visionary with a clear belief that a multidisciplinary partnership was needed between clinicians and educationists to advance scholarship in teaching and learning. As is so often the case when a new and unique concept is supported by leadership and given an opportunity to become reality, 'seed money' was found to cover the essentials such as salary support and operational expenses, allowing the work of the Centre for Education to commence.

Shortly after the establishment of the Centre for Education, the department hired a business manager with experience in supporting academic medicine at the departmental level. Providing support to the Centre was one component of the established role. While the concept of integrating scholarship into a clinical department was new to the business manager, the need to provide infrastructure support was not. Given the initial success of the Centre within a very short period of time and the desire by academic leadership and other stakeholders to build from the initial successes, the manager was faced with a series of critical business questions that had not been previously considered, with the answers considered key to sustain the efforts of both the clinicians and educationists – *How can a*

L.A. Matheson
Department of Medical Imaging, University of Western Ontario,
Ontario, London, ON, Canada
E-mail: lori.matheson@lhsc.on.ca

Radiology Education. R.K. Chhem et al. (Eds.)
DOI: 10.1007/978-3-540-68989-8, © Springer-Verlag Berlin Heidelberg 2009

business plan be developed to support the vision for the future? What needs must be met to ensure this educational endeavour will succeed? Where and how can funding be secured? What infrastructure support is required to sustain the foreseen growth?

17.2
A Review of the Literature

Very little has been written addressing the need for the development and implementation of support for ongoing and expanded medical education outside of that existing within the formal structure of undergraduate education offered by medical schools and formalized residency training in academic clinical departments. As such, it is not surprising that even less has been published addressing the needs from a radiology education scholarship perspective. According to Cohen et al. (2005) "medical education…has become, in many institutions, somewhat of a by-product of [the] principal business lines of research and clinical service delivery… [and] the principal challenge to academic leaders is staying true to the academic mission, recognizing equal importance for its three components of education, clinical and research". With this recognition, it follows that the development of solutions that address the need for infrastructure support must be explored and articulated should radiology departments be committed to responding to educational needs and advancing scholarship.

As articulated by Cohen et al. (2005), leadership needs to continually strive to elevate the status of education in departments. To do so presents what may be realistically termed as a significant challenge, especially in an environment in which resources and funding are limited and not easily accessible. It becomes even more difficult for physicians and educators to address the logistical needs given the time, effort and expertise that are required to explore funding options, locate and secure space, handle human resource matters and build a stable information technology infrastructure. The expertise and efforts of physicians and educators are required elsewhere and when it becomes necessary for them to take on the responsibility of forming a business enterprise to support their educational efforts, the risk of being viewed as perpetual parasitic components of departments, continually seeking money and support from their clinical enterprise (Cohen et al. 2005), becomes very real.

There is significant value and long-term benefit in engaging physicians in implementing innovative educational approaches rather than requiring them to focus on funding, space, information technology and other infrastructure needs required to support their activities. Equally important, although not addressed in the literature, departments and institutions must recognize that the critical business component of education requires attention and they must be willing to broaden the team of experts gathered to include the business manager or other such qualified individual. Just as the radiology department referred to earlier brought together clinicians and educationists in the recognition that both content and process expertise were required to advance scholarship in teaching and learning, the inclusion of a resource/infrastructure expert is vital to address the issue of sustainability of the team's efforts.

17.3
Establishing the Right Team

Building a strong foundation to support the activities of physicians and educationists in their teaching endeavours needs to be the foremost consideration of any business manager. The efforts of physicians, researchers and educators are best focused on activities such as curriculum design, promoting innovative learning models and, ultimately, establishing a learning culture within a radiology department. However, the first challenge is requiring academic physicians to articulate their vision and actively discuss the direction they envision their initiative moving towards. While ideally such discussions and the opportunity to gather a team together should occur in the infancy of a programme, this is not always possible. As was our experience, initiatives had already commenced and the opportunity for input and detailed planning regarding resources and infrastructure followed at a later date. Regardless of the timing, the opportunity for such discussions is essential in order to develop a business plan.

It is suggested that a discussion of this nature involve all members of a multidisciplinary team. The notion that collaboration relating to the advancement of radiology (or any medical speciality) education scholarship is only that of the interest of physicians and faculty members needs to be challenged. While this approach may have worked traditionally, the complexity of sourcing today's infrastructure requirements and accessing available funding requires business knowledge and input. By gathering medical professionals, educators and business managers together, it allows not only the articulation of the vision, but also provides the opportunity for the exploration of avenues and options that may not be considered by a group with expertise in one discipline. Just as a community is essential to foster collaborative learning (Garrison and Arbaugh 2007), the formation of a similar group from various disciplines and with differing areas of expertise responsible for laying the foundation for educational scholarship is what will position radiology departments for success.

The role of the business manager within a clinical academic radiology department that is focused on creating a learning culture and fostering educational scholarship requires specific qualifications, experience and skills. Just as careful deliberation goes into bringing together the team of medical professionals and educators, thorough consideration of the skills of a potential business manager is also required.

Hiring an individual with experience in academic medicine with a solid understanding of the needs of clinical departments is vital. An individual with strong financial management skills with the ability to ensure the efficient and effective use of resources and the ability to prioritize the department's needs and align these needs with the vision and mission of educational scholarship is paramount. The manager must have the ability to implement the administrative components of strategic plans focused on the expansion of radiology education scholarship and must be able to collaborate with the physician leadership group to develop processes and policies that meet the needs of the centre or division of education as applicable. The individual must also be a proven and effective leader, able to assist in developing effective administrative support systems and contribute business expertise to an established team.

While difficult to quantify, the interpersonal skill set of a business manager must also be given careful consideration. Physicians and educators have a very different focus and approach to radiology education scholarship and the business manager must have the ability to not only recognize their scholarly focus but he or she must be able to translate their articulated vision into a business plan containing very specific details. In doing so, the business manager provides concrete mechanisms that can be utilized to support and attain the academic mission. On the manager's part, this requires a keen awareness of the different approaches between clinical academics and educators and what is required from a business perspective. The business manager must be able to facilitate ongoing discussions to draw out information from the other team members, thus ensuring the efforts and focus from a support and infrastructure perspective continue to provide a solid platform and meet the operational requirements for medical imaging education scholarship.

17.4
Infrastructure and Support Considerations

As articulated by Rethy Chhem in Chap. 2 in this volume, the expansion of scholarship in medical imaging education will occur when both physicians and educationists have the opportunities to discuss programme expansion, engage medical students and residents in changes, redesign curricula and conduct research. In understanding the mission and vision of radiology education scholarship, it is possible to define the infrastructure and support that is required. These considerations can be organized into three main categories: space, information technology and human resources.

17.4.1
Space

Our experience was that creating a space for the Centre for Education separate from the clinical activities of the department was necessary. Doing so not only provides a space for physicians, educationists and support staff to work, but it also provides a location for both formal and informal sharing amongst scholars. The creation of separate space elevates the status of the team's efforts and offers a clear indication to other academic leaders, faculty members, medical students and residents that leadership is committed to fostering and supporting the endeavours of the group.

The location and proximity of office space is also an important consideration. While not always possible, especially as is the case in most hospitals and universities, where space is always at a premium, ideally, the centre for education or division of education needs to be easily accessible by medical imaging physicians and students. Clinicians do not have the freedom to be too far from their clinical activities. Having the ability to conduct urgent consults and read results by ensuring a picture archiving and communication system (PACS) is available in the centre is vitally important for the continued functioning of the radiology department and for patient care. The centre also needs to be visible to others who may not need to attend the office on a regular basis but who practice within the radiology department and who will indirectly become part of and benefit from the culture of learning that is developed.

Finally, addressing the need to have consumable supplies available and general office infrastructure support needs to be included in the business plan. Items such as supplies, fax and photocopying equipment and telephone extensions should all be considered in the planning process.

17.4.2
Information Technology

Just as the emerging of information technology such as imaging informatics is one of the reasons it is necessary to expand scholarship in radiology education, the establishment of a centre for education or separate education division requires strong and stable information technology to support its administrative activities and the teaching and learning mission. Consideration should also be given to the development and maintenance of a website that reflects the values of radiology teaching and scholarship. As we learned from our experience, there is a need to plan for and build information technology into a business plan so that the administrative operations of the centre or division are not adversely impacted when aging technology fails or new technology is required.

After only about 7 months in the role, we became aware that the administrative support staff person in the Centre for Education had an older personal computer that, while still functioning, did not allow the individual to work optimally. When the Centre was established, there was opportunity to use some of the existing technology from the department where the Centre was located. Having very limited funding and not knowing the exact requirements of the role of the support staff, the Centre's leadership felt fortunate to be able to leverage what was available. The issue of having to potentially upgrade existing technology was not considered at the start and the challenge that both the Centre and the business manager had to face was how a new computer could be sourced. In this instance, the purchase of a new personal computer was made possible with the input from qualified information technology staff and the leveraging of funds from within the radiology department. However, this was an unforeseen expense and an issue that could have been dealt with proactively through planning. Having to replace the personal computer did provide the opportunity to assess future needs within the Centre and in doing so ensure that a replacement and upgrade programme was feasible and included as part of the business plan.

In Chap. 12 in this volume, Richard Rankin expertly articulates how the introduction of digital imaging and the use of PACS as well as teaching and learning software have changed the way clinical practice is performed and how the possibilities for the advancement of educational scholarship have developed. From this teaching and learning perspective, it follows that a centre or division of radiology education must be one of the key stakeholders in advancing the notion of lifelong learning and scholarly advancement. There is great opportunity for the structuring of both formal and informal teaching and learning sessions and the development of an innovative curriculum for students and residents. Support to radiologists in their continuing professional development and continuing medical education endeavours is also possible with the guidance of educationists.

From a business-planning perspective, consideration should be given to how to incorporate the advanced teaching and learning technology available with the vision and mission of radiology education scholarship. Considerations such as having PACS available within a centre for education, ensuring server and network access in conference and teaching rooms and having Internet access on all workstations are items that need to be assessed and built into the detailed planning process.

One of the most important projects initiated in the early development of the Centre for Education was the establishment of a website. Creating a link to the Centre directly accessible through the radiology department's website allowed the articulation of the vision, mission and purpose of the Centre and reflected the high value placed on medical imaging scholarship and education by the chair of the department. This was not only positively received by the local clinical and university community, but it also provided the mechanism for global outreach. Website development and maintenance needs to be included in a business plan. Ensuring the opportunity for all stakeholders to have input and share their expertise to make the website a lively reflection of the work of the centre or division of education requires planning to ensure a stable platform is utilized, that regular maintenance and changes can be implemented and that there is consideration given to expansion and growth of the website to become interactive in nature.

17.4.3
Human Resources

Without qualified, dedicated and enthusiastic individuals capable of supporting radiology education scholarship, the vision and mission of a centre or division of education will never be realized. As such, a key consideration in the development of a sound business plan is that of staff, namely physicians, educationists, research and administrative support staff. It may also include planning for information technology staff and language translation expertise required occasionally in support of the main activities of the centre or division.

The reality that many, if not all, medical imaging departments face is that staff are not necessarily available to engage in the activities of advancing radiology education scholarship on a full-time, dedicated basis. Many of the physicians need to maintain their clinical practices as this is the area where revenue is generated and hiring full-time educationists who are not already committed to other academic endeavours within their own faculty may be quite difficult. Other challenges such as developing detailed role descriptions and hiring qualified administrative support and research assistants all point to the complexity of the academic environment that departments need to function within.

When the Centre for Education was established, the physician leader, who was also the chair and chief of the radiology department, hired two part-time educationists with PhDs with other responsibilities in their own faculty to work as a team to first establish the Centre and then carry out the vision and the mission. This example is a clear indication of the reality that many departments at various institutions will face. The ideal staffing complement may not be attainable, but that is not to say that other approaches will not be just as viable. The willingness to be innovative is paramount when making staffing decisions.

As part of the development of a business plan, a human resource planning document should also be developed that details the role responsibilities and qualifications required of the educationists, research and administrative support staff who will work within the centre or division. The delineation of duties and the development of job descriptions need to directly relate to and support the vision, mission and purpose of the centre or division of education. Specifically, as was experienced in the development of the Centre for Education, there was a need to have an educationist fulfil the role of education project coordinator and there was also a requirement for curriculum and pedagogy support. Responsibilities such as working with clinical faculty to develop curricula that fosters active and self-directed learning, developing case studies and manipulating content materials for pedagogical purposes ensuring they are easily updated, portable and flexible are three examples of duties that the educationists may perform in their respective roles. From an administrative support perspective, duties may include establishing and updating a Web presence, conducting literature searches and creating annotated bibliographies, formatting research papers, formatting effective presentations and scheduling and supporting meetings, conferences and other events. The identification and formalization of roles and responsibilities will assist not only in the hiring of professional and support staff, but will also allow for the budgeting of salaries for the required positions.

Related to human resource planning is the requirement to build into a business plan the opportunity for practitioners, scholars and support staff to attend and present their experiences at relevant conferences both nationally and internationally as well as to attend educational courses and seminars. Conferences and other symposiums provide the platform for stakeholders to share their experiences and discuss the expansion of medical imaging education and scholarship and, whenever possible, radiology departments need to make these opportunities accessible.

17.4.4
Overview of Business-Planning Considerations

Tying into and leveraging what is already available within the larger institution, whether that is an affiliated hospital or a university or a combination of both, may be very helpful for radiology departments. There may not be a need to develop a completely separate and distinct infrastructure especially if there is the opportunity to share and use available resources. This is where discussions amongst the multidisciplinary team will be valuable in that it is through the sharing of ideas and knowledge exchange that avenues can be explored.

The considerations and items that need to be incorporated into a business plan are varied in nature but each is vitally important to the success of the educational and teaching endeavours. After developing the vision and mission for expanding radiology and medical imaging scholarship, each department will need to identify and assess its own needs and develop a plan that adequately addresses the requirements identified. As Cohen et al. (2005) recognized, there are no simple single solutions, and each institution will find its own unique approach.

17

17.5
Funding and Budgeting

It is a widely accepted truth that the educational mission is expensive (Cooke et al. 2006) as it is one of the activities that physicians engage in that does not generate income. Since teaching and education are not revenue-generating activities, it is very unlikely that radiology departments will have separate funding sources on which they can draw. As such, it follows that funding educational and scholarly activities is one of the most significant challenges that radiology departments must deal with once they have made a commitment to the pursuit of expanding educational scholarship.

We continue to address the need to identify funding sources that are available to sustain the efforts of the Centre from a short-term, medium-term and long-term perspective. Each department will need to be creative and innovative in its approach to procuring funding for radiology education scholarship, as it is an area that is relatively new and has not been formally funded by universities, hospitals or research granting agencies. This does not mean that money is not available, but it is absolutely necessary to be able to define the needs and explore all potential opportunities.

When applications for research grants are developed, it is the ideal chance to determine if there is an opportunity to secure funding for items such as personal computers, research assistants or support staff salaries, and conference presentation funding. Researchers and scholars should be encouraged to work with the business manager in the development of their applications so that the need for funding for particular items can be clearly and realistically detailed in their submissions and so that the valuable link to the vision and mission of the centre or division of education can be addressed as appropriate.

Developing very specific and detailed budgets and managing these budgets in support of radiology education scholarship are the two areas where a business manager should spend most of his or her time. It is absolutely necessary to be able to quantify what the need is from a financial perspective if a radiology department is committed to expanding medical imaging education scholarship. Budgets will need to be established initially for relatively short periods of time and will need to be actively managed. Monitoring and strict control of expenses will need to be an ongoing part of the duties of the business manager along with regular reporting to the chair and the other stakeholders involved in the centre or division of education.

In developing a budget for a centre or division of education, the priority for allocation of funds must first address human resource needs. The majority of funding will be spent on the salaries and benefits of professional and administrative support staff and it is essential to protect this funding and keep it separate from all other sources. The cost of other operational expenses such as information-technology, office and infrastructure-related items will vary and will be dependent upon the unique needs of each institution or department.

17.6
What has been Learned

After supporting the radiology department for more than a year now, we have been able to reflect on the progress made in the Centre for Education. The Centre has far surpassed the expectations of the stakeholders and the opportunity for continued growth and expansion is significant. The notion of a learning culture has taken hold and the linking of all activities to educational scholarship has become commonplace. Formalized business planning has been successfully implemented and unforeseen management and financial issues, while challenging, have and will continue to be addressed appropriately.

Three significant lessons have been learned as a result of establishing the Centre. The first is that there is a need to build a strong and dedicated multidisciplinary team willing to share their expertise and knowledge. It is vital that this team be composed of radiologists and educationists, ensuring content and process expertise are available. Secondly, support and infrastructure needs will only be looked after with the active involvement and input from a business perspective. As such, the third member vital to the team is a business manager. Finally, while it is never too late to implement business-planning and financial-management practices, doing so proactively at the start of the establishment of a centre or a division of radiology education is very wise.

17.7
The Vision for the Future

The foremost purpose of sharing our story in this chapter and detailing the business-planning process was to increase the realization that it is possible to create, build and sustain a centre or division of education focused on advancing medical imaging education scholarship. The secondary goal was to encourage dialogue amongst colleagues, scholars, educationists and other stakeholders on a national and international level related to this topic. Thirdly, it was to challenge other radiology departments to engage in the development and realization of their own goals related to educational scholarship. Fourthly, but certainly not last, we strove to raise awareness that the business planning piece of scholarship in teaching and learning needs further exploration as it is an area that could clearly benefit from extensive research.

There is a responsibility that comes with implementing change to ensure the lessons learned and the knowledge gained are not wasted especially if others could benefit from the experiences such as those articulated in this chapter. As educational scholarship expands and takes root in centres in many countries, there is the opportunity for significant trans-formation within medical imaging as a whole with the potential that the changes made locally will permeate systemwide. Potentially, the foundation that is built in radiology will become the benchmark by which all other medical specialties will base their own educational scholarship endeavours upon in the future.

References

Cohen MD, Gunderman RB, Frank MS, Williamson KB (2005) Challenges facing radiology educators. J Am Coll Radiol 2:681–687

Cooke M, Irby DM, Sullivan W, Ludmerer K (2006) American medical education 100 years after the Flexner report. N Engl J Med 355:1399–1344

Garrison DR, Arbaugh JB (2007) Researching the community of inquiry framework: Review, issues and future directions. Internet High Educ 10:157–172

Shih-chang Wang

18.1
Introduction

A young physician from the city of Kuching in eastern Malaysia on the island of Borneo wishes to become an interventional radiologist. She applies to the Ministry of Health in the capital Kuala Lumpur, in western Malaysia, a peninsula of the Asian mainland. Radiology is an extremely popular discipline, and she is nervous about her chances. Miraculously, she is invited to attend for interview by the Joint Central Committee, which oversees radiology training. From an interviewed group of 150 applicants, she is shortlisted with 35 other trainees, and the Ministry of Health approves her government-funded training position. She is assigned to work and train at the University Sains in Kota Bharu, capital of the Islamic state of Kelantan in northern peninsula Malaysia, as there is no training centre in eastern Malaysia. Her 40 fellow trainees are supervised by ten consultants, and there are two trainees from Iran, working under an agreement between Islamic governments. After 4 years of training and experience, she has passed the two sets of examinations and completed a project-based thesis on fluoroscopic radiation doses to staff in interventional radiology, and she returns home to work in the main government hospital in her hometown.

A year later, she applies for funding to be trained in interventional radiology, and after finding a host department in Melbourne, she embarks on her advanced subspecialist training 12 months later. She returns to government service in the main general hospital in Kuching after a year of what has been fruitful experience and training, enthusiastic about developing new interventional services. There, she finds that the scanners and interventional

Shih-chang Wang
Parker-Hughes Chair of Diagnostic Radiology, Discipline of Imaging, University of Sydney,
Department of Radiology, Westmead Hospital, Westmead NSW 2145, Australia
Email: swang@med.usyd.edu.au

Radiology Education. R.K. Chhem et al. (Eds.)
DOI: 10.1007/978-3-540-68989-8, © Springer-Verlag Berlin Heidelberg 2009

18

equipment are suboptimal and frequently malfunction. On enquiry, she finds they cannot be replaced for another 4 years because of budgetary constraints, even though a brand-new hospital with state-of-the-art radiology facilities is being built only 10 km away. Despite several attempts to change the situation, there is no progress, and she becomes frustrated. After her government bond is served, she leaves for a better-paid position in a new private hospital, to do general radiology on the latest-generation computed tomography and MRI scanners, and occasional interventional procedures.

This scenario contains several elements common to radiology education and training in most of the countries of Southeast Asia. Firstly, entry to the programme is by centralised application and interviews, with training positions being granted through direct government funding. There are only a small number of institutions that are accredited to train radiologists, and most have a large trainee-to-consultant ratio. Assessment includes an intermediate examination barrier to progression, a final examination, and often a research-oriented project culminating in a dissertation or long essay for summative assessment. There is a mixture of entry requirements for the training programme, and foreign-trained physicians may be admitted under special circumstances. Even when international subspecialist training is undertaken through a nationally funded initiative, day-to-day clinical practice in public hospitals is constrained by sometimes severely limited financial resources. There is a tendency to favour construction of new hospitals rather than injecting recurrent funding to improve older institutions. Many of the best-trained young radiologists leave public hospital service as soon as they can for the more up-to-date practice environment and higher levels of equipment and salary to be found in the private sector, and the national goals of building radiological expertise for the development of public healthcare are impeded.

This chapter focuses on specialist postgraduate radiology education and its array of pedagogical approaches and outcomes across Southeast Asia, including early postqualification subspecialist training. Continuing professional development in radiology and undergraduate radiology education are major topics for discussion in their own right, but are outside the scope of this chapter.

18.2
Regional Overview

Southeast Asia is a huge geographic region lying between China to the north and Australia to the south, and the Indian subcontinent to the west and the Pacific Ocean to the east. With 568 million people (10% of the global population) scattered across some 29,000 islands, it has the third-largest regional population in Asia, after China and India. The proportions of national populations greater than one million are shown in Fig. 1. The sociopolitical, economic and healthcare factors in each country differ enormously, and range from one of the richest countries per capita in all of Asia (Brunei) to the poorest in the world (Laos), and from one of the smallest countries in the world (Singapore) to the fourth most populous and world's largest archipelagic state, with 17,500 islands, 6,000 of which are inhabited (Indonesia).

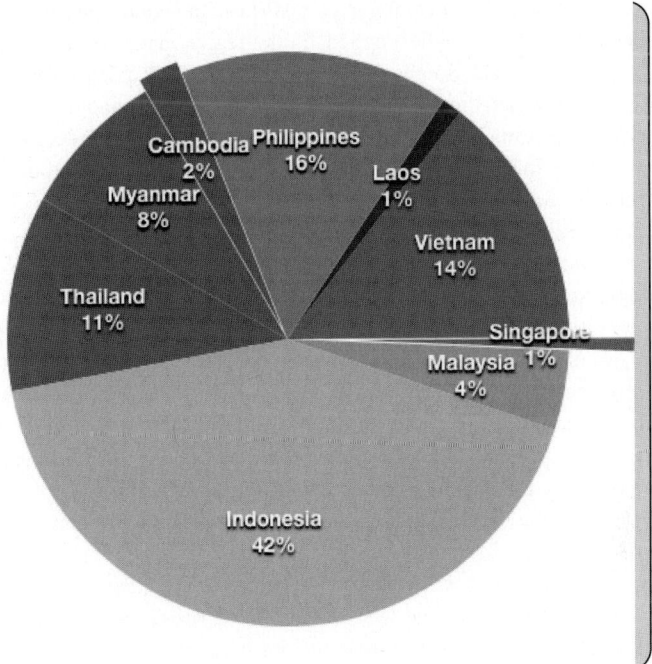

Fig. 1 Population of Southeast Asian nations expressed as a percentage of the entire region's population of over 500 million people. Brunei (350,000) and Timor-Leste (one million) have populations too small to show on this chart

A feature common to all Southeast Asian nations is the large gap in services and expertise between the often very large and densely populated cities, and the generally very poor rural sector with very limited infrastructure and expertise. It can be expected then that the technologically dependent discipline of radiology will be highly concentrated in major urban centres. For example, it has been estimated that 50% of all radiologists in the Philippines work in and around Manila and nearby Quezon City, leaving the majority of its 85 million citizens from some 4,000 inhabited islands with poor access to radiological services. This situation is repeatedly found in every Southeast Asian nation except Singapore, which by dint of being extremely small and a city state with no rural hinterland, is the only nation in the region that has almost equal access to high-level radiological services for all its inhabitants.

For much of the last 200 years, most of this region was under colonial rule or Western influence. Medical education was introduced by foreign powers in the late nineteenth and early twentieth centuries. In general, each country adopted the medical education systems of its colonial ruling powers at the university level (Amin 2003). Today, approaches towards specialist training across Southeast Asia in some way reflect this colonial past: Laos, Vietnam and Cambodia are still influenced by the French; Myanmar, Malaysia and Singapore by the British; Indonesia by the Dutch; the Philippines by the USA; and Thailand,

18

which was never colonised, by a combination of British and American influences. Brunei and Timor-Leste, two of the smallest nations in the region, have no training programme in radiology. In addition, each Southeast Asian country has had quite different systems of government over the last century. The governments have always had direct influence on medical specialist training as a policy of strategic national importance, and generally exert control both by influencing professional bodies to follow specified national guidelines and through direct funding of specialist training both locally and overseas.

These differences in geography, history, demographics and politics result in each country having a unique system for radiology training, assessment and accreditation. Nevertheless, some commonalities in pedagogical approach and philosophy are present.

There is no peer-reviewed literature that covers the spectrum of specialist radiology education in Southeast Asia. There has been no formal survey of Southeast Asian national training programmes other than in occasional unpublished conference reports. In compiling information for this chapter, I explored national radiology association websites, used Web searches, and developed a written survey of radiology education programmes that was conducted amongst senior radiologists from the region. Formal documentation from the various national training programmes was generally not available in English.

Of the countries surveyed, written responses were received from Thailand, Malaysia, Singapore, Indonesia and Myanmar, and questions that arose were clarified by e-mail. From these survey responses, most of these nations have a number of factors in common in relation to the practice and status of radiology as a profession:

> The radiology workforce is much smaller relative to the population than in most industrialised nations.
> Procedural and interpretation workloads are often much higher per radiologist per year than for industrialised nations, even in leading academic centres.
> Radiology as a discipline varies widely in popularity amongst medical graduates, and generally does not have a high profile amongst medical specialties.
> The radiology workforce is much smaller relative to the population than in most industrialised nations.
> Procedural and interpretation workloads are often much higher per radiologist per year than for industrialised nations, even in leading academic centres.
> Radiology as a discipline varies widely in popularity amongst medical graduates, and generally does not have a high profile amongst medical specialties.
> Radiologist's incomes tend to be similar to or sometimes lower relative to those of other specialties, even in the private sector. This may in part explain the lower popularity of radiology in some countries; notably radiology tends to be most popular in the nations where most radiologists work in the private sector.
> Radiology practice models are highly variable, though in general public hospital practice is much less well funded and equipped than in the private sector.
> True subspecialisation is rare, even in the most developed nation in the region (Singapore).

18.3
Socioeconomic and Political Factors

Medical education does not occur in a vacuum. The level of radiology in a country strongly reflects the technical expertise, economic performance and national training policies of the nation, and these are in turn closely determined by the political environment, socioeconomic status and the degree of urban and rural development in each country.

To say that medical training in Southeast Asia has had a troubled past is an understatement in many cases. A number of armed conflicts across the region as part of power struggles between Communist and Western ideologies, nationalist and colonialist forces, and guerrilla and government armies for much of the twentieth century has left many countries' medical manpower severely depleted in the aftermath. As an extreme example, it has been estimated (Gollogly 2005) that after the murderous Khmer Rouge regime in Cambodia was interrupted by the Vietnamese invasion and decade-long occupation after 1979, there were only 20 physicians left in the entire country, eight of whom subsequently left. Rebuilding of medical manpower, expertise and infrastructure did not begin in earnest until the country was returned to democratic rule in the 1990s.

Southeast Asian countries have experienced a wide range of different governmental systems over the last century, from full-blown colonial rule until soon after the Second World War, to periods of open warfare, occupation and liberation, freeform and sometimes chaotic democracy, to authoritarian or dictatorial quasi-democratic governance, to hereditary royalty, military juntas and communist governments, sometimes swinging abruptly from one form of government to another (e.g. the Thai military coup d'état of 2006 that displaced the popularly elected government without warning).

In such rapidly changing political climates, there is a strong tendency to centralise the management of many aspects of society, including medical specialist education. Such centralisation acts to protect professionals against the vagaries of the government of the day, and can remain relatively stable even as governments rise and fall. While this centralisation is attractive to governments, particularly in the name of cost-effectiveness and optimal allocation of training resources, it can have its pitfalls. Projected workforce requirements for specific specialties can be badly miscalculated, leading to either undersupply or oversupply over time; because of the prolonged nature of postgraduate specialist training, it takes at least a decade to correct any such miscalculation once the impact has been felt in the community. For example, Singapore's government decided to constrain radiology specialist training in the early 1990s, and was quite unprepared for the rapid growth in medical imaging that has become pervasive in modern medical practice. By the late 1990s, the resultant marked shortage of radiologists (about 20 full-time-equivalent radiologists per million population in 1998) finally led to policy changes to address this situation, but only in the last few years has this shortfall even begun to catch up to the growth in imaging workload, through a combination of increased local training numbers and active recruitment of overseas-trained radiologists.

Although the opening story spoke of the all-too-common situation of expert radiologists leaving an ailing public sector healthcare system for private practice, a phenomenon not unknown in Western countries, this type of brain drain is at least internal. Prolonged poor socioeconomic conditions in a country can lead to medical staff emigrating overseas to work, even without a war or refugee crisis. This is particularly acute in the Philippines and Myanmar today; many Filipino physicians even retrain as nurses to work in the West for much higher salaries than they can earn as medical practitioners at home. Most Filipino radiologists work in more than one medical centre or hospital most days, to earn what they consider a reasonable income. Physicians are leaving Myanmar to work and train overseas, often on their own initiative and without government support, to seek better opportunities for themselves and their families. A number of Myanma radiologists have sought alternative employment or retraining in radiology in other Southeast Asian nations. Thus, the system of medical specialist training for any discipline can be thrown into disarray by socioeconomic and political factors; intrinsically, the pedagogical aims and outcomes of any radiology training programme are highly dependent on sustained socioeconomic development and predictable political conditions.

18.4
Regional Pedagogical Approaches

Radiology training in the region is usually coordinated through a centralised national system by an organisation such as a college, society or chapter of radiologists, or in some countries by academic institutions or universities. Because Southeast Asian governments directly fund specialist training positions, such organisations usually work very closely with the Ministry of Health, appointing a central committee that typically governs the training programme and policies for radiology. The specialist qualification is usually awarded by the national college or university, and sometimes even the Ministry of Health itself. Some smaller nations (Singapore, Brunei) rely on external qualifications and examinations. In addition, many of the regional governments directly fund newly qualified radiologists to undergo advanced subspecialist training through fellowships in leading international centres. The administrative approaches and the qualifications obtained by radiologists in the surveyed countries are listed in Table 18.1. From the survey responses tabulated, it can be seen that there are a range of pedagogical approaches to specialist training in Southeast Asia (Table 18.2), and while there are several common factors, every programme differs somewhat in the curriculum and execution of radiology education and assessment.

Most programmes require that trainees have some hospital-based clinical experience before entry into the radiology training program, following the principle that expert radiologists need a good understanding of clinical medicine. Although trainees may enter directly after medical school in some programmes (Malaysia, Vietnam, Indonesia), in practice this is not common and most trainees will have at least undertaken their first internship year. Uniquely, Myanmar dictates that not only must all trainees have at least 2 years of initial clinical experience, but that all trainees must also spend their mornings attached to clinical teams to conduct ward rounds and case discussions (postings to neurology, surgery, medicine, paediatrics, orthopaedics, and obstetrics and gynaecology departments are mandatory), returning to the radiology department in the afternoons to perform examinations and interpret studies.

Table 18.1 Training administration and qualifications awarded

Country	Oversight	Qualification awarded and minimum duration of training
Singapore	Centralised Specialist Training Committee, appointed by Ministry of Health	Fellow of the Royal College of Radiologists (3 years) Master of Medicine (3 years) (National University of Singapore) Specialist in Diagnostic Radiology (5 years) (Specialist Accreditation Board)
Malaysia	Centralised Conjoint Training Committee, appointed by Ministry of Health and Universities	Master of Radiology or Master of Medicine (Radiology) (4 years) (awarded by one of three universities)
Indonesia	Centralised Training Committee, appointed by Indonesian College of Radiology	Postgraduate Specialist in Radiology (3 years) (awarded by the Indonesian College of Radiology)
Thailand	Centralised Training Committee, appointed by Royal College of Radiologists of Thailand	Thai Board in Diagnostic Radiology (3 years) (awarded by the Medical Council of Thailand)
Myanmar	Centralised Training Committee, appointed by Ministry of Health	Diploma in Medical Radiodiagnosis (2 years) (awarded by Institute of Medicine, Yangon) Master of Medical Science (2 years) (awarded by the Institute of Medicine, Yangon or the Defence Services Medical Academy)
Cambodia	Centralised Specialist Training, jointly organised by the University of Health Sciences and Coopéra-tion Français	Certificate d'Étude Specialisé (3 years in Cambodia, 2 years in France) (awarded by the University of Health Sciences and Coopération Français)
Vietnam	University training programmes	Master in Radiology (3 years) and Doctor of Radiology (2 years) (awarded by Ho Chi Minh City University and Hanoi University)
	Hospital training programmes	Radiologist Grade I (3 years) and Grade II (2 years) (awarded by the Ministry of Health)

All the programmes surveyed have a significant didactic component, with both structured and unstructured teaching in many elements of radiology knowledge considered essential, especially physics, anatomy and imaging instrumentation. In addition, all programmes rely heavily on formal tutorials, case-based small-group teaching and clinicoradiological rounds as part of the learning environment. Two countries – Brunei and Timor-Leste – have no medical specialist training programmes at all, and rely on other countries to train such specialists. Brunei has an intergovernmental agreement to train radiologists in Singapore. Indonesia has a structurally seamless programme that lacks intermediate barrier

Table 18.2 Pedagogical approach to radiology training and assessment by country

Country	Training	Assessment
Singapore	Mandatory tutorials, lectures and unrostered study time	6-monthly progress report
	Clinicoradiological rounds	3-monthly mini-CEX and DOPS
	Formal teaching of physics, clinical radiology, instrumentation	FRCR Parts 1, 2A and 2B examinations
	Seamless, continuous programme	MMed examination
		Unlimited examination attempts
		Exit interview, logbook/portfolio and training review
Malaysia	Tutorials, lectures	Regular progress reports
	Clinicoradiological rounds	Year 1: examination including essay, MCQ, film reading and viva
	Formal teaching of physics, anatomy, clinical radiology, instrumentation and pathology	Year 3: examination including MCQ, film reading, viva voce
	Intermediate barrier examination	Year 4: rapid reporting, project thesis assessment, viva voce
		Up to 3 attempts per examination
		Final review of progress reports and logbook
Indonesia	Tutorials and lectures	Regular progress reports
	Clinicoradiological rounds	6-monthly mini-CEX and DOPS
	Formal teaching of physics, anatomy, clinical radiology, instrumentation, pathology and research methods	Year 3: examination including MCQ, film reading, viva voce
	Seamless, continuous programme	Up to 2 attempts for examination
		Final review of progress reports and logbook
Thailand	Tutorials and lectures	Regular progress reports
	Clinicoradiological rounds	6-monthly DOPS
	Formal teaching of physics and clinical radiology	Annual MCQ and film reading tests (internal)
	Seamless, continuous programme	Year 3: final national Board examination
		Up to 3 attempts at the examination
		Final review of progress reports and logbook
Myanmar	Tutorials and lectures	Regular appraisals by supervisor
	Clinical attachments	Year 2: DMRD examination
	Clinicoradiological rounds	Year 4: MMedSc examinatoon
	Formal teaching of physics, anatomy, imaging techniques, clinical radiology, pathology and research methods	Up to 2 attempts per examination
	Intermediate barrier qualification	Year 4: thesis examination
		Final review of thesis, progress reports and logbook plus viva voce

mini-CEX mini clinical examinations, *DOPS* directly observed procedures, *FRCR* Fellow of the Royal College of Radiologists, *MCQ* multiple-choice questions, *DMRD* Diploma in Medical Radiodiagnosis, *MMedSc* Master of Medical Science examinations, relying on a combination of progress reports, mini clinical examinations (mini-CEX) and directly observed procedures (DOPS) for regular formative assessment, on an annual basis. The Thai programme uses internal examinations at the end of the first and second training years to assess trainees, alongside the usual annual progress reports. The other training programmes surveyed have barrier summative examinations taken in the first 2–3 years of training, either as an intermediate qualification (e.g. Diploma in Medical Radiodiagnosis, DMRD, in Myanmar, Grade 1 Radiologist in Vietnam, Fellow of the Royal College of Radiologists, FRCR, in Singapore) or else as the first in a series of examinations in the roadmap to the local specialist qualification (Malaysia).

All countries have a final formal summative assessment at the end of the training period, based on an interview and review of the trainee's progress reports, case logbook, courses attended, examinations passed, and any publications or the formal project-based thesis mandated by some programmes. In Malaysia, Thailand and Myanmar, this review is paired with a final viva voce examination. Indonesia and Thailand add an additional objective structured clinical examination (OSCE) style film reporting examination as well. Although none of the programmes use a formal portfolio-based assessment, most of the elements needed for portfolio assessment are obtained and reviewed. Of the countries surveyed, Singapore, Brunei and Cambodia rely heavily on a "foreign" qualification and examination system; for radiologists in Singapore and Brunei the key qualification is the FRCR from the UK, and the final specialist accreditation (Certificate d'Étude Specialisé) in Cambodia is French. All the other Southeast Asian nations have their own national qualifications.

These differences in national approaches to specialist medical education can be viewed in two ways. On the one hand, it is desirable for radiologists to have an internationally recognised and highly portable qualification, even though national training and especially assessment is then potentially hostage to external changes and policies; and on the other hand, it is politically desirable for a country to have direct control over its own national specialist qualifications and training.

18.5
National Radiology Education Programmes

18.5.1
Singapore

The Republic of Singapore is a tiny island nation of four million inhabitants, a former British colony, under what has been described as a highly paternalistic and modestly authoritarian system of government since its independence in 1965. About 70% of Singaporean radiologists work in the public sector in large general hospitals, and 80% of Singaporeans seek their healthcare in that sector. The public sector hospitals regularly review their salaries to reduce the gap between private and public specialists. With few exceptions, private radiology centres are funded by businesses, and most radiologists in private practice are salaried associates; thus, for most radiologists, the disparity in income between the public and private sectors is relatively small.

18

Singapore has the highest number of radiologists and training centres relative to the population of any Southeast Asian country (Figs. 2, 3) and also one of the lowest number of trainees per centre in the region (Fig. 3). The ratio of trainees to supervising consultants in a hospital is limited by Ministry of Health guidelines and funding. Despite region-leading workforce statistics, the utilisation of medical imaging in Singapore is high, and per-radiologist workloads are higher than for most industrialised nations. Although the Ministry of Health has determined that maximum caseload per teaching hospital radiologist is 12,000 examinations per year, this is exceeded in all hospitals other than in the national centres for cancer and neurosciences, which perform very little or no general radiology.

Singapore has the lowest radiology manpower relative to population of any developed economy, and additional strains are being placed on the existing workforce by the government's target of one million health tourists per year by 2012 (Straits Times 2008). A very high proportion of these foreign patients need imaging services, usually delivered in a very short timeframe, so this rising influx of foreign patients effectively increases the utilisation of imaging much more than the equivalent growth in resident population. In short, Singapore must continue to aggressively recruit and train more radiologists to maintain healthy workloads, especially in teaching hospital practice.

All medical specialty training in Singapore is overseen by the Joint Committee for Specialist Training (JCST), which is jointly led by the Ministry of Health and the Division of Graduate Medical Studies (DGMS), an offshoot of the School of Medicine at the National University of Singapore. Discipline-specific specialist training committees (STC) are appointed by the JCST to coordinate and execute medical specialty training. The radiology STC has representatives from all the departments accredited to train radiologists. At the time of writing, the established Singapore Radiological Society and the recently formed College of Radiologists of Singapore, an offshoot of the national Academy of Medicine, have no direct role to play in coordinating radiology training. Nevertheless key members of each organisation are consulted or represented on the national STC.

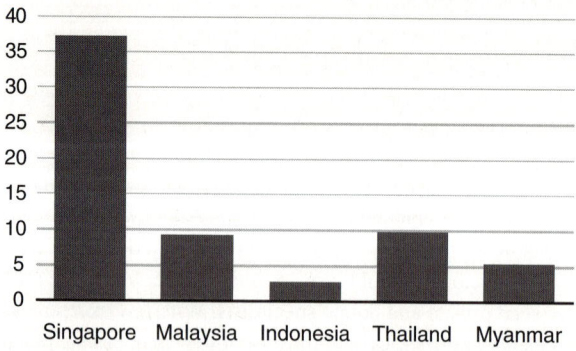

Radiologists per Million Population

Fig. 2 Population per radiologist in the countries for which figures were available from the survey responses. Longer bars indicate a greater radiology workforce

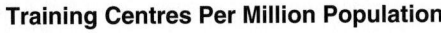

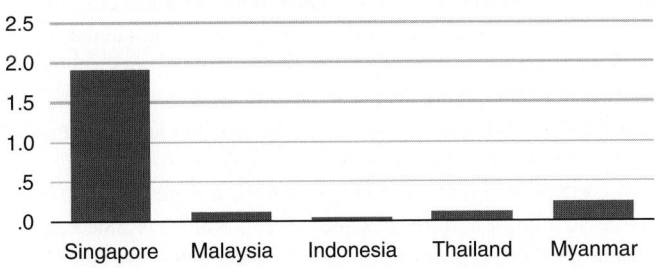

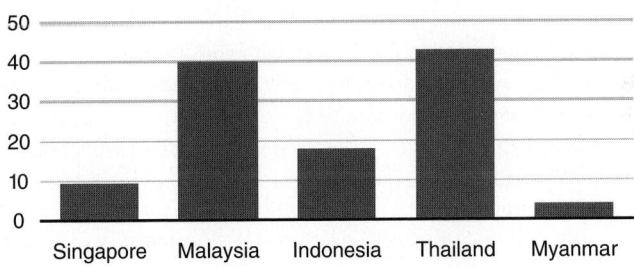

Fig. 3 Training centre statistics for surveyed countries. (**a**) Number of accredited radiology training centres in each country per million population. (**b**) Number of radiology trainees per centre. Shorter bars tend to indicate a higher level of consultant supervision for trainees

Radiology is not very popular as a training specialty among young Singaporean physicians, and typically for every vacant training position there no more than 1.5 applicants each year, even though the training programme is recognised to be of high quality. However, this is not uncommon in the region, and may reflect the typically average level of income, fewer business opportunities and thus lower economic status of radiologists (compared with some medical disciplines at least) in most Southeast Asian nations rather than the reputation of the discipline and training programme per se.

Because of the high regard most Asians have for Singapore's training programmes, the scarcity of radiology training positions in many Western nations and the relative ease with which good candidates can get access to radiology training, about one third of all radiology trainees in Singapore have medical qualifications from other countries; most commonly these are Singaporeans or Malaysians with medical degrees from the UK, Ireland or Australia. Furthermore, Singapore permits overseas-trained radiologists to enter into its advanced specialist training (AST) programme directly, provided they have undergone radiology training previously and have passed all the FRCR examinations. A number of Indian-trained radiologists have recently joined the Singapore radiology workforce under this provision.

All applicants are interviewed by a central panel appointed by the radiology STC. No examination or other barrier is required for entry into radiology. After the interviews, all

18

candidates shortlisted by the STC must be approved by the JCST. Currently, the Ministry of Health pays 40% of the salary of each trainee to the hospitals that employ them. All trainees undergo training compatible with the FRCR curriculum and assessment for the first 3 years of basic specialist training (BST), after which most trainees successfully complete the FRCR examinations and enter a 2-year AST programme that currently depends on 3-monthly subspecialist training rotations under accredited supervision in a more advanced range of postings than for basic training.

A number of structured courses are run by the STC, and are delivered in various series of weekly lectures to trainees at different stages of their training. Trainees are progressively rotated between hospital departments and subspecialty areas after the first year of training.

Assessment is progressive, formative and summative. Progress assessment takes the form of 6-monthly progress reports by department heads of training (recently modified by the introduction of a bidimensional five-point rating scale incorporating knowledge and competence domains, as well as a detailed checklist for radiological knowledge and competence), 3-monthly mentorship discussions with consultant supervisors, and regular logbook entries for each posting. In addition, the STC has recently added 3-monthly mini-CEX and DOPS evaluations. These were introduced to improve the quality of formative and progress assessment, and to enable the programme to move to a continuous ("seamless") training system in the near future. Summative assessment at the intermediate training level is through the FRCR examinations.

Singapore is a regional examination centre for the written FRCR Parts 1 and 2A examinations, so Singapore-based trainees only have to travel overseas for the FRCR Part 2B examination. In addition to the FRCR, diagnostic radiology also has its own specialist qualification, the Master of Medicine (MMed), awarded by the DGMS of the National University of Singapore. Currently, this is virtually identical to the FRCR Part 2B examination, is largely optional and has been used by trainees to enter AST if they fail the FRCR Part 2B examination itself. A final face-to-face interview is conducted with an examination panel, with review of the trainee's experience, learning activities, case logbook, progress evaluations, at least one peer-reviewed publication and evidence of compliance with national training programme requirements. Once training has been deemed complete, the trainee is exit-certified by the STC and placed on the Specialist Register by the Singapore Medical Council's Specialist Accreditation Board.

All junior consultants can then take advantage of the national Healthcare Manpower Development Programme to develop advanced medical specialist skills. Successful applicants are funded to go to major medical centres (usually in North America or Europe) to train in subspecialist fields for at least 6 months. The training programme is in a state of change at the time of writing. National medical specialist workforce needs are growing rapidly, with new hospitals being built and a large influx of medical tourists seeking advanced specialist care. In early 2008, the Ministry of Health secured a large amount of funding (more than US $1 billion) over 5 years to hire and train hospital medical staff at all levels, and has urged all specialties to move towards a more streamlined system of training to satisfy the demand for more specialists. From 2008, 76% of the salary for each new trainee will be funded directly by the government.

Radiology has a so-called exclusive track, where trainees who join remain in the programme fully until exit. Such programmes have been urged to move in the near future to a so-called seamless system where training progression is not impeded by an intermediate barrier examination, so long as the required examinations have been passed by the end of the training period and other training requirements have also been achieved. This should improve the current situation, where a number of trainees that have failed the FRCR examinations remain "stuck" at the BST level for 1, 2 or more years.

Under such a seamless system, the significance and nature of the MMed qualification must change as its current role as an alternative entry point into AST will no longer be required. Conveniently, in late 2007 the Ministry of Health explicitly recognised that clinical research is not only desirable, but is also a crucial component of an advanced healthcare system, and critical to Singapore's generation of new economic wealth through a combination of advanced biomedical research and development as well as medical tourism. This is a major shift in healthcare policy, as previously healthcare was largely regarded as a drain on the public purse. As a result, specialist training programmes have been urged to explicitly incorporate and mandate some research into their training. Diagnostic radiology has been planning for this change for some time, and all trainees entering training from May 2007 onwards are deemed to be in this new seamless programme. Progression from year 1 to year 5 will be through a newly developed formative assessment system. The MMed will become a project-based dissertation conducted in the second half of the training programme, and will satisfy university requirements for a master's level degree, including an approved project, named supervisor, written dissertation and formal examination of the dissertation. Exit specialist certification will depend on trainees progressing satisfactorily through all required elements of the training programme, completing the MMed dissertation to the required standard and undergoing final review of their virtual portfolio, including a logbook of case experience, records of courses and conferences attended, presentations and publications, as well as passing all the required FRCR examinations.

18.5.2
Malaysia

Malaysia is a multiracial multicultural developing nation of almost 25 million people, comprising a peninsula in the west, an eastern part on the island of Borneo, and numerous inhabited small islands. It is a former British colony, and specialist training was once closely aligned to UK-based Royal College programs. However, in the 1980s this situation changed as social, economic and political factors led to each specialist discipline developing independent national training programmes and qualifications.

Malaysia currently has about 230 qualified radiologists (crude rate of about nine per million people or 111,000 people per radiologist), with about 120 trainees nationally, and 35–40 new training positions vacant each year. The training programme is coordinated by the Conjoint Training Board of Radiology, under the auspices of the College of Radiologists, Malaysia. Currently only three hospitals, all university teaching hospitals in peninsular Malaysia, are accredited to train diagnostic radiologists. Expansion of training is occurring. There has been an increasingly large number of trainees per centre, and more centres are being accredited for training; two more non-university government hospitals have recently been accredited for radiology training from 2009.

Radiology is one of the most popular specialties in Malaysia, and entry is quite competitive. Most applicants must first complete at least 1 year of clinical experience prior to entry; the exception is trainee lecturers who apply directly to the universities for junior academic appointments. Applicants submit their curriculum vitae and application forms to the Ministry of Health and the Ministry of Education and are shortlisted for interview by the proposed training departments. Recommendations from departments are then resent to the ministries for approval, and after some last-minute negotiations, the applicants are informed whether they have been successful, and what department they will be working in.

There is no structured rotation programme, and the vast majority of trainees stay in the same department for the duration of their training. Trainees receive formal teaching in physics, anatomy, imaging instrumentation, clinical radiology and pathology during their training. At the end of the first year, an examination comprising an essay, multiple-choice questions (MCQ), film reading and viva voce is taken. A project is commenced in the second year, and in year 3, trainees will complete their intermediate-level radiology examination, comprising multiple-choice questions, OSCE-style film reading and reporting, and a viva voce. At the end of year 4, trainees undergo a final summative assessment, including rapid reporting similar to that used in the FRCR Part 2B examination, as well as evaluation of their written project and a final viva voce. After all elements have been passed, the candidate is awarded the Master of Radiology or the MMed in Radiology, depending on the university. At this time the College of Radiologists of Malaysia does not directly organise the programme, examinations or the final certification, but instead acts to coordinate the training and assessment used by the three training centres.

After completion of training, some Malaysian radiologists are sent to centres overseas for subspecialist training through government-funded programmes. In the past, UK centres were preferred. However, changes in EU regulations have essentially reduced the ability of physicians from Asia to train and work in the UK, and so many are turning to the USA, Canada, Australia and even Singapore as alternatives. The Malaysian government has recognised the need to greatly increase its national radiology workforce. More centres are being planned for radiology training, a larger number of trainee positions are being funded and limited rights of private practice have been introduced into the public sector. The Malaysian Association of Government Doctors has been particularly active in promoting these changes in recent years. In addition, there has been a national recognition of the need to develop research in radiology, and major infrastructural facilities for imaging research are being planned, alongside proposals to improve the standard of research and research expertise nationally. However, there are major constraints, and the coordination of increased training, increased research infrastructure and appropriate funding support is not very well developed at the time of writing.

18.5.3
Indonesia

Indonesia is the third-most populous nation in Asia, and the fourth-most populous in the world. In a nation of some 17,508 islands with 235 million inhabitants across a huge geographic area, any attempt at a tightly controlled, centrally coordinated national training programme would be a logistic headache at the least. At this time there are some 650 registered specialists in radiology in Indonesia, a crude rate of three radiologists per million population, or over 333,000 people per radiologist.

There are 14 nationally accredited training centres for radiology, mostly on the island of Java. Each year up to 45 trainees are taken in, and there are about 160 radiologists in training today. There are very few training centres relative to the population, as well as a low number of trainees per centre (Fig. 3). Training programme guidelines are developed by the Indonesian College of Radiology, which awards the qualification of Postgraduate Specialist after successful completion of the 3-year training programme. Entry into the programme is by direct application and interview by heads of department of various training centres. Although physicians may enter radiology training directly from medical school, the majority have at least 1–2 years of clinical exposure before entering the programme.

There is a planned rotational programme within each hospital department, coupled with structured teaching in anatomy, physics, imaging instrumentation, pathology, clinical radiology and research methods. Assessment is mostly formative, with progress reports, logbooks, mini-CEX and DOPS assessment over the first 3 years. A final examination comprising multiple-choice questions, OSCE-style film reading and interview is conducted in year 3. Trainees have up to two attempts to pass this examination. Many Indonesian radiologists go on to further subspecialist training, often in the Netherlands or elsewhere in western Europe, a long-held tradition for many disciplines. This situation may change with new EU regulations that prevent non-EU citizens from readily working in EU countries.

18.5.4
Thailand

Thailand, with a population of 61 million people, has about 600 practicing radiologists, giving a crude rate of ten radiologists per million people, or 100,000 people per radiologist. Radiology is one of the most popular specialties in Thailand. Government hospital radiologist incomes are relatively low, about the same as those of other disciplines in public service, private radiologist incomes are higher than those of many other private physicians, and are considerably greater than for public hospital radiologists. It should come as no surprise to learn that a large number of Thai radiologists work in private practice.

Radiology training is conducted at major urban centres across the country, in the seven major university teaching hospitals. Currently, there are about 300 radiology trainees, and about 100 new trainees are taken in per year. This increased intake has been the result of government recognition of a national workforce shortage. However, this apparently large number is deceptive; Thailand has a very low number of trainees and training centres per million population (Fig. 3). The training programme is centrally coordinated by the Royal College of Radiologists of Thailand. Application to the programme is to the national training committee within the Royal College, which shortlists candidates and conducts selection interviews. Trainees usually need a minimum of 1 year of clinical experience before joining the radiology training programme.

The programme contains structured teaching in physics and clinical radiology, with intradepartmental planned rotations during training. Written examinations set by each department are conducted at the end of the first and second years. After a mandatory project, a thesis is submitted in the last year. The final exit examination is a formal assessment of the trainee's progress reports, thesis and case logbook, as well as a final barrier Board examination comprising multiple-choice questions, OSCE-style film reporting and a case-based viva voce, set and examined by the Royal College. On successfully completing the examinations and training programme, the trainee is awarded the Thai Board of Diagnostic Radiology by the Medical Council of Thailand.

There are three centres in Thailand accredited to train in five subspecialties through 2-year fellowship programmes: body intervention, neurointervention, body imaging, women's imaging and neuroimaging. After completion, a subspecialist certificate is awarded to the radiologist. Some Thai radiologists go overseas for advanced training, usually at US academic medical centres, in particular for subspecialties for which no centre is recognised in Thailand. This long-pursued strategy has been beneficial for Thailand both from a professional and from a financial viewpoint; most physicians will publish for the first time in English after such training, and US-trained Thai physicians have not infrequently become key service providers in the booming Thai medical tourism industry.

18.5.6
Myanmar

Myanmar has an estimated population of 47 million people. Under military rule for most of the period since 1962, it has a mixed system of medical specialist training that is unique. A former British colony, it developed its own system for specialist training after independence. For radiology the programme has remained little changed for decades, apart from the recent introduction of radiology training in the military hospital system.

There are about 250 radiologists practising in Myanmar, giving a crude rate of five radiologists per million population, or 200,000 people per radiologist. At this time 11 centres (five university and six non-university) are accredited to train radiologists, and each takes on average one trainee per year for the 4-year programme; thus, there are about 44 trainees in radiology at any given time. Although the oversight of medical specialist training is centrally coordinated by the Ministry of Health, the training is planned and delivered by the teaching hospitals. Entry to the programme requires at least 2 years of clinical experience, and all would-be applicants must first sit for and pass a national specialist entry examination in basic medical sciences (anatomy, physiology and pathology). If successful, they may apply for specialist training, and for radiology are interviewed by a national panel and then by the respective heads of departments that trainees indicate a preference for.

Structured teaching in physics, anatomy, imaging techniques clinical radiology and pathology is given, and there is a structured rotation system during training, both within departments and between accredited training centres. Uniquely, all trainees must be attached to clinical units during their training. There are mandatory postings to neurology, obstetrics and gynaecology, paediatrics, medicine, surgery and orthopaedics clinical services, with radiologists typically attending ward rounds and clinical meetings in the mornings and returning to the radiology department to perform and report studies in the afternoons. Although all radiology training programmes emphasise the importance of understanding the needs of the clinical team, this programme is unique in mandating explicit direct daily contact and shared responsibility between clinical teams and radiology trainees.

After 2 years, trainees take an examination comprising a rapid reporting session, a series of short cases with OSCE-style film reporting and a long-case viva voce and inter-view with examiners. Once this barrier has been passed, trainees are awarded the DMRD by the Institute of Medicine in Yangon. After the DMRD, trainees usually go on to the second phase of their training, the 2-year Master of Medical Science programme, which requires a project to be conducted and a thesis to be submitted. The thesis is examined in conjunction with a similar examination to the DMRD, but at a higher level of difficulty with up to two long cases in a viva voce setting, as well as a review of formative progress reports and a logbook. For both this and the DMRD examinations, up to two attempts are permitted to pass them. Success results in award of the Master of Medical Science, either by the Institute of Medicine in Yangon for civilian trainees, or the Defence Services Medical Academy for military trainees.

Finally, after exit certification as a specialist, consultant radiologists are encouraged to consider doing a postgraduate degree, the Doctor of Medical Science. This is a PhD-equivalent research programme that takes 3 years to complete, and that requires submission and formal defence of a thesis, similar to PhD programmes in other disciplines.

18.5.7
Other Countries

Vietnam is a country of 80 million inhabitants along the narrow coastal eastern strip of mainland Southeast Asia. It has had a history of prolonged armed struggle for much of the last 100 years, first against French colonial rule, and then famously against the USA during the 1960s and early 1970s. It is now unified under communist rule, and there has been a progressive growth and development of the economy and the health system since the early 1990s, in parallel with the liberalisation of communist China's economy under Deng Xiaoping. The rapid resultant increase in economic trade and development and the increased openness to Western technologies and training have led to a resurgence of the Vietnamese medical system. Although it is still highly centralised (like most Southeast Asian nations), there has been major growth and development of medical and technical expertise in radiology in the last decade.

According to Hoang (2003), the Vietnamese health system in 2000 had 230,548 medical doctors and higher graduates; approximately 5% of them designated as radiologists. It is highly unlikely that this number could have been fully trained in the way understood in the West, and this is probably analogous to the situation in China, where most "radiologists" are more like technicians or physicians who have undergone very short or limited training, and who practice only a limited range of medical imaging. In such a system, only a small minority have undergone comprehensive formal training in all radiological imaging.

Vietnamese radiological education is performed mostly in Hanoi and Ho Chi Minh City at the university faculties of medicine. After finishing 6 years in the faculty of medicine, a student can follow on immediately to take a 3 year study programme in what is termed the practice training system to obtain the Radiologist Grade I qualification, or complete a

5-year programme to obtain the Radiologist Grade II qualification. Parallel to the practice system, one can follow the academic system through the universities to get a master's degree (3 years) or a doctorate (5 years) in radiology. In general, very few Vietnamese radiologists are subspecialised; virtually all work as general radiologists.

There is little publicly available information on radiology training in Cambodia. However, there is some information on medical specialty training in general, and it is likely that radiology training follows a framework similar to that of other medical disciplines. According to Gollogy (2005), postgraduate medical training is under the auspices of the University of Health Sciences, and partly funded by Coopération Français to provide the French specialist qualification, Certificate d'Étude Specialisé. This programme requires 3 years of postgraduate training in Cambodia, an additional 1 or 2 years of training in France, and is assessed by examinations and a thesis.

This French government initiative, starting from 1991, has a mission to train medical specialists in six disciplines: surgery, obstetrics and gynaecology, anaesthesia, internal medicine, paediatrics and radiology. French expatriate supervisors based in Cambodia act to oversee the programme, and by 2005, 220 Khmer physicians had finished training across all specialties, with all returning to Cambodia to work, but virtually all of these practising in the capital Phnom Penh. No information about specialist training in Laos was available at the time of writing.

Brunei, a small oil-rich state in northern Borneo, has about 350,000 people. Currently there is no training programme for radiology, and would-be radiologists are funded to train in Singapore under a government-to-government agreement.

Timor-Leste is the newest and one of the smallest nations in the region, with a population of one million people, a troubled birth and ongoing political difficulties. Medical specialist training is not organised in this country as yet, but is highly likely to be dependent on the Indonesian system in the future.

18.6
Pedagogical Challenges in Radiology Education

Clearly in such a diverse region, with its enormous range of geographical, economic and sociopolitical factors influencing the delivery of healthcare and medical education, any attempt to provide a unified view of the whole will inevitably suffer from oversimplification.

Nevertheless, it is clear that Southeast Asian nations share many aspects of radiology pedagogical approaches to training and assessment, even though the training influences and drivers differ in major ways from country to country. All countries have centralised planning to try to ensure some control over candidate selection, and standardisation of curriculum and assessment. There is a trend to mandating a project and dissertation. Final assessment always involves review of the trainee's logbook, training records and progress reports. All programmes have a form of barrier examination that is heavily based on theoretical knowledge. Most programmes rely on various forms of viva voce examination, to evaluate the image interpretation and analysis skills of the candidate, even though this type of examination has only modest reliability and reproducibility. The fact that all these programmes use multiple approaches to education and assessment indicates recognition that the expertise to be evaluated in a specialist radiologist is not one-dimensional.

In the main, despite a variety of planned programmes, progress assessment, formative assessment tools, summative examinations and even graduate research theses, radiology education in all countries still largely follows an apprenticeship model, which is still probably appropriate given that much of radiology is a practical clinical discipline where expertise comes largely from high-volume experience in day-to-day clinical imaging and interpretation across a very wide range of medical conditions. It is simply not possible for anyone to become a competent, safe radiologist solely through didactic teaching and reading, even though this base is essential for core knowledge. It is even more difficult for a radiologist to become truly expert in one or more subspecialty areas without serious commitment to integration with clinical practice within such an area, and ongoing continuing medical education over some years. Recognising the difficulty in obtaining such expertise locally, almost all Southeast Asian countries directly fund at least some of their junior specialists to go overseas for advanced subspecialist training, as a strategic approach to enhancing advanced medical expertise in their home country.

Interestingly, Malaysia, Myanmar, Vietnam and in the next 3 years Singapore all have a requirement for advanced trainees to complete a project-based dissertation for submission, examination and eventual award of a higher degree such as a master's or a doctorate. This formal approach to foster research skills is rare in training programmes for radiology; although Sweden has long required all radiologists to obtain a PhD, this requirement is absent in virtually all Western training programmes (many European nations do not even conduct examinations).

So does this approach lead to good-quality radiology research from these nations? Regrettably the answer is by and large no, at least at the time of writing. Developing good research projects and publications requires far more than mandatory projects and university degrees. Job-related incentives such as promotion and salary, strong academic career structure, active mentoring and academic support, a high-quality practice environment with state-of-the-art equipment, as well as a work environment that explicitly develops and supports research after specialist certification are far more important influences on whether good research will emerge from any specialty.

Of all the Southeast Asian countries, only Singapore has so far explicitly recognised research in medicine as a crucial activity for strategic and economic growth, through a coordinated government strategy with appropriate academic incentives, investment in national research imaging infrastructure, collaboration with a leading imaging equipment company and research grant funding explicitly for imaging research. The necessary imaging equipment, world-class scientific personnel and the integration of clinical and research imaging for both animals and humans will be developed over the next 5 years. Whether this approach, in conjunction with mandatory and integrated research skills training, will lead to productive high-quality research-oriented radiologists remains to be seen.

The major challenges for radiology education in the region are thus not so much pedagogical as socioeconomic and logistic. The various bodies responsible for radiology training across Southeast Asia have quite similar approaches and attitudes to this education overall, but often lack enough centres with sufficient numbers of expert teachers to develop the specialty to the level desired. There are a disproportionately low number of suitable training

18

centres in most countries, and public institutions where such training takes place are often underequipped and underresourced. The number of radiologists in the workforce is low by industrialised nation standards, and subspecialist practice is rare, even in Singapore, which has the most developed radiology environment overall.

Nevertheless, a few examples notwithstanding, significant strides have been made in radiology education in the region over the last 40 years. Standards expected in training programmes, from governance and oversight to teaching and learning, are steadily improving. Countries that once had a few radiologists now have hundreds. More and more high-end imaging equipment is being purchased for major urban teaching hospitals every year. To some extent, the gap between private and public radiologist incomes is narrowing in some countries. Training numbers have increased greatly across the region, even though the gulf between current and ideal workforce numbers remains very large.

In general, the trend towards increased quality and quantity of radiology education across the region has paralleled the economic development of each nation. Wherever serious socioeconomic downturns or major geopolitical strife has occurred, medical specialist training has ground to a halt or gone in reverse as physicians have left for better climes. When economies, even communist state-run systems) have grown rapidly, radiology has also grown in tandem. Clearly the advancement of radiology in this part of the world has not depended so much on political governance but rather on the socioeconomic development of the country. Much has been done, and there is much to do.

Acknowledgements

Information about national professional radiology training programmes in various Southeast Asian countries was provided by senior radiologists either in charge of or closely associated with their national radiology college and its central training committee. The assistance of these radiologists is gratefully acknowledged, and this chapter would be much the poorer without their contributions. They include Basri Johan Jeet Abdullah from Malaysia, Daniel Makes from Indonesia, Chamaree Chuapetcharasopon from Thailand and Thazin Han from Myanmar. The author was responsible for the responses from Singapore and information from other Southeast Asian nations. Any errors are the responsibility of the author.

References

Amin Z, Khoo HE (2003) Basics in Medical Education, World Scientific, Singapore
Gollogly J (2005) The Role of NGOs in training Cambodian Surgeons. Powerpoint presentation, [www.utoronto.ca/ois/BRT/2005/Gollogly_2005_NGO.pdf] Accessed 28 February 2008
Hoang DK (2003) Vietnamese Radiology. Diagnostic Imaging, Special Edition: Global Face of Radiology – Asia Pacific. [http://www.dimag.com/globalfaceofradiology/world/?id=47901946] Accessed 28 February 2008
Straits Times (2008) More doctors, nurses for public hospitals in next 5 years. [www.Straitstimes. com] Accessed March 4 2008

Training of Ultrasound Doctors and Educational Reform in West China Hospital of Sichuan University, China

19

L. Yan

19.1
Introduction

Imagine the following scenario. Long lines of customers waiting from early morning every day, rooms of equipment buzzing and flashing here or there, a couple dozen operators bustling about and streamlining customers through various machines. Can you imagine where this is? An indoor Disney-like theme park? Or a testing field for a hot new toy? Neither! It is actually an ultrasound department in a hospital! (Fig. 1)

These pictures illustrate a typical day in an ultrasound department of West China Hospital of Sichuan University: 25 doctors, 25 ultrasound machines, 1,000 patients. The ultrasound examination includes contrast-enhanced ultrasound, intraoperative ultrasound, ultrasound-guided biopsy, and high-intensity focused ultrasound. We are often asked if we work 24-h days given the demands of our patient load. In fact, we generally work 8 h per day, but this means that we must complete the scans very quickly and arrive at a diagnosis quickly as well. For example, we typically examine about 40 general patients and perform about 20 Doppler examinations each half day. We issue ultrasound reports to patients within 10 min of finishing a scan. Doctors participate in the entire process, including the scanning, diagnosing, and reporting. No wonder the doctors depicted in Fig. 19.1 appear so tired. We sometimes joke that our workplace is more like a factory than a hospital. Perhaps this is one of the special characteristics of Chinese ultrasound doctors.

On the other hand, as a Chinese ultrasound doctor, it is often hard for me to answer the question posed by my foreign peers: "Are you a radiologist or a cardiovascular specialist?" Neither description is accurate. The response "I am an ultrasound doctor" may confuse them. The distinction is due to differences in the medical and ultrasound education systems

L. Yan
Ultrasonic Diagnosis Department, West China Hospital, Sichuan University, China
E-mail: luoyand@hotmail.com

Radiology Education. R.K. Chhem et al. (Eds.)
DOI: 10.1007/978-3-540-68989-8, © Springer-Verlag Berlin Heidelberg 2009

19

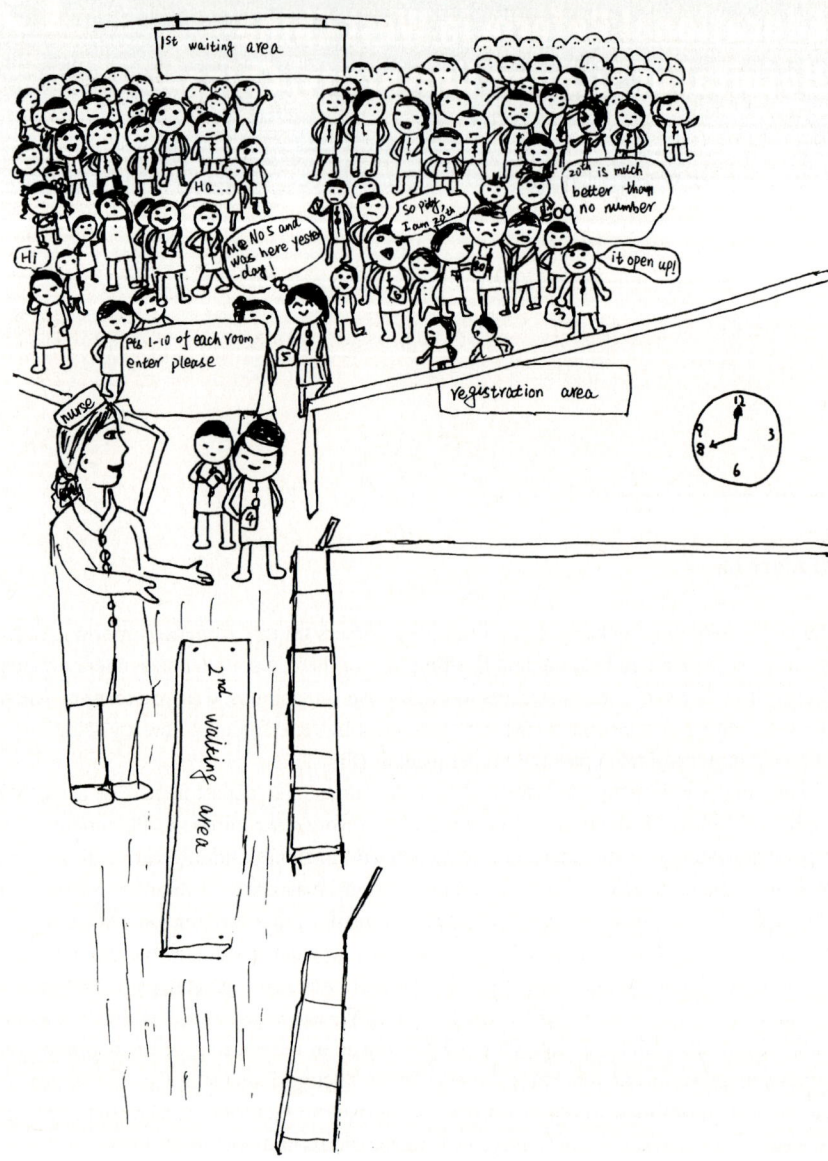

a

Fig. 1 One day in the ultrasound department of West China Hospital of Sichuan University. (**a**) At the beginning of the day, the doctors are high-spirited, the patients are waiting in a long line, and the hospital is crowded. (**b**) During the day, doctors keep busy as they scan, diagnose, and issue reports. Patients pass through the examination room one after another. (**c**) By the end of the day, patients all leave with their reports and doctors are exhausted. (Pictures courtesy of Li Liu)

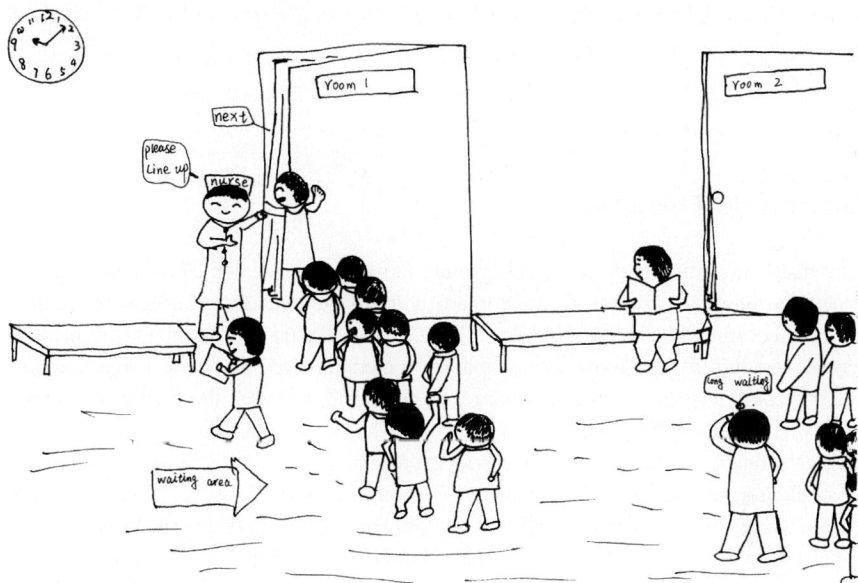

b

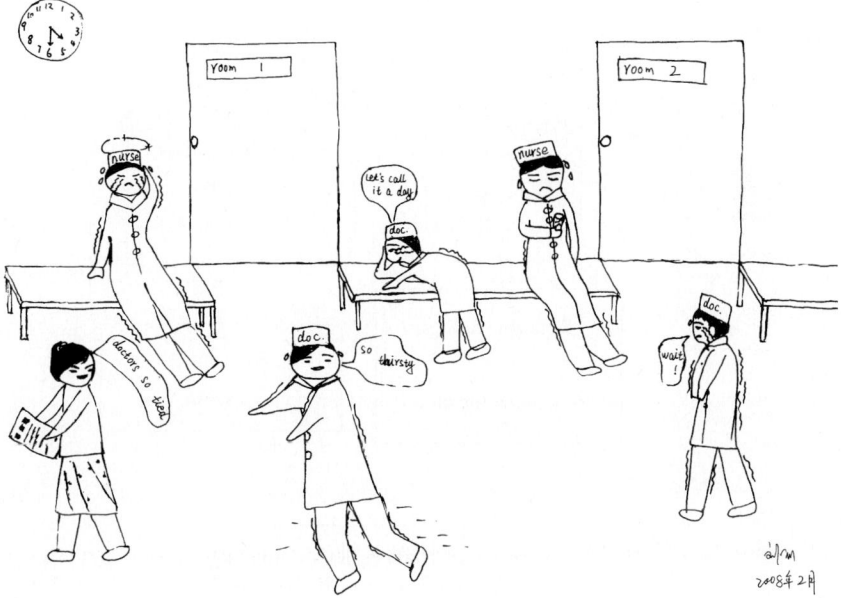

c

Fig. 1 (continued)

between China and the rest of the world. Currently, there are more than 150,000 ultrasound doctors like me working in China.

19.2
Chinese Medical Education

Like many academic medical systems around the world, Chinese medical education has undergone reform. At present, the mainstream model of Chinese medical education and doctor training can be illustrated as shown in Fig. 2. Usually, after 5 years of study in medical schools, graduates may find a job in smaller or medium-sized hospitals. Large hospitals and university hospitals typically require a postgraduate degree at the master or doctoral level. Compared with Western medical education, Chinese medical education takes a different educational path. First of all, high school graduates can apply to medical school directly. Secondly, medical school graduates may be employed as residents and become formal staff of the hospital. Furthermore, doctors employed by one hospital are typically not allowed to practice in other hospitals. However, they can practice at other hospitals on a short-term basis (varies from 3 months to 1 year) for continuing medical education (CME) in large-scale hospitals or university hospitals. Thirdly, there is no standard national resident training program and the resident training varies greatly between hospitals.

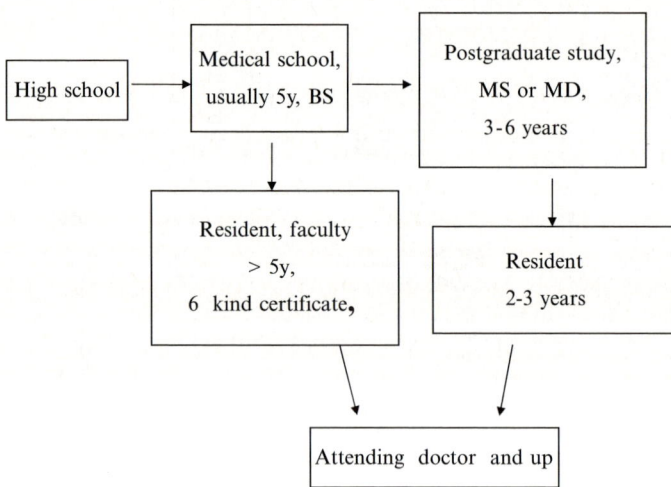

Fig. 2 Medical education and training model in China

A mainstream training program of ultrasound doctors in China is demonstrated in Fig. 3. In China, ultrasonic medicine does not belong to radiology. Instead, it is treated as an independent subject. On the other hand, specially trained sonographers are not available. Under such circumstances, there are many differences between the training programs of Chinese ultrasound doctors and Western radiologists. Firstly, Chinese ultrasound doctors are specialized in ultrasonic medicine only and are usually not permitted in radiological practice. Some may not have much radiological training at all. Secondly, medical school graduates can apply to work in the ultrasound department as ultrasound doctors. Because undergraduate education teaches little about ultrasonic medicine and provides no specific training, these graduates have to begin their systematic study of ultrasonic medicine after they join the ultrasound department. Thirdly, a registered ultrasound doctor requires a license for medical imaging and a certificate for color-Doppler imaging. In other words, physicians and surgeons cannot legally perform ultrasound scanning or sign ultrasound diagnosis papers. Finally, all ultrasound scanning is done by ultrasound doctors instead of sonographers. Here we may draw the conclusion that every ultrasound doctor is a sonographer plus an ultrasound diagnosing physician, as shown in Fig. 4. So the correct answer to the often-asked question of "Are you a radiologist or a cardiovascular specialist?" is that I am neither a radiologist nor a cardiovascular specialist.

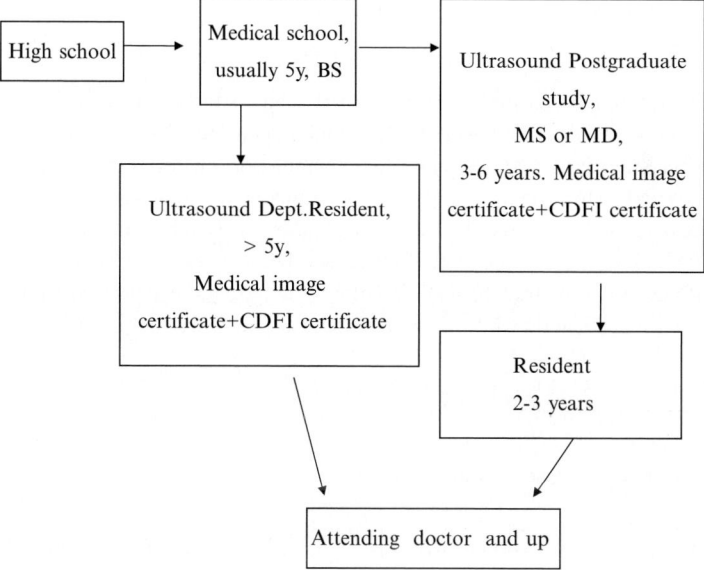

Fig. 3 Educating and training protocol of Chinese ultrasound doctors

19

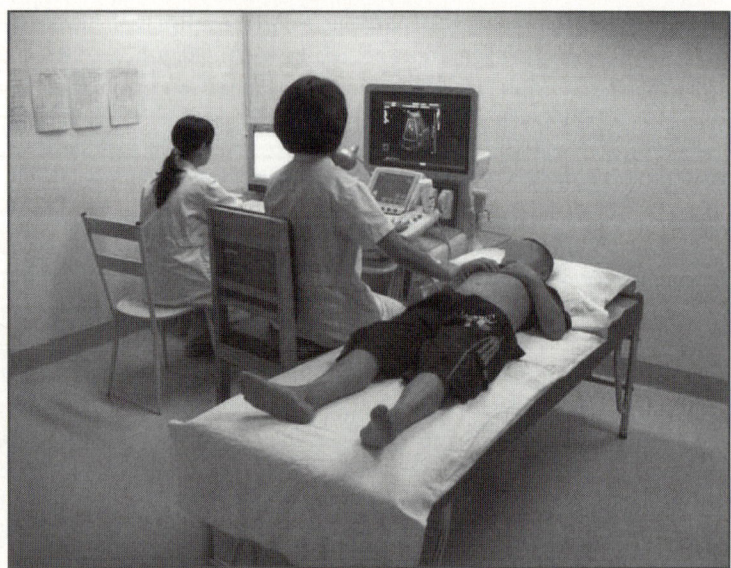

Fig. 4 Chinese ultrasound doctor's work mode. As shown, scanning and diagnosing is done at one place. Images are archived in a mini picture archiving and communication system (PACS) or a PACS. The computerized examination reports are ready in less than 30 min and the report will be connected to the hospital information system

Obviously, through this kind of training, ultrasound doctors are practiced in ultrasound scanning and have rich experiences in ultrasound diagnosing. This fact makes it possible to cope with the massive volume and timely completion of ultrasound examinations in Chinese hospitals. However, spending too much time on scanning and having insufficient knowledge in related disciplines limits the development of scholarship for ultrasound doctors. It also hinders the development of ultrasonic medicine as a whole. As such, Chinese ultrasound education and training demands reform. It needs to keep pace with international medical imaging education while at the same time accommodating our specific situation.

19.3
Reforming Chinese Medical Education

Some Chinese university hospitals have begun exploring new training programs for medical imaging doctors.[1–7] Sichuan University, affiliated with West China Hospital (SUWCH) located in Chengdu, is one of these pioneers. As a well-known medical school and the biggest general hospital in China, SUWCH is dedicated to medical education and research as well as reform.[8–13] In terms of ultrasound education, on the one hand, we continue to carry on traditional Chinese academic education including degree programs and CME courses as detailed later. On the other hand, we have established the first 5-year standard ultrasound (imaging) resident training program in China. We are also the first medical center devoted to exploring the education and standard training of medical imaging technicians (including sonographers). In the following sections a brief introduction of our education and training programs is provided.

19.3.1
Degree Programs

> Undergraduate education: There is no specific curriculum of ultrasonic medicine for undergraduate medical students. The introduction to ultrasound is found in textbooks of medical imaging, and includes radiology, ultrasound, and nuclear medicine. Usually, 6–18 school hours are required for a brief introduction of the basic principles and indications of ultrasound in order to give students some ideas of the merits, disadvantages, and clinical applications of ultrasound examination.
> Postgraduate education: During 3 years (master) to 6 years (doctor) of postgraduate study, the curriculum includes basic ultrasound theories and ultrasound-related fundamental knowledge. Training in related departments and orientation in ultrasound submajors are also prerequisites before doing a graduation thesis.

19.3.2
Continuing Medical Education

> Short-term CME includes specific subjects such as the clinical application of ultrasound enhancement agents and three-dimensional ultrasound. We normally offer four to six such courses per year and each course usually takes 1–5 days.
> The refresher program is a 3–12-month program hosted by large or university hospitals and is normally offered to ultrasound doctors from medium-sized or small hospitals. This program can focus on general ultrasound education or on a submajor of ultrasound medicine such as echocardiography or ultrasound for obstetrics and gynecology.

19.4
Training Program for Ultrasound Residents in West China Hospital, Chengdu, China

19.4.1
General Information

This program is the first one of its kind in China and was initiated in 2003. During the 5 years' training, residents are trainees instead of employees of the hospital.

19

19.4.2
Current Training Plan

> › Year 1: To rotate in related clinical departments, including two internal medicine departments and two surgical departments. At the end of this stage, trainees should pass the national medical licensing examination.
> › Year 2: To rotate in imaging departments, including 6 months in a radiology department, 3 months in an ultrasound department, and 3 months in a nuclear medicine department. A basic understanding of these three imaging modalities, their clinical applications, as well as the advantages and disadvantages of each area is required.
> › Years 3–5: Ultrasonic medicine training. To rotate within submajors of ultrasound, including abdominal ultrasound, echocardiography, ultrasound for obstetrics and gynecology, vascular ultrasound, small-parts ultrasound, and interventional ultrasound. Junior attending doctor's level is the goal for this stage of training. Trainees should also pass the licensing examination for Doppler ultrasound imaging. At the end of the fifth year, trainees are encouraged to attend the examination for attending doctor hosted by the Ministry for Public Health.

Meanwhile, trainees should also take some elective courses such as evidence-based medicine, teaching-method training, and research training such as literature searching and paper writing.

19.4.3
Challenges

There is no existing ultrasound resident training model to copy; therefore, it is not clear how to design our training program to meet international standards and also, at the same time, to meet the demands of our situation in China.

19.5
Medical Imaging Technician Education and Training Program at Sichuan University Affiliated with West China Hospital

19.5.1
Background

Supported by the Chinese Medical Board, the first department of undergraduate education for allied health professions in China was established in West China Hospital in 1999. The goal of this program was to cultivate high-standard medical technicians. The submajors of the allied health professions included: medical imaging technician (including X-ray, computed tomography, MRI, nuclear medicine, and ultrasound), clinical nutriology, rehabilitation, respiratory therapy, and ophthalmic optician. After 4 years' study, a bachelor of science degree is awarded.

19.5.2
Present Status

More than 200 students have graduated from this department in the past 5 years. Our graduates are welcomed by hospitals owing to their high-quality performance. The growth of the department of the allied health profession is obvious. The submajor of rehabilitation has already expanded into the rehabilitation department. The future of the submajor of medical imaging technician has also been prosperous. The academic education of this submajor includes X-rays, computed tomography, MRI, nuclear medicine, and ultrasound. Hospitals, especially large ones, need a large number of imaging technicians to do the examinations. West China Hospital also has a 2-year medical imaging technician training program for the graduates before they are employed as a radiography technician, sonographer, or nuclear medicine technician. Training more sonographers will greatly enhance the scholarship of our program. These highly trained sonographers are able to perform ultrasound scans and make preliminary diagnoses under the surveillance of doctors upon the completion of their training. Ultimately, this will eventually free up some time for physicians to participate in research or teaching. At this time, however, scanning methods are not standardized; therefore, the sonographers that are trained within the individual hospitals cannot offer their service to other hospitals or physicians. We will need to focus on improving the training of diagnostic medical sonographers.

19.6
Conclusions

China has the biggest population in the world and, therefore, the largest number of patients. China is also short of health resources. With the widespread demand for ultrasound examinations and growing awareness of its role in detection and diagnosis, it has become one cornerstone of the new "three routine examinations" along with blood tests and chest X-rays. Opportunities and challenges coexist, but we continue to focus on how to meet international standards while simultaneously meeting the needs of our situation in China.

Acknowledgments

Many thanks to my colleagues Qiang Lu for his great efforts with the English translation and Li Liu, who painted the cartoons for this chapter.

19

References

1. Chen F, Zeng Z, Lu B (2005) Consideration of integrating education in all-around university with global standard. Chin Med Eng 13:330–331
2. Chen H, Li L (2004) A comparison between different higher medical education systems in Hong Kong and that of the mainland. Res Educ Tsinghua Univ 25:30–34
3. Li K (2001) The consideration on reformation of education and training about medical imaging doctor in China. Chin J Med Imag Technol 17:3–4
4. Li P, Chen G, Li F (2003) The study of ultrasound doctor training program in new circumstances. Shanghai Med Imag 12:158–121
5. Li Y (2003) The global standards on quality improvement for the WFME the medical education of the postgraduates (after graduation.) Med Educ (China) 23:45–51
6. Wu R, Wang X, Hu T (2007) The reflection and countermeasures of further perfect the standardized training for resident doctors. Contin Med Educ 18:22–25
7. Zhang X, Li X, Wan X (2004) Attitudes of Chinese medical students towards the global minimum essential requirements established by IIME. Teach Learn Med 16:139
8. Deng H, Wan X, Chen G (2002) About "Global minimum essential requirements in medical education". Educ Rev 4:96–98
9. Guo X, Ang X, Ao Y et al. (2004) the discussing of the strategies for the existing problems in the resident training program. Chin Hosp Manag 24:42–43
10. Huang L, Wang X, Shu M et al. (2005) To improve the system of residency training program. Mod Prev Med 8:992–993
11. Wan X, Zhang Z, Li G et al. (2005) "Global minimum essential requirements in medical education" and its experimental implementation in China. Med Educ (China) 25:11–13
12. Wang X, Yi J, Shu M et al. (2005) The comparison of resident training program and global minimum essential requirements in medical education. Mod Prev Med 32:367–368
13. Wang X, Yan Z, Shu M et al. (2007) A survey of resident doctors: evaluation of the practical value towards the global minimum essential requirements in medical education. Chin J Evidence-Based Med 7:99–103

Teaching Radiology at the Angkor Hospital for Children in Siem Reap, Cambodia

20

M. Fortier

I walked up to the gate and one of the security guards recognized me.
He welcomed me back for this my second year.
Again there were over 300 patients waiting in the courtyard, patients with pneumonia,
malnourishment, dehydration, and infections such as malaria. This scene is not unique
and is repeated in clinics throughout the developing world.
Days later, part of my experience was accompanying a home care nurse.
We ventured out into the countryside to attend to HIV-positive children.
I met courageous children struggling with poverty and social stigma as well as their disease.
One 12-year-old girl was managing to care not only for herself but also
for her ailing grandfather.

20.1
The Community

As a radiologist, my job was primarily focused on the teaching the local radiologist but also on participating in teaching other physicians in this hospital. The following is my journey as a student as much as an educator at the Angkor Hospital for Children (AHC) in Siem Reap, Cambodia.

During a series of trips to Angkor Wat, New York City photographer Kenro Izu saw children in need and was moved to action. In 1995, Izu created Friends Without a Border, a nonprofit organization. AHC opened its doors January 14, 1999 and is funded entirely by the financial support of this organization.

This is a teaching hospital situated in the heart of Siem Reap in northern Cambodia. Its mission is to provide nurturing pediatric care, medical education, and community reach. It fulfills this mission through many services and it is so much more than just hospital care. As of January 2008, the total numbers of patients through AHC were 517,245 outpatients, 22,767 inpatients, 82,222 emergency visits, and 10,524 home visits. The needs are extensive.

M. Fortier
Department of Medical Imaging, Schulich School of Medicine
and Dentistry, University of Western Ontario, London, ON, Canada N6A 5C1
E-mail: marielle.fortier@lhsc.on.ca

Radiology Education. R.K. Chhem et al. (Eds.)
DOI: 10.1007/978-3-540-68989-8, © Springer-Verlag Berlin Heidelberg 2009

243

The infant mortality rate is 56.69 deaths per 100,000, whereas in Canada this rate is 5.08 per 100,000 (Wikipedia 2008). The major causes of death under the age of 5 years are neonatal causes (30%), pneumonia (21%), and diarrhea (17%) (WHO statistics report of 2007). The major burden of disease is related to HIV-AIDS, malaria, and tuberculosis. Programs at AHC are not only about acute care, but also include teaching families about nutrition and follow-up care on home visits. AHC not only provides a wide scope of patient services, but also has teaching of health care professionals as an integral part of its mission. After the Khmer Rouge regime, only 40 physicians remained in Cambodia in 1979. There has been much rebuilding of medical education since then. There is a two-pronged approach to medical education at AHC: provision of knowledge and skills for current practice, and development of medical teachers for the future.

AHC is just a few kilometers from Angkor Wat. The archaeological site of Angkor Wat has been designated a World Heritage Site by UNESCO, but people live in poverty in the neighboring villages. AHC ensures that children of these communities have access to health care.

20.2
Health and Imaging Needs of the Community

The health needs in developing countries are at times overwhelming. Provision of public health measures such as safe drinking water and mosquito nets could prevent illness for a larger target population. However, my expertise lies in specialized diagnostic skills and not public health. Nonetheless, it is important to acquaint oneself with the prevalent diseases facing the local physicians and aid in diagnosis with available resources. For example, tuberculosis is unfortunately common in the patients being seen at AHC but is a rare entity in my tertiary teaching practice. Common reasons for requesting an X-ray at AHC include pneumonia and trauma. Ultrasound is required to assess for adenopathy, abscesses, and cardiac disease, to name only a few indications. Ultrasound is preferable to computed tomography (CT) in assessing most pediatric problems given that no radiation or sedation is involved. However, CT would be more complete in dealing with cases of severe trauma.

Roadblocks that can be encountered are numerous. The practice of diagnostic imaging requires sophisticated equipment. There are often issues regarding this equipment in the context of a developing country such as delivery, ongoing maintenance, and availability of "consumable" supplies (Stark and Fortune 2003). For example, ultrasound examinations require the use of gel and the availability of this resource would definitely affect the ability to perform this test. For plain films, one needs processing with chemicals or a "dry" processor. CT and magnetic resonance imaging have the additional requirements of complex equipment and also technical staff with the necessary training to operate this equipment.

20.3
Implementation-Transition

How can and should we teach in developing countries? Some key points are:

1. Awareness of learning needs
2. Teaching outside the box
3. Future implications

Important considerations include meeting learning needs, being creative, as well as being culturally and community sensitive. Traditional methods in radiology are one-to-one teaching with review of films and discussions. This is not always feasible owing to the remote location and time constraints on visiting faculty. However, many methods are available. The Internet enables access to international literature as well as consultation with other radiologists worldwide. This assumes the availability of computers and Internet services. The World Library and Information Congress held August 2005 in Oslo, Norway, focused on the issue of the "digital divide" – that is, the divide between those that do and those that do not have access to communication technology. (World Library and Information Congress 71st IFLA Conference 2005) Some health care workers in developing countries must rely on Internet cafes to avail themselves of the current literature. Computers with Internet access capability should be available in the hospital or clinic and ideally in the immediate working environment of these workers. This enables not only access to knowledge but also immediate translation into practice.

Acquisition of skill could be addressed by having the students spend time with staff in centers willing and able to provide this experience. However, funding is an issue to contend with.

Teaching should also be tailored to what examinations can be done with the local resources. It would pointless to teach biopsy techniques if there is no existing mechanism to have pathological review of the specimens. But this does not preclude developing new or established techniques in developing countries. Basic fluoroscopic or ultrasound procedures could be performed. For example, intussusception reduction is possible under ultrasound rather than with fluoroscopy but as always necessitates backup by surgery in the case of perforation. Abscess aspiration drainage could be done with sonographic guidance and may reduce the need for surgical intervention. Brant et al. describe work in Nepal where nephrostomy drainage was done with a feeding tube or angiographic catheter (Brant et al. 1996). New techniques could be developed by rethinking common approaches.

Currently, ultrasound is performed by physicians in many parts of the world not only in developing countries. In North America, trained sonographers perform the scan but this process is supervised and interpreted by radiologists. The latter results in an efficient means of caring for more patients. This method could be implemented in developing countries but would require organized training of sonographers. This can be done in the context of existing programs but may necessitate establishing new programs. Ferraioli and Meloni organized a sonographic training program at a district hospital in Pemba island, Tanzania (Ferraioli and Meloni 2007). Ultrasound can be made more available and is safe without the use of radiation (Mindel 1997).

In addition to establishing initial competency, measures should be put into place to ensure continued education and acquisition of skills.

Continuing education can be pursued by means such as teleconferencing. This reinforces previous training and can impart new knowledge (Pradeep et al. 2007). Teleconferencing provides face-to-face interaction by video. This affords more opportunities to students with access to faculty and experts more often.

It is important to be cognizant of what the students need and to engage them. This ensures inclusion of relevant material to the local practice (Bates et al. 2007).

20.4
Providing Opportunities To Make the Transition

Medical education in the developing world should not be seen as a Band-Aid measure but rather as an investment. It is inadequate to only supply resources. We need to provide for information transfer and development of local talent. Although we are dealing with globalization, some action must be taken for investing in local "human capacity" as well as increasing collaboration across regions (Sadana et al. 2004).

Diverse groups and agencies have participated in health care in developing countries. Many provide clinical care and expertise. Some, such as the World Federation of Societies of Anaesthesiologists, assist in setting up worldwide standards of care (Enright 2007). Others embark on personal rather than group experiences. Individual physicians can participate and play an integral role in medical education in developing countries. Ecclersley and Tan spent a year teaching at the Mbarara University of Science and Technology in Uganda (Eccersley and Tan 2005). Their work included a list of activities similar to those of medical faculty members in North America: formal lectures, ward rounds, teaching clinical skills, but also some administration and research commitments. Their frustrations are different from those encountered in the developed world, namely, lack of investigations, unique barriers to care, and cultural differences.

This raises the question of how can we best take action. Awareness of learning needs of health care providers as well as the prevalent health issues is pivotal. Training of physicians can be done not only with traditional measures but also with Internet access and teleconferencing. We must rethink established processes. Our aim should be to not uniquely contribute to a developing country but rather to work in a remote and resource-poor environment. This has implications much beyond the so-called developing countries to areas with third-world conditions in the developed world.

Inasmuch as we are educators, we are also perpetual students. Learning from physicians in a developing country not only broadens experience but enhances performance back home in the developed environment (Eastwood et al. 2001).

One can incorporate this experience into teaching our trainees. This has enhanced not only my teaching file but also my approach to instruction. For upcoming teaching sessions, I recognize that essential components include assessment of learning needs, program expectations, and ability to adapt to various working environments. My enthusiasm for teaching has been renewed by promoting learning in two very different environments. This experience has better enabled me to deal with the challenges put forward by my students. My commitment to teaching at AHC is ongoing. When I do return to Cambodia, I plan to help organize an electronic file of interesting cases and to expand ultrasound services not only at AHC in Siem Reap but hopefully in other Cambodian communities. This could serve as a model for providing ultrasound services to remote areas in my own country.

References

Bates I, Ansong D, Bedu-Addo G, Agbenyega T, Yaw Osei Akoto A, Nsiah-Asare A, Karikari P (2007) Evaluation of a learner-designed course for teaching health research skills in Ghana. BMC Med Educ. doi: http://www.biomedcentral.com/1472-6920/7/18

Brant WE, Budathoki TB, Pradhan R (1996) Radiology in Nepal. Am J Roentgenol 166:259–262

Eastwood JB, Plange-Rhule J, Parry V, Tomlinson S (2001) Medical collaborations between developed and developing countries. Q J Med 94:637–641

Eccersley L, Tan L (2005) Teaching medicine in a developing country. Br Med J 331:130–131

Enright A (2007) The World federation of societies of anaesthesiologists: Supporting education in the developing world. Anaethesia 62 (suppl 1):S67–S71

Ferraioli G, Meloni MF (2007) Sonographic training program at a district hospital in a developing country: Work in progress. Am J Roentgenol 189:W119–W122

Mindel S (1997) Role of imager in developing world. Lancet 350:426–429

Pradeep PV, Mishra A, Mohanty BN, Mohapatra KC, Agarwal G, Mishra SK (2007) Reinforcement of endocrine surgery training: impact of telemedicine technology in a developing country context. World J Surg 31:1665–1671

Sadana R, D'Souza C, Hyder A, Chowdhury AMR (2004) Importance of health research in South Asia. Br Med J 328:826–830

Stark P, Fortune F (2003) Teaching clinical skills in developing countries: are clinical skills centres the answer? Educ Health 16:298–306

Wikipedia (2008) List of countries by infant mortality rate (2005) http://wikipedia.org/wiki/List_of_countries_by_infant_mortality_rate(2005) Accessed 28 April 2008

World Library and Information Congress 71st IFLA General Conference and council. "Libraries – a voyage of discovery" August 14–18, 2005 Oslo Norway. Access to electronic health care information resources in developing countries: experiences from the Medical Library, College of Medicine, University of Nigeria. http://www.ifla.org/IV/ifla71/Programme.htm Accessed April 28 2008

21.1
Narrative

I must have looked suspicious to the customs people when I arrived in Lima with my large bulk on wheels in 1985. I was very protective of it and would not allow anybody to handle my boxes. Of course, I was singled out by the airport customs people and they insisted on knowing what was I carrying. When they finally peered inside, they were somewhat astonished that all I had in those boxes were carrousels loaded with hundreds of slides. They asked me what my lectures were about so I took the time to explain to them in some detail. Suddenly an inquisitive crowd formed around me. Everyone, it seemed, had a family member with seizures or a parent with dementia, while some of them suffered from severe headaches. Before I had even left the airport I had several people consulting me about their neurological problems. They all wanted my professional card and asked if they could attend my lectures. When I was finally released, they apologized profusely for delaying me.

The lecture I was to present was organized by the Department of Internal Medicine, Universidad Peruana Cayetano Heredia, University Hospital, Lima, for their Medical Grand Rounds. Attendance at these rounds can be quite substantial. My talk was about the importance of imaging in diagnosing neurological diseases. It was a broad topic and addressed mainly nonradiologists. Addressing your former teachers, classmates, and others can be both exhilarating and also somewhat intimidating.

Since 1980, neuroradiology has been my exclusive practice, beginning with 1 year of fellowship and then joining University Hospital as a specialist. In 1987, I was given an opportunity to work at the Montreal Neurological Hospital and Institute, where most of my time was spent in the MRI section. The magnet was newly installed as the first in Canada.

R. DelCarpio-O'Donovan
Professor of Radiology, Department of Neurology and Neurosurgery, McGill University Health Centre, Montreal, QC, Canada
E-mail: raquel.delcarpio@muhc.mcgill.ca

Radiology Education. R.K. Chhem et al. (Eds.)
DOI: 10.1007/978-3-540-68989-8, © Springer-Verlag Berlin Heidelberg 2009

21

Since there were no local experts who could teach me how to use it, I learned on the job. It was an exciting challenge. Most patients we examined had positive findings. I started accumulating substantial teaching files, which I have shared with the young residents at McGill University and later in various parts of the world.

21.2
Language as a Cornerstone of Cultural Teaching and Learning

When the invitation to lecture at my alma mater came, the first challenge was to make the presentation in Spanish. Although it is my mother tongue, it was many years before that my medical and radiological language became English. I knew that when Peruvian professors (who trained and worked abroad) went back and gave their conferences in English, they were frowned upon. I had been a harsh critic myself. "Cultural competence" is a concept that has been re-energized during the past decade. Language is certainly the cornerstone of culture (Betancourt 2004). Even with translators, unless these professionals are properly trained in the medical/radiological lingo, interpreter errors can play a significant role in making mistakes (Early 2003).

Keeping these things in mind, finding the appropriate terms in Spanish was essential. Not many MRI textbooks had been translated yet, no papers were being published yet and no MRI scanners were in general use in Spanish-speaking countries for enough time to allow for publications. I believe, however, that the effort to do the translation was not only appreciated but also resulted in lectures that were more easily followed and understood by my audience. In Peru, medical students, residents, and the attending staff have a wide spectrum of English comprehension: few are completely unable to follow a lecture, few are perfectly at ease, and a large number can understand enough to get some benefit from an English presentation. Asking questions to the lecturer, on the other hand, is a significant challenge that only a minority are prepared to face. When a lecturer presents in his/her native language, and particularly if somebody as distinguished as Donald Resnick is the speaker, the attendees busily take notes, photographs of his slides, or record his lectures. Resnick is a master of interesting and didactic presentations. However, if a native Spanish speaker were to present in another language, the audience would not be as readily forgiving, even if the speaker were a gifted lecturer.

A group of specialists that would be totally excluded from English lectures would be technologists as these professionals rarely have a working knowledge of a second language.

21.3
Technology: The Necessity for Adaptability

When I first began lecturing in Lima – after that first invitation, many more arrived from various places in Peru – the lectures were presented using slides mounted in bulky carousels and using projectors that were not always reliable. At times, the local projectors did not take carousels but some outdated devices. I had to remove all the slides from the carousel they had traveled in and make them conform to whatever contraption was provided. Those invaluable slide trays were never checked in as luggage with the airlines, even if they were cumbersome carry-ons that you never parted with.

Most of my presentations were done with dual projectors. Sometimes I would arrive for the lecture and find there was only one projector (this was before e-mail, and preliminary exchanges were made by expensive phone calls and the messages were not always transmitted correctly) or we would start with two projectors and then one light bulb would blow without there being a spare. Thus, the lecture had to struggle on with half of the material originally prepared. The other half had to be imagined by the audience. Subsequently, I learned to travel with my own spare light bulb.

Today, most facilities in Peru, even when I lecture in smaller cities, have state-of-the-art computers and LCD projectors. Prior to giving my talks, I download my lectures onto their hard discs and leave them there in case someone wishes to use them at a later date. The customs people do not bother with the tiny USB memory device I now carry for my lectures.

On a few occasions I had to give the lectures in bright, sunny rooms with no blinds on the windows! Hospital bed sheets (that someone ran to get) were not ideal for darkening the rooms. So, like a good trooper I worked with what was provided. At the end of the presentations many of those in attendance (and this has happened in several countries) would ask me to leave them my slides, always claiming they were to be used for teaching purposes. Making the slides had been a major enterprise for me and rarely had I two identical copies. Parting with my slides, which I did exceptionally, was quite painful.

21.4
Considering Your Audience

21.4.1
Medical Students

A most important consideration is the audience – if they are medical students, the themes are more generic and the purpose of the presentation mostly stresses the importance of imaging in the diagnosis and management of diseases. My aim is to sell the specialty so that enough students will eagerly apply to the radiology residency programs and the bank from which to choose will be bigger and more competitive.

An interesting socioeconomic aspect of radiology in Peru (and other developing countries) is that most radiologists will need a significant amount of capital in order to start a private practice. Most specialists work half days in government agencies, the armed forces, municipal health care facilities, or some form of public hospital where the equipment and personnel are provided. The radiologist receives a fixed salary for his/her work. (These salaries tend to be quite low.) The serious income is earned in private facilities, or *clínicas*. Usually a small group of physicians – not necessarily radiologists – and often businessmen raise enough money to buy equipment for these private outfits.

Radiologists who do not have enough capital at the beginning of their career have to make do by working in a hospital and working for a colleague or the owners of equipment in the *clínicas*. This factor deters some bright but impecunious students from going into radiology as a specialty. On this issue, I try to encourage radiology students by telling them that the gains made from working as a radiologist far outweigh the difficulties needed for their initial investment.

Another goal I have when lecturing to medical students is to entice them to do elective periods in radiology so that they are better educated in this specialty and to get them more sensitized to what various imaging studies offer the patient.

When the students rotate in radiology, they learn about the difficulties; for example, an already weakened patient that has to drink 1 L of bitter-tasting fluid before an abdominal computed tomography (CT) scan, or how hard it is for an elderly person with back pain to lie still for half and hour on the MRI table.

Students should learn early in their career how to request the most effective tests for the most accurate diagnosis, particularly when they deal with a population of scarce financial resources. Therefore, in my lectures to students I emphasize:

1. The importance of imaging for obtaining a diagnosis
2. The progress of the specialty, thanks to new technology: computers, ultrasound, magnets, catheters, filters, etc.
3. The importance of the radiologist as a member of the team treating patients and the need to change the old attitudes that considered radiologists as second-class specialists.
4. The importance of choosing the best test for the most accurate diagnosis without exhausting the patient's limited financial resources.
5. Radiology as a fulfilling career choice that allows a wide spectrum of subspecialties, where one can always access cutting-edge technology and where radiologists can make an enormous impact on patient management considering the amazing medical and technological advances in recent years pertaining to patient treatment.

In many developing nations, radiology is practiced (thankfully less and less) by untrained medical staff (Curso Refresco 2007) and this creates a serious problem that gives a bad name to our specialty. The unorthodox practice of self-referrals by neurosurgeons or gastroenterologists (who sometimes own and use this equipment on patients) creates havoc to the patients well-being when these procedures are done by physicians who do not have the complete training and knowledge of stringent radiation principles. These "radiologists" are known for their "heavy foot" on the fluoroscopy pedal as well as unnecessarily repeating radiation procedures on children or young adults. This creates a mindset to the untrained eye that dictates "*If you have a hammer then everything looks like a nail.*"

In my professional opinion, the aforementioned guidelines are so basic and yet so crucial to the diagnosis and care of patients and yet all too often not taught in medical school. As a result, I have taken all lecturing opportunities to enlighten my students in these matters.

21.4.2
Radiology Residents

When teaching radiology residents, the content of the lectures is mostly academic. An effort is made in presenting subjects or themes in depth, underlying the differential diagnosis, the advantages of one imaging technique over another, and bringing up the most recent medical advances.

When instructing this audience, I will invariably stress the importance of the radiologist as a consultant, "the doctor of doctors." Our job is not just producing a report (Dalla Palma 2006), we also have to become an integral part of the medical team and communicate promptly with our consultant by phone, or e-mail, by demanding more clinical information, by recommending an alternative, more efficient-effective study, by suggesting a follow-up, and by always being honest and transparent. If we want respect as professionals we have to earn it by our ethical behavior.

With the advent and present widespread use of picture archiving and communication systems the images are available to the clinicians. Some medical professionals assume that is all they need, images that they think they can interpret, with, at times, disastrous consequences for the patient as in the example of a neurosurgeon interpreting an amyloid angiopathy bleed for a ruptured arteriovenous malformation. The management is different for each entity.

On the other hand, the diagnostic possibilities have now been expanded to subcellular level and the radiologist will have to train in molecular imaging, optical imaging, and nanotechnology (Dalla Palma 2006). For the Peruvian radiology residents, the concept of subspecialization is not yet familiar. Most aim to be polyvalent, "jacks-of-all-trades" in the human anatomy and in the technical skills. They are familiar with reading CT scans of the brain, mammograms, pediatric plain films, performing obstetrical ultrasound, arthrograms, and peripheral angiograms. Some are extraordinarily gifted and competent but have no choice but to practice in remote or small towns. In the larger universities or specialized hospitals, some create a niche with the greater part of their activity in a specialized field, while in the *clínicas* they tend to multitask. Presently there are only two trained neuroradiologists in Lima.

At the end of my talks, many radiology residents have approached me and asked for the opportunity to spend some time in my radiology department at the McGill University hospitals (some medical students have done the same). At least a dozen young Peruvian men and women have done rotations with us. My colleagues in Montreal, quite generously, have accepted these residents and students and have not only given them the opportunity to radiology but they also have served as role models in professionalism, in ethics, in teaching, and in research. If fact, it is known that those physicians exposed to the "developed world" training programs are more prone to apply research and teaching when they go back to their respective countries (Harrington et al. 1991).

21.4.3
Nonradiologists (Other Physicians)

If my lectures are directed at other specialists, neurologists, neurosurgeons, ophthalmologists, endocrinologists, oncologists, etc, extreme care must be paid in expressing, without compromising the basic principle, that radiology should be practiced by radiologists, not by those who own the machines.

I have to make it clear that their reputations are best preserved if they do what they are trained to do and they serve their patients better by allowing the experts to do their work. Turf battles can be nasty and the best way to win them is by striving to be the best in one's own specialty.

One point I emphasize to our referring colleagues is the importance of giving us pertinent information that will allow us to perform the most appropriate study. I suggest they cultivate a working relationship with the radiologist so that the request is more a consultation, never an order. It is important to always keep in mind what is best for the patient, the least expensive, least invasive method to reach the proper diagnosis.

21.5
Topics and Border Crossing

When lecturing in Peru, I used to feel hesitant as to whether I should mention diseases rarely or never seen there. The opposite occurred to me when lecturing in industrialized countries: Should I show infectious cases that are rarely seen? With the world getting smaller all the time, infections never heard of in Canada are now always included in our differential diagnosis. People travel much more today than when I started teaching and all diseases types are seen everywhere. When I studied medicine, I never encountered a case of multiple sclerosis. It was said that multiple sclerosis did not occur in Peru. Today my neurology colleagues do not see those cases frequently, but often enough to think of it in certain cases. Also, there were disease processes we never learned in medical school. For example, cavernous angiomas of the CNS. Even in developed countries this was a hardly known entity, a rare autopsy finding, Since the advent of MRI, cavernous angiomas are easily identified and in fact not that uncommon. So, cases like this are useful for emphasizing the importance of imaging in the acquisition of knowledge about certain diseases.

Again, instead of presenting a list of diseases or lesions of a certain nature (i.e., tumors of the posterior fossa) to a group of surgeons, I present a mixture of surgically correctable abnormalities. The idea is to keep the audience interested and it will certainly happen if they can relate to the subject presented. For the rheumatologists, I prepare a lecture on CNS manifestations of rheumatic diseases with several examples of the complications we see on CT scans or MRI images. They appreciate this effort. And so on for the various subspecialties.

21.5.1
The Power of Humor

Not to sound too dramatic, I include relevant humor in these talks. Humor as we know can be a minefield. It is a treacherous affair. There is ample literature on the use of humor in the teaching of medicine (Fry 1994; Robinson 1991; Ziegler 1998) although its place seems paradoxical. Trying to introduce humor requires not only mastering the language but also the culture: a most delicate balance.

21.5.2
Reciprocal Learning

In all my years of lecturing in Peru, I have been humbled several times. I have been shown cases, often acquired with great effort by the residents (who go out to the *clínicas* and sometimes beg on behalf of their patients to have the studies done gratis or significantly discounted) or by the patient's relatives, who with great sacrifice pay for the studies. Some of these images I had never seen before and the best I could do was give a differential diagnosis. There are, mainly infectious, diseases that we do not see in developed countries, so I learn from them. Often, minimal imaging has been performed on their patients but frequently, when the final outcome is fatal, there will be an autopsy. Years ago I met a neuropathologist from the Neurological Hospital in Lima. He was incredibly generous. He showed me his department's specimen collection, he opened many of his glass containers, and with reused disposable gloves took out lovingly, one by one, many brains from their formalin bath. He would recount the patients' clinical history, evolution, surgery, and the final diagnosis. I was deeply moved by his love for his specialty and what seemed a passion for his carefully collected brains. He offered me and delivered to photograph many of his brains, particularly those that resembled cases I had previously shown, but only with CT or MRI. I now have fabulous image–disease correlations thanks to him.

It is also admirable how specialists in third-world countries counterbalance their scarce resources. I recall a Caribbean country where they were recycling the helium for their MRI scanner. They had a huge bag occupying an entire large room where they recovered and "treated" the gas to make it reusable. Space is cheaper there than new helium.

21.6
Recommendations

1. International elective rotations for radiology residents as a choice should be encouraged. Several programs through the Colegio Interamericano de Radiologia are now available for residents. There is no doubt that exposure to large, often richer, and

21

better equipped facilities has a positive impact on the young students. I have been receiving many of my compatriots for elective periods in my department. With the help of other institutions, I could extend the project.

2. Form subspecialists mainly for large teaching institutions This concept, widely accepted in academic centers, has proven very valuable mainly for difficult diagnoses but also for the better teaching associated with it. As a neuroradiologist, neurologists and neurosurgeons respect my opinion; we share the same scientific interest.

3. Discourage the practice of the specialty by nontrained radiologists. In developed countries, the training period to become a radiologist is 4 years. For a clinician, trying to interpret images without appropriate training is preposterous. It may be a lucrative practice, but in the end is not best for the patient.

4. Encourage visiting professors programs. The Peruvian Radiological Society can apply to have these professors sponsored by several international organizations. For example, the Radiological Society of North America has a most interesting International Visiting Professor Program through its Committee on International Relations and Education. Likewise, the International Society of Magnetic Resonance in Medicine generously supports visits by MRI authorities to developing countries and the Colegio Interamericano de Radiologia sponsors several Latin American radiological societies every year, paying travel expenses for experts in various fields of radiology.

21.7
Summary

Teaching radiology in Peru has been an enriching experience. I look forward to my next presentation and I take great pride in preparing my lectures in Spanish. My greatest satisfaction derives from the great changes I notice: more young people aiming for subspecialties, many requesting elective periods in developed countries in well-recognized training programs, and more interest in publishing articles on radiology. Recently I have started to work with the Department of Tropical Medicine of the Universidad Peruana Cayetano Heredia. Here we are reviewing unique cases of amebiasis in the CNS. My intention is to link young researchers in medicine and in radiology and try to come up with some outstanding publications. I have been traveling to Peru and teaching at least once a year for the last 23 years. I hope I will continue for several more. With luck, I will be able to give back to my compatriots after having received so much in my youth.

I have come to the realization that as a teacher I myself need to continue to learn. Nowhere has this become more apparent to me than in the classroom every time I conduct a lecture, whether it is here or somewhere abroad. The more I read on a given subject, the more fascinated I become by how much knowledge advances or how explanations of a given phenomenon evolve. Repeating a lecture in exactly the same way over long periods could be risky if changes have occurred in the interim. "Fusing" old concepts with the new ones requires an alert mind that lends itself to creativity at times.

An essential aspect of teaching and lecturing is respecting the audience and recognizing they expect valuable information in exchange for the time they give us. Being prepared and presenting the latest information in an interesting fashion conveys this message to the audience, thus creating respect that is reciprocated. The enthusiasm of the teacher is also something readily recognized by the students. A seamless presentation is the result of thorough preparation. I repeatedly tell my residents and colleagues *"unless you are obsessive in the preparation of your lectures, do not expect to have an acceptable final product."*

In conclusion, key elements for a successful talk are as follows:

1. Knowing your subject inside out
2. Updating the contents
3. Giving serious attention to what kind of medium you will be using
4. Knowing how to address a specific audience
5. Using humor in appropriate dosage and fashion
6. Respecting the time allotted

I believe with a little practice and dedication on the part of the student, a lecture can go from mundane to magnificent.

Acknowledgments

I must acknowledge the work done by my academic assistant, Tanya Chernishov, who aided in the editing and translating of, and conceived many creative ideas for, this chapter.

References

Betancourt JR (2004) Cultural competence – marginal or mainstream movement? N Engl J Med 351:10

Curso Refresco, Foros, Foro de discussion del 2do Congreso Virtual de Radiologia CIR, Dic 2007, 23:53

Dalla Palma L (2006) Tomorrow's radiologist: what future? Radiol Med 111:621–633

Early PJ (2003) Language barriers lead to medical mistakes HealthLink Med College of WI {http://healthlink.mcw.edu/article/1031002276.html}

Fry WF (1994) The biology of humor. Int J Humor Res 7:111–126

Harrington WJ Sr, Gotuzzo E, Vial S, Restrepo J, Baldi J, Young PM, deFillo M, Guderian R, Harrington WJ Jr (1991) Estimating impacts on developing countries of the decrease in U.S. training opportunities for foreign medical graduates. Acad Med 66:707–709

Robinson V (1991) Humor and the health professions. Slack, Torofare, NJ

Ziegler JB (1998) Use of humor in medical teaching. Med Teach 20:341–348

Using the World Wide Web to Develop Competencies Around the Globe

22

C. Daniels

22.1
Introduction

Medical education is in a revolution. Increasing social, scientific, and technological pressures are causing a shift toward the delivery of radiology learning initiatives that are more effective and efficient. Distance education and computer based teaching through the use of multimedia CD-ROMs, for example, are amalgamating through the increasing integrating power of the Internet (Ruiz et al. 2006). Using the World Wide Web to develop and assess radiology competencies presents an valuable opportunity to evolve radiology education.

There are several factors which influence distributive learning and competency assessment in radiology. These include (1) the ubiquitous benefits of incorporating Web-based educational tools into a more traditional radiology instruction, (2) the need to re-evaluate and expand the role of educators in radiology, (3) the development of effective and efficient learning and assessment resources is time-consuming, (4) defining the balance between distributive and traditional learning methods, and (5) radiology is a technically demanding specialty which put stresses on the distribution infrastructure, particularly in some technology-challenged global communities. However, distributive learning has the potential to enhance personal learning and evaluate competencies owing to (1) its nonlinear structure, (2) its potential highly interactive capability, (3) its feedback potential, and (4) its rich media capability. Also, such digital resources present a practical means of incorporating the conceptual structures surrounding the complexities of educating adults into radiology education. We will discuss all of these issues and determine the state of distributed learning in the progression of radiology education and toward the development of competencies throughout our global community.

C. Daniels
Diagnostic Medical Physics Division, Department of Radiology, Dalhousie University, NS, Canada
E-mail: cupido.daniels@gmail.com

Radiology Education. R.K. Chhem et al. (Eds.)
DOI: 10.1007/978-3-540-68989-8, © Springer-Verlag Berlin Heidelberg 2009

22.2
Effectiveness of Digital Radiology Learning Resources

Many surveys have been conducted to determine the interest in and use of Web-based learning tools for medical education. In one such survey, Kitchin and Applegate (2007) found that Websites were called on as a first-line resource by radiologists, residents, and technicians to answer questions. A recent publication by Rowell et al. (2007) reported that 97% of respondents rely on Web-based radiology education, with 88 and 42% of respondents reporting using the Internet at least once a week and once a day, respectively, for radiology education. However, Internet material is not as readily accepted as peer-reviewed print material (Grunewald et al. 2006; Rowell et al. 2007). Users tend to have less confidence in Web content than in academic journals and textbooks.

Rowel et al. (2007) analyzed five studies comparing Web-based learning with other more traditional educational methods, including printed materials, courses, case discussions, and workshops, which exposed several advantages of Web-based learning. All of the studies revealed an equal gain in knowledge and equal or more efficiency compared with traditional education. Interestingly, learner satisfaction for Web-based learning was higher than for traditional methods for three out of the four studies which looked at this parameter and was equal in the fourth. One study evaluated the impact of the educational methods on patient care (Fordis et al. 2005). Because the goal of medical education is not to increase the knowledge base as much as it is to improve skill sets for enhanced patient care, this is an interesting assessment to consider when evaluating educational methods. In this study in which patients' medical charts were compared before and after the Web-based educational intervention, there was an increase in appropriate treatments for high-risk patients (Fordis et al. 2005). The long-term effect of this learning intervention was not assessed.

22.3
The Educational Framework

Radiology learners are generally of an age during which the principles associated with adult education apply. To develop effective and efficient Web-based learning material for radiology education and to evaluate competency requires knowing the target audience and understanding the principles associated with adult education.

Adult learners are a diverse group. They differ in their goals for learning and their personal characteristics, such as personal organization, open-mindedness, and prior education experiences. The reasons why adults choose to learn are different among individuals and within an individual's life cycle. These reasons include fulfilling a job requirement, addressing a limitation, personal interest, distraction, or to meet new people. In the case of radiology education, more often than not, the motivation falls more into the first three reasons listed. However, these various motivations affect the type of experience the learner has from an educational intervention and should be kept in mind when creating education for adults. Likewise, the reasons why adults choose not to participate in continuing education are also varied and include factors such as finances, geography, lack of time, or personal esteem. Another factor which influences the effectiveness of digital learning resources in particular is digital fluency. Digital fluency refers to the ability to retrieve, understand, and use digital information in an effective and efficient way. Younger radiology learners are generally members of the *iGeneration* or NetGen, those who spent their formative years during the rise of the World Wide Web (Oblinger and Oblinger 2005). However, digital fluency among older learners in radiology is also generally high owing to the specialty's rapid evolution into the digital realm over the past decade. Nevertheless, this is factor than can limit some radiology professionals from seeking Web-based learning opportunities.

22.4
Practical Measures

Further to understanding the audience, it is important to transform the principles associated with an adult educational framework into practice and to consider the technological infrastructure. In the following sections we will consider various features of Web-based learning and how these features can practically address some important principles in adult education.

Adults learn best through materials which represent real-life situations. One of the major benefits of using the Web in radiology education is the ability to incorporate multimedia. Besides text, the Internet allows an integration of other material, such as still images, audio, animation, and video (Fig. 1). This integration is intuitive for an educational

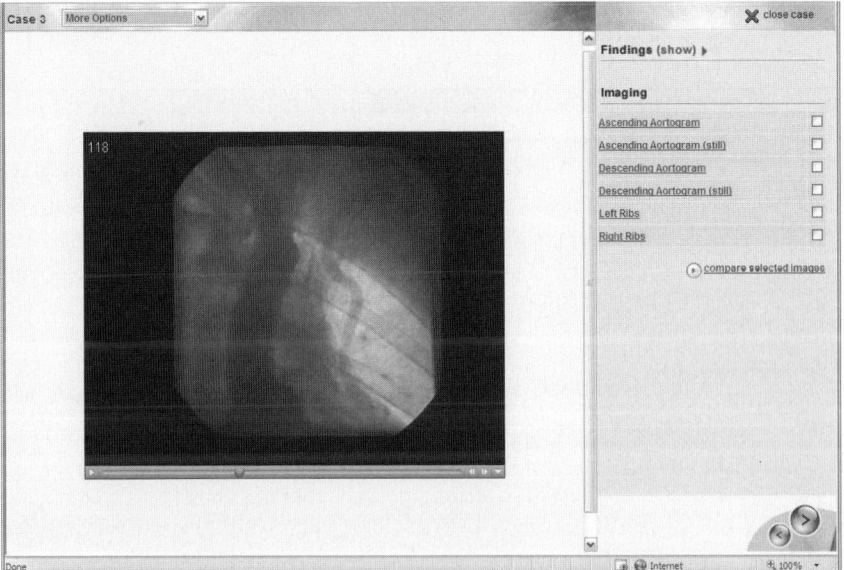

Fig. 1 Multimedia. A video illustrates a real-life technique and addresses visual learning

program especially in areas of diagnostics such as radiology, which calls for visualization of pathological findings (Curran 2000; Zajaczek et al. 2006; Kalb and Gay 2003; Hoa et al. 2006). Adults are unique in the ways they learn compared with other individuals and throughout their own lives. Learning styles have many sources and have an impact on the way education is experienced. Addressing different learning styles is often a great challenge in delivering education to a large audience. The incorporation of multimedia into learning can impact the gaps left by traditional learning. Also, by presenting content through various media, we are encouraging learners to learn concepts from diverse perspectives. In general, those in scholarship in radiology lead complex lives, of which learning is only a part. Real life often distracts even the most motivated adult learner. Multimedia presents a means of engaging learners and stimulating interest in the subject by infusing freshness and entertainment into the experience of learning. The case-based format of many Web-based radiology education resources holds special significance (Fig. 2) (Zajaczek et al. 2006; Hoa et al. 2006; Halsted et al. 2004). This format emphasizes problem-oriented, active, and interactive learning. Case-based learning presents situations close to real life, which helps with contextualization and application of acquired knowledge. A Web-based learning program also lends itself well to multidisciplinary information (Fig. 3) (Halsted et al. 2004). Because radiology is an area of medicine that liaises with many other specialties, this quality helps imitate the real-life situation facing radiologists and adds relevancy to adult learning.

Adults have a vested interest in their learning activity and their active participation in the design develops a sense of ownership, which enhances the learning activity. This is also consistent with the principle that adults should be treated with respect and be acknowledged for their knowledge and experience by allowing them to express opinions. It is wise to conduct an assessment or survey of the intended audience prior to Website creation to determine their needs and design preferences (Grunewald et al. 2006; Curran 2000). Websites can be continually updated according to user preferences (Curran 2000). This

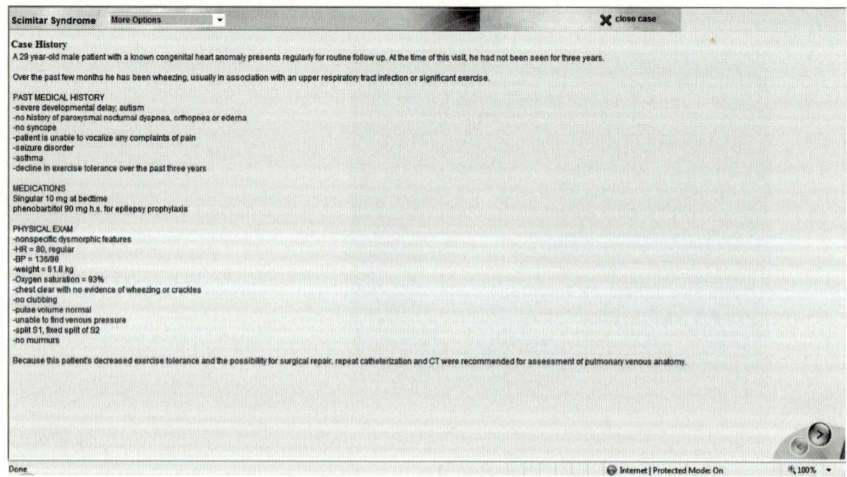

Fig. 2 Case-based learning. A case history is central to case-based online learning

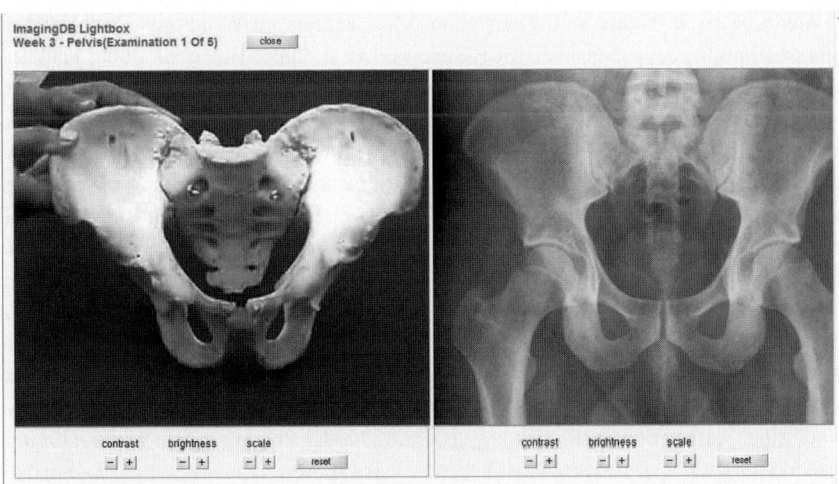

Fig. 3 Multidisciplinary. Anatomical and radiological images

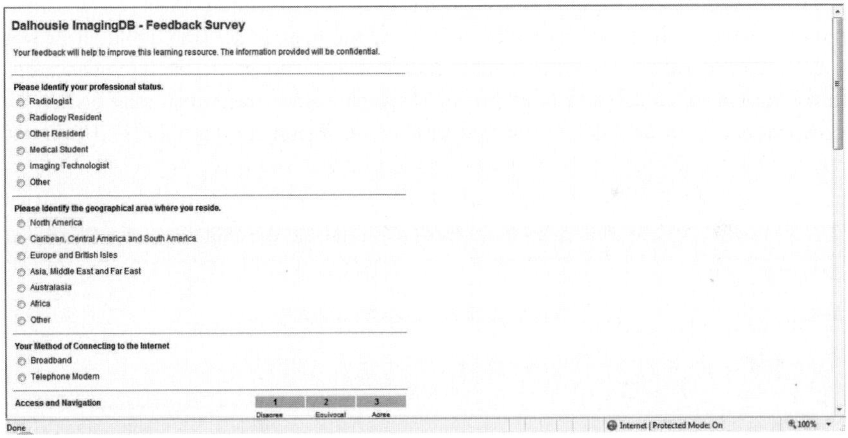

Fig. 4 Feedback. A feedback survey is used to involve learners in the ongoing development of a Web-based-learning site

can involve cooperation of the audience in the form of feedback given through surveys and questionnaires provided on the Website available at any time (Fig. 4) (Curran 2000; Grunewald et al. 2006). An important way that education can promote participation of adult learners is by involving them in the creation and continuing development in the form of representation on steering committees, questionnaires, and feedback on educational tools. Also, by incorporating continual feedback from users, an educational tool is better able to adapt to a changing and broadening audience.

Adults learn anywhere and at any time. Most authors on Web-based learning highlight accessibility as a major benefit (Grunewald et al. 2006; Hoa et al. 2006; Kalb and Gay 2003; Zajaczek et al. 2006). This is discussed in terms of unlimited, international, free, and fast globalization of information. The feature of accessibility can present major benefits for underdeveloped countries and/or learners with fewer resources for continuing education (Kalb and Gay 2003; Hoa et al. 2006). An important addition to making these Websites available internationally is to register them with major search engines (Fig. 5) (Kalb and Gay 2003).

The delivery of educational material via the Internet is "anywhere, anytime." The Internet can be accessed at the workplace or at home. A quick survey of residents revealed their top sources of information to be http://www.statdx.com, http://www.emedicine.com, http://www.e-anatomy.org, http://radiographics.rsnajnls.org, and http://www.wikipedia.com. A Web-based course can be accessed throughout the workday or at a designated time. In addition, learning opportunities are becoming harder to come by for some radiology residents as work hours are limited and there is less opportunity to observe cases (Sparacia et al. 2007).

It is not essential that learners and educators be in the same location, but it is critical that there is a harmony between technical infrastructures which may be dependent on remoteness of any party throughout the learning process. When considering Web-based medical education, it is crucial to look at the technical infrastructure available to the learners in order to realize the benefits of accessibility via the Internet (Curran 2000; Grunewald et al. 2006). Herein lies one of its weaknesses for users who access the Internet via dial-up connection, often referred to as plain old telephone service, which may or may not be dependable (Curran 2000; Grunewald et al. 2006; Pallof and Pratt 2003). Bandwidth

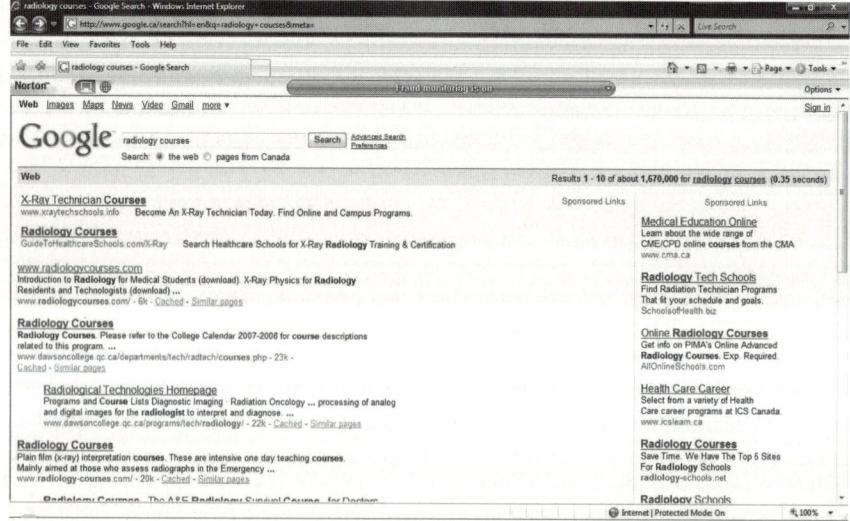

Fig. 5 Global access. A Web-based-learning site registered with a major search engine encourages global accessibility

becomes an issue when considering transfer speeds of text, but more so for multimedia such as images, sound, or video. One solution to this could be to provide downloadable versions that can be downloaded over the requisite time and then accessed whenever learning is scheduled. Educators should also consider their technical situation as a barrier to the distributive learning. The ability to communicate either synchronously or asynchronously often establishes a level of comfort for an adult learner to know that "there is somebody on the other side." Educator involvement is required throughout the learning process and poor Internet connectivity presents a potential significant roadblock to program delivery and maintaining contact.

Just as technology affects our day-to-day lives, so too will it have an impact on our education. Advancements in technology mean increases in access to education and improvements which allow us to simulate real-life situations. Economics must be considered when providing adult education since personal finances and government support of educational programs may have a significant bearing on whether or not an adult chooses to participate in learning experiences and the way he or she accesses education. One advantage of using a Web-based program is that we are able to address some of these factors through personal computers and distance education, which reduce the cost of transportation, instructors, etc.

Adult learners lead busy lives. As a result, flexibility is a fundamental factor in adult education. Time for education is often restricted or sporadic and a useful learning tool fits into a realistic schedule. Physicians today around the world are a heterogeneous group – and this group continues to diversify. An effective learning tool will allow users of different gender, family structure, religion, and lifestyle to access learning opportunities at personally suitable times and locations. Adults are busy and have wide responsibilities that can easily distract them from learning. Activities which encourage participation, collaboration, and real-life problem-based learning tend to capture the interest and attention of adults best.

Adults generally prefer self-directed, individualized learning activities. Much of the literature on the subject of Web-based learning discusses self-directed, individualized learning as one feature (Curran 2000; Halsted et al. 2004; Davis et al. 2005; Zajaczek et al. 2006; Kalb and Gay uj; Scarsbrook et al. 2006; Grunewald et al. 2006; Hoa et al. 2006). An interactive, Web-based learning format offers the possibility for learners to direct their own learning in terms of pace and content. For example, users can choose to cover units of material on the basis of their individual needs, they can have control over how much information they access before an attempt at diagnosis, and can choose optional tutorials within a module (Fig. 6). Because educational activities must fit into a busy life schedule, adults tend to be responsible for scheduling, doing, and evaluating their individual education.

Adults usually learn by choice; therefore, they have more control over when and what they learn. Adults, when seeking to learn, are driven by relevancy and the opportunity to individualize learning for specific weaknesses.

Adults bring experience to the learning activity. An interactive, self-directed educational activity acknowledges prior experience and is designed in a way that will accommodate different backgrounds and connect background knowledge and life experience to the task at hand. Moreover, this customizability of many Web-based learning programs supports the notion of lifelong learning (Zajaczek et al. 2006) by catering to an individual at many points in his or her education. The interactive character of Web-based learning tools is

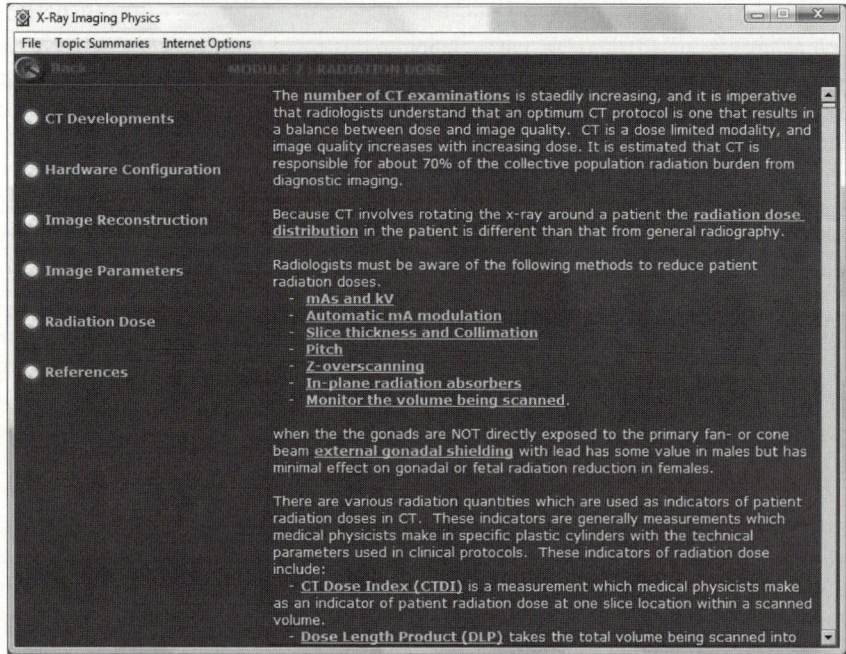

Fig. 6 Self-directed learning. Flexibility of content choice offers various topics and links within topics to allow personalization of learning

essential to consider when creating education for expert learners as often between and within specialties there can be extreme variation in experience (Halsted et al. 2004).

Interactivity is key in shifting the education of adults to learner-centered rather than instructor-centered or content-centered (Ruiz et al. 2006). Rather than the instructor or the content directing learning via traditional methods of teaching such as lectures and textbooks, respectively, allowing students to direct their own learning means a focus on the learner.

Adults are goal-oriented. Adults choose learning experiences which show clear objectives of things they will gain through participation. This affects how adults view the experience and how they implement learned concepts. Adults choose learning experiences that present immediate practical applications. Practical learning presents the possibility of influencing their lives. By using case-based problem solving, learners access performance/skill-based content that can directly influence the way they practice. In addition, adults learn effectively through active rather than passive learning.

Adults prefer immediate feedback. Rapid performance evaluation is often related to users' perception of effectiveness and learning outcomes (Hoa et al. 2006; Curran 2000; Halsted et al. 2004). Correspondingly, education providers need to supply evaluations and timely feedback for learners (Fig. 7). This is used by learners to assess their grasp of the material and make choices about how they learn in the future. Tracking users' learning through evaluations is also useful for providers to gauge effectiveness and steer continual development.

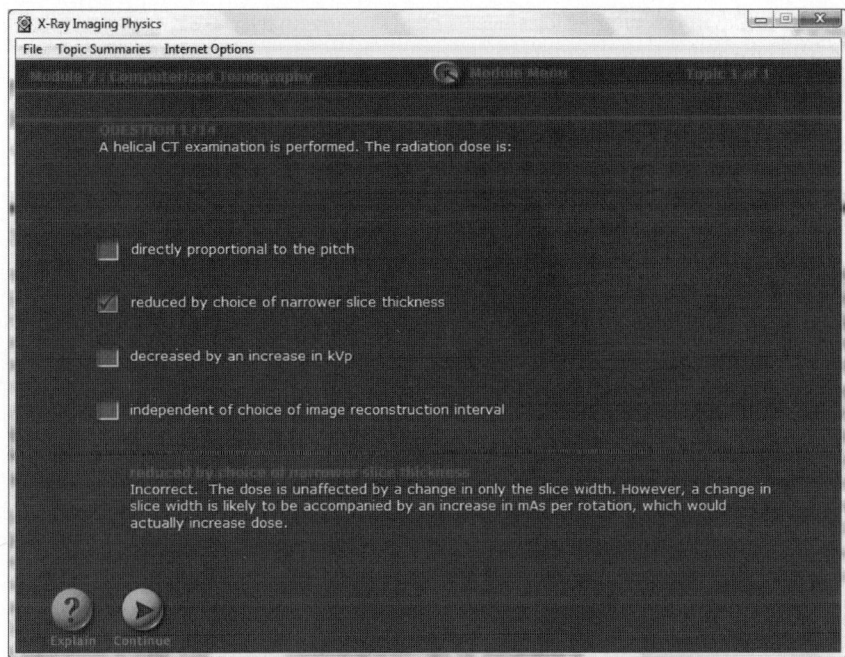

Fig. 7 Evaluations. Evaluations in the form of quizzes or tests can provide quick feedback for learners and even offer learning for incorrect answers as shown in this screenshot

Adults relate best to instructors who are keen, competent, and available. This also applies to Web-based learning. Distributed learning encourages an expanded role of educators and education providers. As mentioned above, learner-centered education (Weimer 2002; Pallof and Pratt 2003) focuses on the student and the learning outcomes and active rather than passive learning. This does not diminish the role of instructors; rather it leads to a shared responsibility for learning between the instructor and the students which encourages interdependence. Educators and students should both feel a degree control over the learning experience, with increased power allotted to students than seen in traditional instructor-led education. As an educator, one way of facilitating this adjustment is to establish learners as co-creators, providing opportunities for students to provide feedback during the instructional process. The instructor can then respond to the feedback and adapt and modify his/her teaching on the basis of what is learned (Pallof and Pratt 2003). Also, by including self-directed learning experiences, students have more choice than ever to participate in the trajectory of their own learning.

The outlook on content must also change if learner-centered education can succeed. Traditionally, there is a focus on quantity rather than quality. With learner-centered education, the role of content has evolved from a transmission model, aimed at filling minds with information, to a constructivist model in which students work together to build on their past knowledge and experience, and develop skills and performance abilities that will help with real-life problem solving. This approach requires that the instructor work to first establish an environment in which students feel "safe" enough to take risks, try out ideas, and both give and receive constructive and critical feedback.

22.5
Implications for the Facilitator of Distributive Learning

Providing radiology education online requires a different kind of commitment from educators, often a larger one. It takes more time from educators because interface and content design are a greater challenge. A simple, intuitive interface is essential because it facilitates efficient and instinctive navigation and makes a site "user-friendly." This has an effect on the user satisfaction with Web-based learning and a positive interaction with the interface increases the likelihood that a learner will repeat use. Regardless of perceived learning outcomes, adult learners have busy lives, and attractive, time-efficient Websites can lure focus. Content, when presented through Web-based learning environments, it is no longer linear. This can present a challenge for education providers. Designing content for a Website calls for creativity and integration of information, often across many topics and levels. Content design also requires a commitment to continual development. Much content will remain accurate across time, but some content changes. Fortunately, Websites are quickly and cost-effectively updatable according to current practice or new knowledge (Kalb and Gay 2003; Reid et al. 2004).

For years, teachers have tended to teach largely in the same way they were taught. The increase in technological innovation over the past decade in particular requires different approaches to teaching. Successful Web-based instructors are innovative and open to expanding their skill set and responsibilities. Some of the major barriers expressed by students learning in virtual environments relate to difficult navigation or poorly organized content (Bennet et al. 2004). Innovative creators and instructors of Web-based learning experiences must continually develop their understanding of learners' needs in conjunction with evolving technological capabilities in order to develop compatible learning tools.

Furthermore, designing education for a global audience puts onus on the designer to acknowledge issues of diversity. Online education for an diverse student population requires good verbal and visual communication by avoiding ambiguity and being sensitive to different cultural interpretations of language and images. Something as simple as time-zone differences can create difficulties for educators and learners if not acknowledged. It may be beneficial when creating an online radiology education program for a global audience to enlist the help of international experts. This can give the learning experience a wider perspective and help cultivate an international user base (Reid et al. 2004).

22.6
The Role of the Sponsoring Organization

The organization supporting adult education should be physically and environmentally, structured to encourage learning. Institutions must recognize the different and intensive commitment required from instructors and support staff of Web-based learning and this must be recognized and appropriately compensated to promote motivated staff. A potential challenge of Web-based learning often overlooked is the lack of accessibility by faculty. As organizations we need to support distributed learning in this respect (Rowell et al. 2007)

22.7
Conclusion

Despite the increase in Internet use in medical education, radiologists still prefer traditional educational resources for clinical information and continuing medical education (CME) (Rowell et al. 2007). Aside from barriers which can be addressed by instructional course designers and organizations, including navigation, content design, support, and access in the workplace, there are other existing challenges. User perception of reliability of online content can be a significant deterrent. This can be dealt with through thorough peer-editing and authorship by experts in the field. In addition, it is important to make authors' names and credentials visible and provide contacts to minimize anonymity of content sources. Cumbersome Websites with slow-loading multimedia can be frustrating when trying to fit learning into a busy schedule. This can be addressed by regular maintenance and the continual advancement of technology. Lack of CME credit has been cited as limiting use of Web-based learning for some professionals in the field of radiology. At this point, however, online CME is viewed as less effective, less efficient, and less preferred than other forms of CME such as institutionally run CME (Rowell et al. 2007). A major goal of CME and medical education as a whole is to ensure the best possible care for patients in terms of practical improvement in diagnosis, management, and treatment. There is a need for further research into the real outcomes of Web-based learning in radiology compared with traditional methods in order to address these perceptions of potential online learners. Portability as a barrier to Web-based learning will gradually be mitigated by the increase in use of laptops, personal digital assistants, and the blooming ubiquity of computer access (Rowell et al. 2007).

The Internet is fundamentally a way to share information to various sites irrespective of time or place. It is this nature which allows Web-based learning to reach a global audience. Simply making radiology education available online does not make it suitable for an international audience. As mentioned earlier, diversity must be considered in all aspects of design, content, and practicalities. Language and general means of communication, access patterns, time zones, and technological infrastructure should all be taken into consideration when creating an effective international online learning tool.

One projected consequence of developing global competencies via the World Wide Web is an international standardized curriculum (Reid et al. 2004). The reality of today's global infrastructure means that there is still inequality to access, with poorer access largely contained in the global south. Distributed learning is a capital-intensive endeavor in terms of setting up access points, support, and necessary equipment in order to practically apply learned techniques and knowledge. This truth means we cannot at this point match capital-rich parts of world with capital-poor ones.

We must recognize that different people learn differently; so, although Web-based learning will take on a larger role in radiology education, it most likely will never replace traditional education, and even online coursework should accommodate different styles of learning. Being able to print course material or notes from a Website accommodates some people who prefer to study and refer back to hard copy. Because Web-based learning is complementary to traditional learning in a distributed learning model, students often feel more comfortable in traditional lectures and are able to focus better on what is being said, knowing that notes and exercises are available online. Distributed learning has the potential to make face-to-face interaction between learner and educator more meaningful.

References

Bennet NL, Casebeer LL, Kristofco RE et al. (2004) Physicians' internet seeking behaviours. J Contin Educ Health Prof 24:31–38

Curran VR (2000) An eclectic model for evaluating web based continuing medical education courseware systems. Eval Health Prof 23(3):318–347

Davis LP, Olkin A, Donaldson SS (2005) Continuing medical education in radiology: A glimpse of the present and of what lies ahead. J Am Coll Radiol 2(4):338–343

Fordis M, King JE, Balantyne CM et al. (2005) Comparison of the instructional efficacy of Internet-based CME with live interactive CME workshops: A randomized controlled trial. J Am Med Assoc 294:1043–1051

Grunewald M, Ketelsen D, Heckemann RA et al. (2006) www.tnt-radiology.de: Teach and be taught radiology: Implementation of a web-based training program based on user preferences as determined by survery. Acad Radiol 13:461–468

Halsted MJ, Perry L, Racadio JM et al. (2004) Changing radiology resident education to meet today's and tomorrow's needs. J Am Coll Radiol 1:671–678

Hoa D, Micheau A, Gahide G (2006) Creating an interactive web-based e-Learning course: A practical introduction for radiologists. RadioGraphics 26: e25; published online as 10.1148/rg.e25.

Kalb B, Gay SB (2003) Internet Resources for Education in Radiology. Acad Radiol (10 suppl 1): S81–S86

Kitchin DR, Applegate KE (2007) Learning radiology: A survey investigating radiology resident use of textbooks, journals, and the internet. Acad Radiol 14:1113–1120

Oblinger D, Oblinger J (2005) Educating the net generation: Educase. Available: www.educause.edu/educatingthenetgen

Pallof RM, Pratt K (2003) The virtual student: A profile and guide to working with online learners. Jossey-Bass, San Francisco

Reid JR, Goske MJ, Hewson MG et al. (2004) Creating an international comprehensive web-based curriculum in pediatric radiology. Am J Roentgenol 18(2):797–801

Rowell MR, Johnson PT, Fishman EK (2007) Radiology education in 2005: World wide web practice patterns, perceptions, and preferences of radiologists. Radiographics 27:563–571

Ruiz JG, Mintzer MJ, Leipzig RM (2006) The impact of e-learning in medical education. Acad Med 81(3):207–212

Scarsbrook AF, Graham RN, Perriss RW (2006) Radiology education: A glimpse into the future. Clin Radiol 61(8): 640–648

Sparacia G, Cannizzaro F, D'Alessandro DM et al. (2007) Informatics in radiology: Initial experiences in radiology e-Learning. RadioGraphics 27: 573–581

Weimer MG (2002) Learner-centered teaching: Five key changes to practice. Jossey-Bass, San Francisco

Zajaczek JEW, Götz F, Kupka T et al. (2006) eLearning in education and advanced training in neuroradiology: Introduction of a web-based teaching and learning application. Neuroradiol 48:640–646

The Role of a Learned Society in the Promotion and Dissemination of Knowledge

P.A. Peetrons

23.1
Introduction

Musculoskeletal ultrasound is a rather new technique of examining muscles, tendons, ligaments, joints, peripheral nerves, and subcutaneous tissues. Although some historical papers and case reviews appeared in French and US literature in the mid to late 1970s (Cooperberg et al. 1978; Duval and Mambrini 1975; Moore et al. 1975; Seltzer et al. 1979), it was really during the early 1980s that musculoskeletal ultrasound was reported as a method able to show muscles, tendons, soft-tissue tumors, and joints (Crass et al. 1984; Middleton et al. 1984; Peetrons et al. 1984; Peetrons et al. 1986; Seltzer et al. 1980). The first book was on cross-sectional ultrasound anatomy of muscles edited by Bruno Fornage, in French in 1987 (Fornage 1987). The first book dedicated to pathology was written in German by Bernd-Dietrich Katthagen and dealt only with shoulder lesions (Katthagen 1988). The first book written in English about the full range of musculoskeletal ultrasound indications and results was edited by Marnix Van Holsbeeeck and Joe Introcaso and was published in 1991 (Van Holsbeeck and Introcaso 1991) and was followed the same year by the first book in French, by Fornage, about all musculoskeletal indications and the results of ultrasound (Fornage 1991).

At the same time, magnetic resonance imaging (MRI) came into business. The indications in musculoskeletal diagnosis were almost the same as with ultrasound. The MRI images were much easier to understand and seemed to be less operator-dependent than ultrasound images. Many radiologists learned rather MRI than ultrasound because ultrasound was much more time-consuming to perform for the radiologist at that time. The learning curve for ultrasound was very long, compared with that for MRI, because ultrasound was

P.A. Peetrons
Department of Radiology, Centre Hospitalier Molière Longchamp, Brussels, Belgium
E-mail: ppeetrons@bigfoot.com

Radiology Education. R.K. Chhem et al. (Eds.)
DOI: 10.1007/978-3-540-68989-8, © Springer-Verlag Berlin Heidelberg 2009

23

a self-performed technique, whereas MRI was an almost completely standardized and somewhat automatic technique performed by experienced technologists.

Musculoskeletal ultrasound was not widely taught in universities because professors were not used to the technique and because many were more involved in the emerging MRI teaching. A consequence was that musculoskeletal ultrasound remained rather unknown, leaving referring physicians skeptical or unsure of the accuracy of the musculoskeletal ultrasound method. However, the manufacturers continued to improve the equipment by developing new high-frequency probes, better spatial and contrast resolution, new pre- and postprocessing software, and smaller and cheaper units. Many people in Europe, more so than in the USA, still believed that there was a place for musculoskeletal ultrasound instrumentation alongside the much larger and considerably more expensive MRI instrumentation.

However, the main problem that remained was achieving the level of competence and a comparable degree of skill among a critical mass of radiologists using musculoskeletal ultrasound, which would lead to increased recognition of the method among both prescribers and the radiologists themselves. Such a level of competence seemed impossible to achieve in the universities, so during the early 1990s we saw an emergence of dedicated learned societies, with the goal of teaching musculoskeletal ultrasound among practicing radiologists (and since the twenty-first century, among rheumatologists as well).

23.2
Musculoskeletal Ultrasound Society

The Musculoskeletal Ultrasound Society (MUSOC) was established in 1991, under the leadership of Marnix Van Holsbeeck, and in collaboration with Michael DiPietro (a pediatric bone radiologist) and J. Antonio Bouffard. The birth of MUSOC followed the publication of Van Holsbeeck and Introocaso's book on the subject. They organized their first MUSOC meeting in Phoenix, AZ, USA. At that time, their conception of teaching was considered revolutionary. It has since been copied by many other societies through the world. They began by asking the industry of ultrasound diagnosis to lend enough machines to allow small groups of attendees participating in demonstration workshops to perform normal examinations. Along with the classic theory courses offered during morning sessions, the faculty taught afternoon sessions in small groups. The demonstrations utilized authentic, practical "hands-on" scans of patients serving as models. This type of active teaching was a relatively new phenomenon in 1991 and has had an enormous impact on the success of MUSOC.

At the inaugural meetings, the majority of the participants had minimal (if any) musculoskeletal ultrasound experience. The focus therefore modeled the procedures for a normal examination, to ensure that all participants understood and could perform the examinations using proper and adequate techniques. A comparison of illustrated anatomy, cadaver dissection, and arthroscopy on one side of the visual presentation "view" and musculoskeletal ultrasound on the other side was stressed in many lectures. This innovative approach was successfully introduced and validated as a teaching method at the 1996 Montreal MUSOC annual course by Germain Beauregard, Rethy Chhem, and Étienne Cardinal. Since then, this method has been adopted worldwide and used at most workshop on musculoskeletal ultrasound.

Today, the meetings have evolved, offering both a "basic" course, dedicated to those with little or no musculoskeletal ultrasound experience, and an "advanced" course for those who seek to improve upon their existing knowledge. The basic course continues to look much like the early versions of the courses started in the early 1990s, featuring anatomical approaches, the orthopedic surgeon's point of view, and an overview of the main joints in dedicated hands-on sessions (shoulder, elbow, wrist, hip, knee, and ankle). Advanced courses now consist mainly of short lectures that highlight new or less known applications of musculoskeletal ultrasound (e.g., nerves, interventional musculoskeletal ultrasound, fingers and toes, dynamic imaging, sacroiliac joints, etc.), followed again by hands-on targeted practice of what was learned in these new applications. Participants may now choose whether to follow an entire course or they may select one of the two subcourses. For example, in a recent meeting in Paris, France, approximately 375 people participated; 250 attending the whole meeting, 35 attending only the basic course, and 90 attending the advanced course exclusively.

The MUSOC codirectors decided at the outset that MUSOC would be inclusive, in order to draw international participation. The first meeting was hosted in Phoenix, AZ, USA, in 1991. The second meeting was hosted in Switzerland (1992), and it has since been held in the USA, Canada, and other countries around the world. To date, the annual meetings of the Society have been hosted in North America seven times, Europe seven times, Asia two times, and South America two times. The internationalization of the meeting served an important purpose, as it was a means of training and educating groups of teachers in each country visited. As local teachers were prepared for the meetings, they were also added to the international faculty, raising the number of people qualified to teach to 32 as of August 2007. Working collaboratively with local teachers also helped establish a consistent standard of examination around the world. Similarly, the number of participants also increased exponentially from less than 100 when we began, to approximately 375 at the 2007 annual meeting. To accommodate the increase in numbers, we needed 32 machines and models. Since participants are interested in having a variety of hands-on experiences with different instructors operating a number of different pieces of equipment, the logistics of planning, organizing, and implementing the workshops has also become more complex.

Participation at the conferences has also reflected the international agenda. At the 2007 meeting, attendees represented 42 different countries, including France, Chile, New Zealand, Canada, and South Africa to name a few, and also included representatives from emerging countries in the Gulf, Central America, and Asia.

In the past, sessions were organized with the help of a local hospital, which brought patients to the hands-on rooms. This practice became increasingly difficult to organize and indeed was not possible in all countries owing to privacy issues despite the overwhelming positive response from participants, who appeared to genuinely appreciate the timely in vivo application of what they heard during the scientific sessions.

In 2000, MUSOC introduced a hands-on version of interventional musculoskeletal ultrasound. This workshop continues today. The organization of this part of the hands-on session allows participants to perform biopsies, cyst aspiration, wire localization, abscess drainage, removal of foreign bodies, and intraarticular corticoid injections under ultrasound guidance. William Shiels initiated this part of the meeting. It requires considerable preparation, as the models for the practical component are whole turkey breasts and pig's feet. The preparation Shiels undergoes to mimic solid tumors in a muscle or intramuscular abscess with a fluid-pus level presents one of the most significant challenges for the organization, but results in one of the most meaningful learning experiences for the beginners in the audience. (To view a sample MUSOC program from Paris 2007, see Table 23.1.)

Table 23.1 Sample program, MUSOC Annual Meeting (Paris, August 2007)

Basic Session		
Saturday		
1:00 P.M.	Introduction	
1:15 P.M.	Shoulder	– Anatomy
		– Normal US
		– Live Demo
		– Common Pathology
2:30 P.M.	Elbow	– Anatomy
		– Normal US
		– Live Demo
		– Common Pathology
3:30 P.M.	Coffee Break	
4:15 P.M.	Wrist	– Anatomy
		– Normal US
		– Live Demo
		– Common Pathology
5:30 P.M.	End of the session	
Sunday		
8:30 A.M.	Hip	– Anatomy
		– Normal US
		– Live Demo
		– Common Pathology
9:30 A.M.	Knee	– Anatomy
		– Normal US
		– Live Demo
		– Common Pathology
10:30 A.M.	Coffee Break	
11:00 A.M.	Musculoskeletal infection in Peds	
11:30 A.M.	Ankle	– Anatomy
		– Normal US
		– Live Demo
		– Common Pathology
12:30 P.M.	Lunch	
2:00 P.M.	Hands On	Shoulder
		Elbow
		Wrist
		Hip
		Knee
		Ankle

(continued)

Table 23.1 (continued)

Advanced session	
Monday	
8:00 A.M.	Brachial Plexus: from normal to pathology
8:15 A.M.	Upper limb nerves: from normal to pathology
8:30 A.M.	Lower limb nerves: from normal to pathology
8:45 A.M.	Contrast media and MSUS
9:00 A.M.	Tendon hypervascularization: why and when?
9:10 A.M.	Subacromial impingement
9:18 A.M.	Posterior shoulder impingement
9:26 A.M.	Anterior instability of the shoulder
9:34 A.M.	Clefts and partial thickness tears of the rotator cuff
9:42 A.M.	Rotator cuff interval
9:50 A.M.	A-C joint instability
9:58 A.M.	Is Us convenient for rotator cuff muscle atrophy
10:06 A.M.	Discussion
10:25 A.M.	Coffee Break and Poster exhibition
11:00 A.M.	Lateral elbow pain
11:08 A.M.	Hand and finger masses
11:16 A.M.	Rheumatoid hand
11:30 A.M.	Scapholunate ligament
11:38 A.M.	Palmar and plantar plates
11:46 A.M.	Pulleys and other retinaculae of the hand and wrist
11:55 A.M.	Discussion
12:20 P.M.	Quiz
1:00 P.M.	Lunch
2:30 P.M.	Hands on
Tuesday	
8:00 A.M.	New advances in MSUS
8:15 A.M.	Elastography: is it useful?
8:25 A.M.	3D and 4D in MSUS
8:35 A.M.	Interventional: tutorials and applications
8:55 A.M.	US treatment of rotator cuff calcifications
9:03 A.M.	Discussion
9:15 A.M.	Lumps and bumps around the knee
9:23 A.M.	Sacroiliac joints
9:31 A.M.	Necrotizing fasciitis
9:39 A.M.	Groin pain
9:49 A.M.	Anterior hip pain
9:57 A.M.	Peritrochanteric pain
10:05 A.M.	Discussion
10:15 A.M.	Coffee Break and Poster exhibition
10:40 A.M.	Sonographic guidance of DDH treatment
11:00 A.M.	Pediatric extremity injury or pain
11:20 A.M.	Pediatric foot
11:40 A.M.	Discussion on Peds

(continued)

Table 23.1 (continued)

12:00 P.M.	Medial ankle pain
12:10 P.M.	Heel pain
12:18 P.M.	Pain in the forefoot and toes
12:26 P.M.	Diabetic neuropthy syndrome
12:34 P.M.	What do we look for if an ankle sprain doesn't heal?
12:42 P.M.	When to perform muscle ultrasound and what are we looking for
12:50 P.M.	Thoracic wall and axilla
1:00 P.M.	Discussion
1:30 P.M.	Lunch
2:30 P.M.	Hands on
	Interventional
	Foot and toes
	Frequently asked questions
	MSK US for technologists
	Muscles of the upper thigh

DDH developmental dysplasia of the hip, *MSUS* musculoskeletal ultrasound, *MSK* musculoskeletal, *US* ultrasound,

23.3
Groupement des Echographistes de L'Appareile Locomoteur

The Groupement des Echographistes de L'Appareil Locomoteur (GEL) functioned much the same way as MUSOC, but in French-speaking countries and regions (France, Belgium, Switzerland, and Quebec). This relatively smaller society began in 1997 and was dedicated to the teaching of musculoskeletal ultrasound through workshops limited to 80–100 people and focusing on a maximum of two joints. The 1-day meetings were divided into sessions on theory, followed by hands-on applications; both lasting about 1.5 h. Like MUSOC, the hands-on sessions were authentic, allowing participants opportunities to handle a transducer, perform live examinations on normal subjects, guided and corrected by experienced teachers. By 2008 GEL had held approximately 20 workshops, at a rate of about two per year.

GEL was founded primarily by Jean-Louis Brasseur and the first president of the society, Philippe Peetrons. Peetrons was succeeded by Stefano Bianchi until 2007. The particular feature of the GEL workshops was that although the meetings took place in France, Switzerland, and Belgium, they generally targeted smaller cities to allow increasing numbers of radiologists to participate in the meetings. Like MUSOC, this outreach strategy led to growth of the faculty membership and of locally qualified teachers. At its inception, GEL had fewer than ten teachers, requiring them to travel a couple of times per year within France or to neighboring countries. Today, there are more than 30 teachers able to spend their time guiding the next generation of musculoskeletal ultrasound practitioners into practice, and perhaps teaching as well. This model of teaching looks very much like the "companionship" that we find, for example, in the world of art. Beginners work with companions as part of the process toward becoming masters. Becoming a master in teaching includes focused time in scholarship (including the theory presented at the annual meetings) combined with practice (application of what has been learned). After 20 workshops to date, GEL has brought this teaching to approximately 2,000 people.

By 2006, GEL had about 1,000 members and was approached by another French-speaking scientific society called Groupe d'Étude et de Recherche Ostéo-Articulaire (GETROA). Both societies realized that they shared many of the same members, resulting in a duplication of membership fees. The societies therefore decided to merge into a single society which they called Société d'Imagerie Muscolo-Squelettique (SIMS), and Jean-Louis Brasseur is currently Chair of the newly merged society. It is the biggest organ-based society in the French-speaking medical community. SIMS amalgamated the two meetings held per year by GETROA with the two meetings per year held by GEL. Members (and nonmembers) can now choose from four meetings per year; two to be held in Paris and two to be held elsewhere in France or a neighboring French-speaking country. Moreover, SIMS is now organizing meetings in other countries where significant numbers of radiologists understand or speak French, such as Canada, Brazil, and Chile. These additional meetings are always linked to a local meeting to ensure sufficient participation.

23.4
Role of the Learned Societies

As mentioned earlier, musculoskeletal ultrasound requires a form of companionship, with experienced teachers guiding and correcting learners in a way that delves into the subject in greater depth than afforded by traditional teaching models. Typical ex cathedra courses are insufficient to teach more sophisticated operator-dependent techniques. In the past, most of the operator-dependent techniques were taught in a hospital setting, with one professor surrounded by his/her assistants (e.g., surgery, endoscopy, laparoscopy, and so on). However, in musculoskeletal ultrasound, this was not possible. It took much too long for a sufficient number of people with sufficient levels of technique, skill, and experience to achieve an acceptable level of accuracy. Since musculoskeletal ultrasound was a new diagnostic tool, too few people around the world, including at universities, were using or teaching musculoskeletal ultrasound correctly or with sufficient accuracy. Traditional teaching of the radiology students included teaching conventional and Doppler ultrasound, but the time and the ability to teach special applications such as musculoskeletal ultrasound were lacking. Moreover, most of the radiologists who had become professors had not been trained in the newer, and at that time, little known technique. In most parts of the world, therefore, the vast majority of radiology students did not have any opportunity to experience musculoskeletal ultrasound during their normal 3–5 years' residency. However, once in their own business in private practice or in clinics, they found increasing demand for musculoskeletal ultrasound from outpatients, athletes, and rheumatoid patients. The realization that their formal university education was not sufficient to prepare them for this practice spawned the role and the format initiated and undertaken by the learned societies.

The societies have met the demand through teaching a combined method of diagnosis in standard format (e.g., the classic meetings and conferences with some live demonstrations), but also through organizing authentic hands-on sessions that allow the participants opportunities to conduct practical examinations on normal or abnormal subjects under the guidance of a skilled teacher. Even experienced participants enjoy this practical application as it allows them to share their experience with other skilled instructors. It offers an opportunity to ask specific questions about any difficulties that they have experienced in their own practice and get an informed response. Annual and biannual meetings also serve to bring instructors together and to share new knowledge and developments generated in their individual practices, thereby creating an additional professional development outcome.

This level of scholarship is mainly targeted at radiologists or other specialists involved in musculoskeletal ultrasound rather than at students in radiology. The collaboration among professionals raises the overall quality of the operator-dependent method of diagnosis while also providing consistency to routine examinations for all parts of the body. This consistency in routine procedure and technique then becomes a standard process for examining patients around the world. The improved accuracy of the techniques used is therefore shared and applied in a similar manner. Moreover, a critical mass of potential teachers is growing throughout the world. Local organizations now rely on these two pioneer societies for direction, further causing an increase in the spread of improved technique. For example, participants of the MUSOC meetings are organizing local meetings in their respective countries, and passing their knowledge and skill on to greater number of colleagues, sometimes inviting experienced MUSOC presenters to attend their local meetings. As we have grown, we have witnessed participants return two or three times to further improve their practice and we have noted significant improvement in their level of skill, knowledge, and technique – leading some to be invited to join the faculty. We have no doubt that this method of "companionship teaching" has contributed to our ability to achieve an improved level of scholarship that translates into better practice, and therefore, improved patient care.

References

Cooperberg PL, Tsang I, Truelove L, Knickerbocker WJ (1978) Gray scale ultrasound in the evaluation of rheumatoid arthritis of the knee. Radiology 126:759–763

Crass JR, Craig EV, Thompson RC, Feinberg SB (1984) Ultrasonography of the rotator cuff: Surgical correlations. J Clin Ultrasound 12:487–492

Duval JM, Mambrini A (1975) Valeur de l'échotomographie dans le diagnostic d'hématome de la gaine des muscles droits abdominaux. Nouv Presse Med 4:349–350

Fornage B (1987) Echographie du système musculo-tendineux des membres. Vigot, Paris

Fornage B (1991) Echographie des members. Vigot, Paris

Katthagen BD (1988) Schultersonografie: Technik-Anatomie-Pathologie. Thieme Stuttgart, New York

Middleton WD, Edelstein G, Reinus WR, Leland Melson G, Murphy WA (1984) Ultrasonography of the rotator cuff: Technique and normal anatomy. J Ultrasound Med 3:549–551

Moore CP, Sarti DA, Louie JS (1975) Ultrasonographic demonstration of popliteal cysts in rheumatoid arthritis: A noninvasive technique. Arthritis Rheum. 18:577–580

Peetrons P, Stienon M, Carlier L, Conrads Y, Jeanmart L (1984) Ultrasonographie des sarcomes des tissus mous. J d'Echographie et de Med Ultrasonore 5:305–307

Peetrons P, Delmotte S, Stehman M, Peetrons A (1986) Lésions de la coiffe des rotateurs: Apport spécifique de l'échographie. Acta Orthop Belg 52:703–716

Seltzer SE, Finberg HJ, Weissman BN, Kido DK, Collier BD (1979) Arthrosonography: Gray-scale ultrasound evaluation of the shoulder. Radiology 132:467–468

Seltzer SE, Finberg HJ, Weissman BN (1980) Arthrosonography, technique, ultrasound anatomy and pathology. Invest Radiol 15:19–28

Van Holsbeeck M, Introcaso JH (1991) Musculoskeletal Ultrasound. Mosby, New York

Radiology Education in the Faculty of Medicine at Cairo University (Kasr Al-Ainy Hospital)

24

S.N. Saleem, Y.Y. Sabri, A.S. Saeed

24.1
Introduction and Historic Background

Medical practice has always been an integral part of the history of Egypt (Todd 1921). Medicine in Egypt dates back to Pharaonic Egypt (Kemet). The Edwin Smith, the Ebers, and the Kahun papyri all witness the academic study and practice of Kemetic medicine (Breasted 1930; Bryan 1930). Egyptian physicians were also influenced by Al-Razi (864–930 A.D.) and Ibn-Sina (Avicenna 980–1037 A.D.), the famous Muslim physicians. The scholars of Islam helped in the transmission of medical science through the dark ages, from the decline of ancient learning to the rise of modern learning (Browne 2002). The hospital was one of the greatest achievements of medieval Islamic society. The medieval Islamic hospital was a more elaborate institution with a wider range of functions than the earlier sick-relief facilities offered by some Christian monasteries. Some hospitals were medical teaching institutions with formal classes. Clinical training at the bedside in a medieval Islamic hospital, whether as an apprentice or through formal instruction, was a part of medical learning for a substantial number of formally trained physicians (Dols and Adil 1984; Savage-Smith 1998).

In modern history, the Faculty of Medicine at Cairo University, established in 1827, continues the glory of medicine in Egypt as one of the biggest and oldest medical schools not only in Egypt but also in Africa and the Middle East. In 1937, the faculty was named after Al-Ainy Pasha, whose palace was originally the school's main building. In fact, "Kasr Al-Ainy" literally means "Al-Ainy's palace" when translated into Arabic. At that time, Kasr Al-Ainy Hospital accommodated 1,500 beds and 300 students who studied seven

S.N. Saleem (✉)
Department of Diagnostic Radiology, Kasr Al-Ainy Hospital, Cairo University, Egypt;
University of Western Ontario (Education in Radiology and MRI), London, ON, Canada

Radiology Education. R.K. Chhem et al. (Eds.)
DOI: 10.1007/978-3-540-68989-8, © Springer-Verlag Berlin Heidelberg 2009

subjects: chemistry/physics, anatomy, physiology, pathology, medicine, hygiene, and pharmacology (Sonbol 1991). Medical education has expanded dramatically since then.

In this chapter we discuss the modern Kasr Al-Ainy Hospital facilities, personnel, equipment, clinical services, education duties, and resources. The current status of the Radiology Department, its relation to the world, and the intentions for the future are also discussed.

24.2
Modern Kasr Al-Ainy Hospital Facilities

Nowadays, Kasr Al-Ainy Hospital comprises six facilities located at Cairo University Hospital: Al Manial University Hospital (1,794 beds); Gynecology Diseases and Delivery Hospital (297 beds); Internal Medicine Diseases Hospital (306 beds); New University Children Hospital (185 beds); New Kasr Al-Ainy Teaching Hospital (1,200 beds); and Out Patient Clinic (receives about 750,000 patients annually). Each of these facilities has a radiology unit that is a branch of the main Radiology Department at Kasr Al-Ainy Hospital. Figure 1 shows an overview of the main building of Kasr Al-Ainy Hospital.

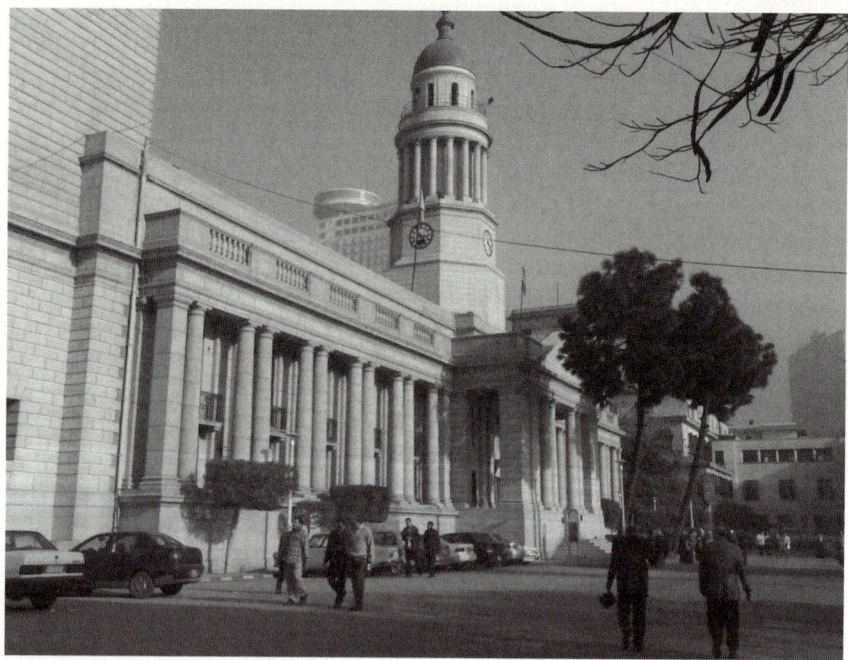

Fig. 1

24.3
Radiology Department of Kasr Al-Ainy Hospital: Personnel, Equipment, and Clinical Services

The working personnel in the Radiology Department (in academic year 2007–2008) are 17 professors, 14 assistant professors, ten lecturers, and 35 assistant lecturers in addition to 40 nurses and 19 nurse supervisors. The nonmedical workers include 75 technicians and 86 clerks. The Radiology Department is formed from nine units that represent different internationally recognized radiology subspecialities, namely, musculoskeletal imaging, neuroradiology, gastrointestinal tract (GIT) imaging, uroradiology, cardiothoracic imaging, vascular and interventional radiology, women's imaging, pediatrics radiology, and emergency radiology. The Radiology Department is well equipped with up-to-date diagnostic imaging machines Table 24.1.

The hospital serves about a million patients annually (a quarter of them are inpatients) from Egypt as well as from other countries and areas in the region such as Libya, Palestine, and Sudan. Table 24.2, shows the reported average numbers of patients served annually in the Radiology Department according to the latest statistics.

24.4
Radiology Department's Teaching Duties

In addition to providing the hospital services, the Radiology Department participates in well-designed undergraduate and postgraduate teaching courses for radiodiagnosis.

Table 24.1 Equipments in the Radiology Department of Kasr Al-Ainy Hospital

Type of machine	Number
Plain X-ray	21
Fluoroscopy and digital radiography	10
Mammography	3
Angiography and interventional radiology	3
Ultrasonography and Doppler	8
Computed tomography	6
Magnetic resonance imaging	3

Table 24.2 Average number of radiological studies performed in the Radiology Department of Kasr Al-Ainy Hospital annually

Imaging procedures	Number of studies
Plain X-ray and radiographic techniques	170,000
Ultrasonography	10,000
Doppler	5,000
Angiography and interventional radiology	1,400
Computed tomography	22,000
Magnetic resonance imaging	10,000

24.4.1
Radiology Education for Undergraduates

Only students who finish their secondary school with high grades (95% or more) are accepted by Kasr Al-Ainy Hospital to study medicine for 6 years. In their final year, medical students study radiology. The radiology teaching course for undergraduates is a 3-week course repeated throughout the academic year for groups of about 100 students. The Radiology Department teaches a total of 1,500 final-year medical students annually.

The curriculum is designed to prepare the medical student for a general practitioner post. The following imaging branches are taught in separate 90-min lectures that cover all of the subspecialties: musculoskeletal imaging, neuroradiology, gastrointestinal tract imaging, uroradiology, chest imaging, cardiac imaging, vascular imaging, women's imaging, pediatrics radiology, and emergency radiology.

At the end of this course, a final-year medical student is expected to recognize the different imaging techniques and their indications, and review and recognize the classic radiological appearance of common diseases in the different systems. All lectures are given using PowerPoint presentations as well as hard-copy film sessions.

The undergraduate students are tested twice to assess their knowledge of radiology. The first time is at the end of the course in the Radiology Department, where an assignment is requested of each student covering one of several preindicated items (e.g., computed tomography, CT, appearance of a brain abscess, plain X-ray findings in emphysema, radiological changes in rickets, etc.). At the end of the academic year the student is examined for the second time in radiodiagnosis as a part of the final examination in surgery, medicine, and pediatrics. The examination consists of both an oral element and spotting to identify abnormal findings on hard film copies. A Bachelor of Medicine and Bachelor of Surgery, or in Latin Medicinae Baccalaureus et Baccalaureus Chirurgiae (MBBCh), degree is awarded on the completion of studies in the medical school. The MBBCh degree is equivalent to the Doctor of Medicine (MD) degree in North America. This is followed by 1 year of obligatory clinical training (internship) in the units of surgery, internal medicine, pediatrics, emergency unit, gynecology, and obstetrics. By completing the internship, the student is licensed as a general practitioner. To attain a residency position in the Radiology Department of Kasr Al-Ainy Hospital, the candidate must have been graduated from the Kasr Al-Ainy Hospital Faculty of Medicine and attained his/her internship at Kasr Al-Ainy Hospital. Applicants with the highest grades are accepted for radiology residency at Kasr Al-Ainy Hospital.

24.4.2
Radiology Education for Postgraduate Studies

24.4.2.1
Residency

The average number of residents accepted annually is 12 candidates. The total number of junior and senior residents in academic year 2007–2008 was 35. The Radiology Department offers 36 months of residency training. Radiology residents spend a period of

3 months in each of the nine subspecialty units in addition to 3 months at New Kasr Al-Ainy Teaching Hospital. This will make a total of 30 months of obligatory cycling, leaving 6 months for reattending subspecialties according to the candidate's preference and the needs of the department.

Throughout the residency training, the students attend a 24-month education program to prepare them for their Master of Science (MSc) in Radiology degree. To obtain a MSc in Radiology degree, the candidate has to sit two examinations (parts I and II) and defend a thesis/essay. The aim of the education program for the MSc in Radiology degree (parts I and II) is to establish a qualified specialized radiologist who will be able to fulfill the following at the end of the program:

> Be aware of current and advanced diagnostic imaging modalities and their applications in medicine for diagnosis and treatment
> Be able to run a radiodiagnostic unit providing the basic and common diagnostic procedures
> Be able to write a comprehensive report on a radiological study with clinical radiological interpretation to deduce the correct diagnosis or the possible differential diagnosis
> Be able to conduct research work and to get benefit from published scientific research, and to present a short talk on an assigned topic
> Be able to communicate and keep pace with radiology practice in other parts of the world (e.g., Europe, North America)
> Be prepared to acquire and apply the recent trends in radiology
> To have sufficient preliminary knowledge about the use of computers and information technology in radiology practice and research

Starting from academic year 2009–2010, a new 5-year residency training system will be applied.

24.4.2.2
MSc in Radiology (Part I): 6 Months

Part I of the education program for candidates of the MSc in Radiology degree is a 6-month course that covers the basic sciences of radiology. During this period the postgraduate student is exposed to the basic radiological information essential to establish his/her career as a radiologist. The following subjects are studied: radiation physics, radiological positions and techniques, radiological anatomy, darkroom principles, radiobiology and nuclear medicine, and medical statistics and computer skills.

Radiation Physics: 20 h

The course covers the physical principles of conventional radiology, ultrasound, CT, magnetic resonance imaging (MRI), and nuclear medicine imaging, with integration of these principles into how an image is produced and comprehension of the effect of the different physical factors on the quality of the image generated and the resultant diagnostic data.

Radiological Positioning and Techniques (30 h)

The course includes how to radiograph anatomic regions in the human body (skull, spine, chest, abdomen and pelvis, upper and lower limbs, etc.) with fair knowledge of the exposure factors and accurate positions of each anatomic part. Full knowledge is required of the different current radiological techniques in conventional and advanced radiology and angiography, including patient preparation, procedure of examination, contrast material used, patient aftercare, and the possible complications of each technique, as well as the management of these complications. Reactions to contrast material and their management as well as the contraindications to specific types of examinations are also topics that are addressed.

Radiological Anatomy (40 h)

Anatomy is studied as demonstrated by different radiological and imaging procedures, including conventional radiography, contrast studies, CT, and MRI. The anatomic regions of interest should cover the following:

- Skull and its contents, including the brain and cerebral vessels, skull base, pharynx, and temporal bone
- Face and facial bones, orbits, sinuses, jaws, and salivary glands
- Neck, thyroid, larynx, and extracranial vessels
- Spine, spinal cord, and meninges
- Musculoskeletal system, including bones, joints, ligaments, and muscles
- Heart and great vessels
- Chest
- Gastrointestinal system, including solid organs such as liver and spleen
- Genitourinary system
- Peripheral vessels and lymphatic system
- Breast

It is to be noted that the following topics are included in part II: CT of complex maxillo-facial anatomy, anatomy of petrous bones, parapharyngeal spaces and mouth floor, breast CT and MRI, MRI of the face and neck, MRI of the joints (except the knee studied in part I), and MRI of the heart.

Darkroom Principles (15 h)

In this course, we focus on darkroom construction, the radiographic film, the film cassette, intensifying screens and the film–screen combination, the processing machine and the processing techniques, film criticism and common faults in film processing, as well as film copy and subtraction techniques.

Radiobiology and Nuclear Medicine (15 h)

The radiobiology course includes radiation effects on normal tissues at different levels (chromosomal, cellular, and subcellular), tissue reactions to radiation, as well as radiation-protection principles. The course in nuclear medicine includes imaging of the cardiovascular system, renal imaging, hepatic imaging, thyroid scan, bone scan, and breast scan. In addition, modes of examination and scanning are also covered and include conventional gamma camera, dual-head simultaneous acquisition gamma camera, theory of positron emission tomography scanning, and the production and utilities of ultra-short-lived isotopes.

General requirements for candidates for the MSc in Radiology degree (part I) include basics of medical statistics, basics of medical research, basics of archiving and computer search, and basics of organization of scientific meetings and conferences.

24.4.2.3
MSc in Radiology (Part II): 18 Months

By the end of this time, the resident should have worked in most of the subspeciality units in the department and is expected to have a fair knowledge in the following diagnostic fields:

- Neuroradiology
- Head and neck radiology
- Musculoskeletal radiology
- Cardiothoracic radiology
- Gastrointestinal radiology
- Genitourinary radiology
- Vascular imaging and intervention
- Doppler studies and CT and magnetic resonance angiography
- Breast imaging

In each diagnostic field studied, most of the pathological entities are expected to be covered, including congenital, traumatic, inflammatory, neoplastic, and miscellaneous conditions.

Candidates for the MSc in Radiology degree should know also the physical principles and clinical applications of the following imaging modalities:

- MRI and spectroscopy
- CT
- Doppler vascular imaging, echocardiography, and endosonography techniques
- Molecular imaging

24

Scientific Activities, Continuing Medical Education, and Credit Hours

Scientific Activities:

1. To fulfill the required credit hours, candidates are expected to attend the following *scientific activities*:
   The scientific meeting of the Radiology Department (once per week): the resident is expected to attend the 2-h meeting, prepare the scientific material, present cases, and share in discussions
   The annual refresher course organized by the Radiology Department (March)
   The annual scientific meeting of the Faculty of Medicine (April)
   Thesis discussions that take place in the Radiology Department
   This is an important prerequisite for the candidate to fulfill to be able to defend his/her thesis.
2. *Technical procedures*: attendance and performance of the different techniques, including angiography, interventional, CT, MRI, Doppler imaging, and digital imaging

Master's Degree Thesis/Essay

To complete the master's degree, a research project is required in the form of a thesis/essay; the chosen thesis/essay topic should have a scientific value. The research is supervised by a senior member of the Radiology Department (an assistant Professor or a full professor) and may be supported by a staff member of a clinical department depending on the research topic selected. To obtain a MSc in Radiology degree, a resident must pass two examinations (parts I and II) and successfully defend the research project (thesis/essay).

After completing the residency, some residents are promoted to assistant lecturers.

Assistant lecturers in the Radiology Department practice radiology as well as carry out academic duties in the different subspecialities while they study for their degree of MD in Radiology. There were 23 candidates for the MD degree in the 2007–2008 academic year, while there were 81 for the degree of MSc in Radiology.

24.4.2.4
MD in Radiology

The requirements for this degree are:

1. A 6-month course in surgery, internal medicine, and pathology
2. A 2-year course in radiology practice and lectures, after which the candidate may apply for the MD examination, which is held twice a year
3. A research project completed by the candidate, supervised by two senior members of the radiodiagnosis unit usually in association with a senior staff member in a clinical department

24.4.2.5
Postgraduate Examinations (MSc Part II and MD)

The postgraduate examinations are held twice a year in May and November.
The examination comprises the following:

1. Four days of written examinations as follows:
   a. Multiple-choice questions for radiology (3 h)
   b. Short questions for radiology (3 h)
   c. Pathology (2 h)
   d. Surgery (1 h) and medicine (1 h).
2. Six days of oral and practical examinations:
   a. Oral radiology examination (1 day):
      i. Four examiners for the MSc in Radiology degree
      ii. Ten examiners for the MD degree
   b. Practical radiology examinations (2 days):
      i. Ten short cases for which to write a diagnosis
      ii. Three long cases to report upon
      iii. Practical ultrasound examination with three examiners
   c. Surgery (1 day): oral and practical examinations
   d. Medicine (1 day): oral and practical examinations
   e. Pathology (1 day): oral and practical examinations

24.4.3
Continuing Medical Education

The residents and assistant lecturers are expected to fulfill the following:

- Attend a once-yearly event (annual meeting). Recent published research work of the department members is presented as short talks and lectures in this meeting by the researchers.
- Attend a weekly conference in the department where cases are presented and short talks are given by different units' members.
- Attend the Journal Club early-morning lectures presented by junior staff during the academic year (September to May). Lectures are presented by the assistant lectures (four times per week); the topics of the lectures are selected and supervised by the chairman of the Radiology Department.
- Attend weekly scientific meetings that are held in the musculoskeletal imaging unit where residents and assistant lectures prepare assignments and short Power-Point talks.
- Attend weekly scientific meetings that are held in the cardiothoracic imaging unit discussing interesting cases from the previous week with residents and junior staff of the department (958 cases were discussed in the 2007). As credit hours are required to succeed in the program, there are usually no problems with attendance at lectures.

24.4.4
Education Resources in the Radiology Department

Radiology education resources are obtained from the Radiology Department's medical library and digital library. Figure 2 shows part of the Radiology Department's medical library.

The Radiology Department's medical library contains two teaching files of hard copies of films: a diagnostic radiology teaching file (composed of X-ray and radiological procedures) that was purchased from the USA, and one compiled in house. The collection is composed of hard copies of conventional and cross-sectional modalities (CT and MRI) of cases collected in the Radiology Department and subdivided into topics (skeletal, gastrointestinal, etc.). The Radiology Department's medical library contains a collection of radiology textbooks and a collection of periodicals. A challenge that we face is that the Radiology Department does not subscribe to many radiology periodicals (hard copy or online) and those that it does subscribe to need to be updated.

The in-house teaching files comprise a medical image database for MRI, CT, and X-rays. The file is subdivided into subtopics and presented either as unknown or by the diagnosis. Each case is provided by a diagnosis and differential diagnosis. There are also digital tutorials available on CDs, covering different subtopics. The library currently contains five personal computers and two data-viewing machines. The limited number of equipped lecture rooms relative to the increasing number of students poses a further challenge.

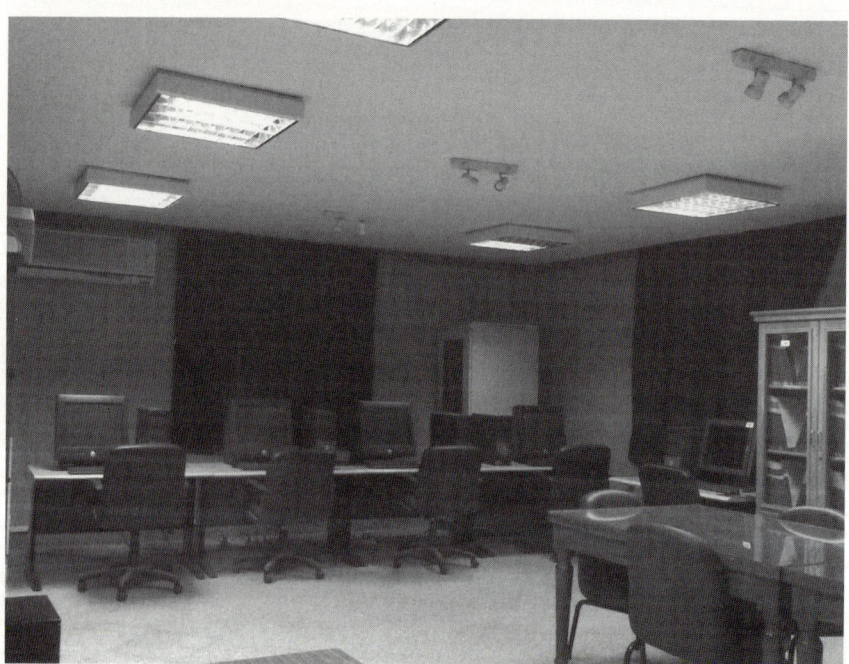

Fig 2.

24.5
Radiology Department of Kasr Al-Ainy Hospital and the World

The radiology education program is well received by the residents as well as the faculty members. The radiology residents are known to be competent and accomplish their clinical duties successfully. The radiology education program at Cairo University has a good reputation. The number of applicants to the program, coming from Egypt and other countries in the Middle East region, increases annually. The graduates of the program are well received in clinical and academic practice nationally and internationally.

Practicing radiology at Kasr Al-Ainy Hospital is not only deeply rooted locally but is also innovative and has its international influence. The ties between radiology practice at Cairo University and international medicine are based on thought, research, and mutual exchange of findings and discoveries. The contribution of researchers from the Radiology Department of Kasr Al-Ainy Hospital to the worldwide knowledge of radiology is innovative. Many articles on research work that took place in the Radiology Department of Kasr Al-Ainy Hospital have been published in prestigious North American as well as European journals; e.g., Aly and Abdel-Atty (1999), Shahin et al. (2001), Saleem (2003, 2005), Saleem et al. (2005, 2007), and Zaki et al. (2008). The Radiology Department is well represented too at renowned international radiology conventions. At the Radiological Society of North America 2007 annual meeting, the department was represented at 13 events, with one of them receiving a cum laude award.

24.6
Radiology Department of Kasr Al-Ainy Hospital: Stated Mission

1. To develop an outstanding, honorable clinician/practitioner, researcher, and teacher capable of offering adequate medical care and following medical ethics
2. To advance the knowledge base of radiology by developing and encouraging scientific research
3. To disseminate knowledge through continuing education of our students, graduates, and colleagues
4. To promote outstanding programs of medical care to serve society and to promote environmental development
5. To maintain the atmosphere of co-operation, peer relation, and mutual respect in the university society
6. To encourage and to foster individual creativity in the university society

24

24.7
Looking to the Future

Starting from academic year 2009–2010, a new 5-year residency training system will be applied. The modified program will dedicate more time for the students to conduct research and to be able to teach those who follow.

24.8
Summary

The Radiology Department of Kasr Al-Ainy Hospital offers education programs for undergraduate and postgraduate students. The program provides the students with the knowledge and clinical experience necessary to serve in medical care in Egypt and the Middle East region. The program is also planned to prepare the students to be scholars and to be able to conduct research and to teach.

References

Aly YA, Abdel-Atty H (1999) Normal oesophageal transit time on digital radiography. Clin Rad 54:545–549

Breasted JH (1930) The Edwin Smith surgical papyrus. University of Chicago Press, Chicago

Browne EG (2002) Islamic medicine. Goodword publications, New Delhi

Bryan PW (1930) The papyrus ebers. Geoffrey Bles, London

Dols MW, Adil SG (1984) Medieval Islamic medicine: Ibn Ridwan's treatise "On the prevention of bodily Ills in Egypt." University of California Press, Berkeley

Saleem SN (2003) MR imaging diagnosis of uterovaginal anomalies: Current state of the art. Radiographics, online 10.1148/rg.e13 http://radiographics.rsnajnls.org/cgi/content/full/e13v1

Saleem SN (2005) MRI features of Neuro-Behcet disease. Neurographics 4:1–36

Saleem SN, Belal A, Elghandour N (2005) Spinal cord schistosomiasis MR imaging appearance with surgical and pathologic correlation. Am J Neuroradiol 26:1646–1654

Saleem SN, Said A-H, Lee D (2007) Lesions of the hypothalamus: MRI diagnostic features. Radiographics 27:1087–1108

Savage-Smith E (1998) Islamic culture and the medical arts. http://www.nlm.nih.gov/exhibition/islamic_medical/islamic_12.html. Accessed 15 April 1998

Shahin AA, Sabri YY, Mostafa HA et al (2001) Pulmonary function tests, high resolution computerized tomography, alpha-1 antitrypsin measurement, and early detection of pulmonary involvement in patients with systemic sclerosis. Rheumatol Int 20:95–100

Sonbol A (1991) The creation of a medical profession in Egypt, 1800–1922. Syracuse University Press, Syracuse, NY

Todd TW (1921) Egyptian medicine: A critical study of recent claims. Am Anthropol (New Series) 23:460–470

Zaki MS, Abdel-Aleem A, Abdel-Salam G et al (2008) The Molar tooth sign: A new Joubert syndrome classification system tested in Egyptian families. Neurology 70:556–565